D1543879

$2.99

Low Back Pain

Low Back Pain

Bernard E. Finneson, M.D., F.A.C.S.

*Chief of Neurological Surgery, Crozer-Chester
Medical Center, Chester; Sacred Heart Hospital,
Chester, Pa.; Taylor Hospital, Ridley Park, Pa.; Clinical
Associate Professor of Surgery (Neurosurgery),
Hahnemann Medical College, Philadelphia*

Illustrations by Barbara Finneson

J. B. Lippincott Company
Philadelphia · Toronto

Copyright © 1973, by J. B. Lippincott Company

This book is fully protected by copyright and, with the exception of brief excerpts for review, no part of it may be reproduced in any form, by print, photoprint, microfilm, or by any other means, without the written permission of the publishers.

ISBN-0-397-50314-8

Library of Congress Catalog Card Number 73-9611

Printed in the United States of America

6   5

Library of Congress Cataloging in Publication Data

Finneson, Bernard E
  Low back pain.

  Includes bibliographies.
   1. Backache. I. Title. [DNLM: 1. Backache.
WE755 F514L 1973]
RD768.F56   617'.5   73-9611
ISBN 0-397-50314-8

To my wife, Barbara,
MEDICAL ARTIST IN RESIDENCE,
*who elegantly illustrated this book
and whose talent is a source of great personal pride*

Preface

This book is an effort to provide a practical and useful guide for evaluation and management of the various forms of low back dysfunction commonly encountered in practice. Although back pain has probably existed from the time the progenitors of man first assumed the erect stance, it is startling to appreciate how meager and rudimentary is our knowledge of the subject.

Low back dysfunction has been my principal medical interest for more than twenty years appropriating a progressively increasing apportionment of my time. At present, I am involved in this work almost exclusively. When I first was exposed to the problem of low back pain, it appeared to be a rather simple mechanical derangement. After having concentrated my interest and time in this field of inquiry, my indisputable factual knowledge of the subject appears much less certain than when I was a neophyte. In most instances, I suppose a conscious fallibility is less damaging than an ill-founded dogmatism in arriving at a clinical decision.

Most of the techniques described are widely accepted, and no claim is made for an "original method" of treatment. However, a number of unique biases that are based on the trials and errors of my personal experience have been insinuated into the text. Foremost is my persuasion that the largest group of treatment failures result either from improper evaluation or an inadequate trial of conservative management.

BERNARD E. FINNESON, M.D.
Neurosurgical Clinic
Crozer-Chester Medical Center

Acknowledgements

There are many persons for whose help and encouragement in my writing of this book I am deeply grateful.

Dr. Ralph Cloward, an outstanding spinal surgeon, has kindly written Chapter 7 in which he describes his technique. A brilliant and innovative pioneer, he is widely known for his fresh approach to old problems. The book is enhanced by his contribution, and I am grateful for his help. This chapter was adapted from monographs originally published by Codman & Shurtleff, Inc.

I wish to thank Dr. Norman Shealy, who was instrumental in the conception and technical development of dorsal column stimulation, for permitting me to use some of his material on this subject. Several of these illustrations and photographs were kindly provided by Medtronic, Inc. Dr. Shealy also provided me with information on the technique of articular nerve rhizotomy, a procedure which he introduced. I wish to express my respect and admiration for Dr. Shealy and believe his understanding of the problem of pain is second to none.

The kindness and generosity of Dr. William Scoville during my all too brief visit to Hartford is most appreciated. It afforded me the privilege of observing a master surgeon.

The W. B. Saunders Company kindly permitted me to adapt several sections from the second edition of my book *DIAGNOSIS AND MANAGEMENT OF PAIN SYNDROMES.* These include sections originally written by Dr. Arthur Grollman of Southwestern Medical School, The University of Texas, and Dr. Martin Meltzer of New York University School of Medicine. I am twice grateful for their help.

I received many suggestions and invaluable support from our neurosurgical nurses, both past and present, Mrs. Ann Bell Shoustal, R.N., Miss Teresa Dye, R.N., Mrs. Julie Fisher, R.N. Miss Ann Nelling, R.N., and Mrs. Linda McCleery, R.N.

I want to express my appreciation to Miss Eileen Parker, Miss Judy Cassidy and Mrs. Marjorie Morris who ably and cheerfully performed the typing and secretarial tasks.

The illustrations were done by my wife, Barbara, a dedicated and skillful professional medical illustrator. I believe they are so fine that any comment by me would be superfluous. To properly visualize the surgery, Barbara would scrub, be gloved and gowned and become part of the "surgical team." Most of my surgery starts at 7:30 a.m., and her willingness to arise at the necessary time to take part in the procedure was truly a labor of love.

Julia Y. Chai, Medical Librarian of Crozer-Chester Medical Center, has been most kind in providing me necessary assistance.

Mrs. Dinetta Palmer of the Crozer-Chester Medical Center Operating Room staff has worked as my instrument nurse for more than 17 years, and I consider myself blessed to have her on my team.

Throughout the years, I have drawn freely upon the expertise and kindness of the radiologists in the three hospitals I serve and am grateful for their help. I am particularly indebted to Dr. Hal Prentiss, neuroradiologist at Crozer-Chester Medical Center, who has been most generous with his time and encouragement.

I have been particularly fortunate to be associated with Dr. Maurice Davidson, a fine physician and one of the kindest men I have known. I thank him for his forbearance in assuming many of the practice burdens during the preparation of this monograph.

I am deeply indebted to the staff of the J. B. Lippincott Company for their support and encouragement. I particularly wish to thank Mr. J. Stuart Freeman and Miss Jean Hyslop for their kindness and help.

BERNARD E. FINNESON, M.D.
Neurosurgical Clinic
Crozer-Chester Medical Center

Contents

1. Basic Science 1

Anatomy of the Low Back 2
   Development of the Low Back 2
      Embryology 2
      Degenerative Effects of Living 6
      Spinal Curves 6
   Lumbar Vertebrae 7
      Vertebral Foramina and the "Lateral Bony Recess" 8
   Sacrum and Coccyx 9
   Articulations and Ligaments of the Lumbar Spine 10
      Vertebral Body Articulation 10
      Vertebral Arch Articulation 13
   Pelvic Articulations and Ligaments 15
      Pelvic-vertebral Articulation 15
      Sacroiliac Articulation 17
      Sacrococcygeal Articulation 17
      Symphysis Pubis 17
   Blood Supply of the Lumbar Spine 17
      Blood Supply of the Intervertebral Disc 17
   Nerve Supply of the Lumbar Spine 18
   Low Back Musculature 19
      Extensors of the Lumbar Spine 19
      Flexors of the Lumbar Spine 20
      Abductors of the Lumbar Spine 23
Biomechanics of the Lumbar Spine 24
   Mobility of the Lumbar Spine 24
   Biomechanical Changes in the Intervertebral Disc 26
   Biomechanics of the Intervertebral Disc 26
   The Skeleton As a Structural Unit 28
   Stress Studies of the Lumbar Spine 28
      Axial Compression 29
      Torsion 30
      Clinical Verification of Stress Studies 31
   Extrinsic Spinal Support 31
   Pressure Measurements in Lumbar Discs 33

2. Evaluation 37

Examination of the Patient 38
   History 38

Sit Back and Listen 38
Low Back Pain 38
Sciatica 39
Motor Impairment 39
Sensory Impairment 40
Sphincter Impairment 40
True Sciatica Versus Musculoligamentous Pain 40
Past Medical History 41
Examination 41
Systematic Approach 41
X-ray Lumbosacral Spine 49
Retrograde Reasoning 49
Equivocal Diagnosis 50
Common Radiographic Abnormalities 50
X-ray Contrast Studies 58
Myelogram 58
History 58
Patient Apprehension 59
Principle of Myelography 59
Myelogram Controversy 59
Indications for Myelography 61
Preparation of Patient 61
Positioning 61
Myelogram Technique 62
Postmyelogram 69
Myelogram Tracing 69
Discogram 69
Basic Principles 69
History of Discography 71
Technique of Midline Lumbar Discography 72
Interpretation of Discogram 74
Lateral Approach 74
Advantages and Disadvantages of Discography 75
Postmortem Discography 75
Role of Discography 76

3. Psychology of Low Back Dysfunction 77

Psychology of Pain 78
Organic Pain and "Imaginary" Pain 78
Pain and the Doctor-Patient Relationship 79
Reactions to Pain 79
Emotions 79
Adaptation 80
Socioeconomic and Cultural Factors 80
Athletics 81
Body Area 82
Psychosis 82
Absence of Pain 82
Pain and Sensory Deprivation 83

Evaluation of Pain 84
   Difficulties in Diagnosis 84
Management of Pain 85
   Overtreatment 85
   Target Fixation 85
Secondary Loss and Secondary Gain 86
   Prolongation of Symptoms and Secondary Gain 86
Placebos and the Placebo Effect 87
   Double-blind Method 87
   Mechanism of Action 88
   "Placebo-Reactor Type": Fact or Fancy? 88
Nonorganic Backache 88
  Apocryphal Diagnosis 88
  Hypochondriac and Malingerer 89
    Hypochondriac 89
    Malingerer 90
  Management 92

4. Conservative Treatment 93

Nonsurgical Management of Low Back Pain and Sciatica 95
  Rest 95
    Limited Activity Program 95
    Mattress 95
    Bed Rest 95
  Traction 97
  Physiotherapy 98
    Heat 98
    Massage 99
  Trigger Points 99
  Manipulation 100
    Maneuvers 101
  Medication 104
    Morphine 105
    Synthetic Derivatives of Morphine 106
    Codeine 106
    Synthetic Addicting Analgesics 106
    Non-narcotic Analgesics 107
    Anti-inflammatory Drugs 109
    Muscle Relaxants 111
    Miscellaneous Drugs 111
  Occupational Changes 111
  Psychotherapy and Hypnotherapy 112
  Activities of Daily Living and Faulty Posture 112
    Standing and Walking 113
    Sitting 115
    Driving 116
    Lifting 116
    Sleeping 116
    Establishing Proper Habits 117

Low Back Exercises 117
  Purpose 117
  Exercises Adapted to the Patient's Specific Needs 118
  When to Start Low Back Exercises 118
  Preexercise Evaluation 118
  Establishing an Exercise Program 120
  Relaxation Exercises 120
  Pelvic "Uptilt" 120
  Exercises for Hip Flexor Elasticity 121
  Low Back Exercises 121
    Phase 1 121
    Phase 2 122
    Phase 3 124
Low Back Supports and Braces 124
  History 124
  General Principles in the Use of Low Back Supports 125
    Low Back Mechanics 125
    Immobilization—Fact or Fancy 126
    Fitting Supports 126
    Purposes of a Spinal Support 126
    Brace Versus Corset 126
  Braces 127
    "Three-Point Pressure" Principle 127
    Knight Spinal Brace 129
    Williams Brace 129
    Taylor Brace 129
  Corsets 130
    Trochanter Belt 130
    Sacroiliac Corset 130
    Lumbosacral Corset 130
    Dorsolumbar Corset 132
  Less Frequently Used Supports 132

5. Lumbosacral Strain 133
  Epidemiology 134
  X-ray Abnormalities 134
  Wastebasket Diagnosis? 134
  Chronic Lumbosacral Strain 135
    Signs and Symptoms 135
    Pathophysiology 135
    Management 135
    Exercise for Shortened Achilles Tendon 136
  Acute Lumbosacral Strain 137
    Signs and Symptoms 137
    Management 137

6. Lumbar Disc Disease 139
  Statistical Analysis 141
  Symptoms 141
    Preexisting Backache 141

Secondary Gain 142
History of Trauma 143
Primary Symptoms 144
Absence of Sciatica 144
Sciatica 145
Sciatic Distribution 145
Activities and Posture 146
Radiculitis 148
Motor Symptoms 149
Sensory Symptoms 149
Scoliosis and Posture 149
Gait 151
Signs 151
Mobility of the Spine 151
Reflex Examination 153
Sensory Changes 155
Motor Dysfunction 156
Straight Leg Raising 156
Consideration of Other Lesions 156
Electromyography 156
X-Ray Findings 157
Vacuum Phenomenon 157
Intervertebral Disc Space Narrowing 157
Vertebral Body Alignment 158
Degenerative Changes 158
Foraminal Root Compression Syndrome 161
Transitional Lumbosacral Vertebrae and Root Function 163
Treatment of Lumbar Disc Disease 163
Conservative Management 168
Rest 168
Traction 169
Physiotherapy 169
Trigger Points 170
Manipulation of the Low Back 170
Medication 170
Occupational Changes 171
Activities of Daily Living 171
Low Back Supports and Shoe Lifts 171
Inadequate Response to Conservative Management 173
Intractable Symptoms 173
Persisting Motor Signs 173
Intermittent Symptoms 173
Subjective Response 173
Lumbar Disc Surgery 173
Indications for Surgery 173
Contraindications for Surgery 174
Normal Myelogram 177
Surgery 177
Historical Development 177
Double-check Side of Lesion 177

Anesthesia 177
Position 178
Surface Landmarks 181
Preparing the Skin and Draping 183
Skin Incision 184
Subperiosteal Dissection 189
Developing the Interspace 192
Interlaminar Surgery 194
Vascular and Visceral Injuries During Disc Surgery 203
Operative Report 204
Postoperative Management 204
Cause of Operative Failure 205
Common Causes of Postoperative Pain 205
Results of Initial Surgery 205
Exceptional Lumbar Disc Problems 205
Cauda Equina Syndrome 205
Transdural Excision of Midline Disc Extrusion 208
The Repeat Operative Procedure 210
Indications for Repeat Surgery 210
Technical Considerations in Repeat Spinal Surgery 211
Reexploration Following Complete Laminectomy 215
Results of Repeat Procedure 215

7. The Cloward Technique 217

Removal of Disc 218
Introduction 218
Operative Technique 219
Position and Anesthesia 219
Skin Incision 219
Fascia and Muscles 219
Ligamentum Flavum and Laminae 220
Disc Removal 224
Discussion 224
Transverse Skin Incision 226
Ligamentum Flavum 226
Use of Chisel and Hammer 226
Articular Facets 226
Disc Removal 226
Intrathecal Cortisone 227
Conclusion 227
Posterior Lumbar Interbody Fusion 227
Introduction 227
Disc Removal 228
Bone Grafts 230
Bone Grafting 231
Wound Closure 233
Postoperative Care 235
Discussion 235
Conclusion 235

8. Analgesic Blocks 237

    Lumbar Epidural Block 238

        Site of Injection 238

        Position 238

        Technique 239

    Caudal Block 240

        Sacral Canal 240

        Sacral Hiatus 243

        Technique 243

        Complications 245

    Paravertebral Block 246

        Indications 246

        Technique 246

9. Posterior Lumbar Rhizotomy 249

    The Patient Selection 249

        Procedure 250

10. Stenotic Lumbar Spinal Canal Syndrome 254

    Stenotic Lumbar Spinal Canal 256

        Historical Data 256

        Cervical Versus Lumbar Spinal Canal Stenosis 257

        Anatomical Characteristics 257

        Radiographic Characteristics 257

        Lumbar Mobility 257

        Clinical Characteristics 259

        Plain X-ray Changes 261

        Myelography 261

    Lumbar Spondylosis and the Stenotic Lumbar Spinal Canal 262

        Lumbar Disc Dynasty 262

        Pathology of Lumbar Spondylosis 263

        Progressive Development of Lumbar Spondylosis 263

            Degeneration of the Nucleus Pulposus 263

            Degeneration of the Annulus Fibrosus 264

            Fibrosis 264

            Complete Fibrous Ankylosis of the Intervertebral Joint 265

        X-ray Changes 266

        Lumbar Spondylosis with Spinal Cord of Normal Dimensions 266

            History 266

            Examination 266

        Lumbar Spondylosis with Stenotic Lumbar Spinal Canal 267

            History 267

            Examination 268

            Treatment 269

        Impacted Spinous Processes 269

    Achondroplasia and the Stenotic Lumbar Spinal Canal 270

        Abnormalities of the Spine 270

        Spinal Degenerative Changes 271

        Achondroplastic Dogs 271

Myelogram 271
Treatment 272
Paget's Disease of the Lumbar Spine (Osteitis Deformans) 272
Pathology 272
Microscopic Changes 272
X-ray Changes 273
Myelogram 273
Signs and Symptoms 273
Laboratory Findings 274
Diagnosis 274
Treatment 274

11. Spondylolysis and Spondylolisthesis 276
Spondylolysis 277
Etiology 277
Clinical Features 279
Treatment 279
Spondylolisthesis 279
Pseudospondylolisthesis 279
Isthmic Spondylolisthesis 280
Classification 280
Mechanical Factors 281
Establishing a Skeletal Weight-bearing Line 282
Causes of Pain Production 284
Signs and Symptoms 284
Physical Findings 285
X-ray Findings 286
Management 286
Reverse Spondylolisthesis 287
Lateral Vertebral Displacement 288

12. Vertebral Osteoporosis and Backache 289
Osteoporosis 290
Known Causes of Osteoporosis 290
Etiology of Postmenopausal (Senile) Osteoporosis 291
X-ray Diagnosis 291
Laboratory Data 292
Signs and Symptoms 292
Differential Diagnosis 292
Treatment 293

13. Infections of the Lumbar Spine 296
Infections Subsequent to Disc Surgery 296
Soft Tissue Infections 296
Signs and Symptoms 296
Management 296
Intervertebral Disc Space Infections 297
Signs and Symptoms 297
Management 298
Refractory Infections 298

Meningitis 298
Infections Without Antecedent Operations on the Spine 299
Nontuberculous Infections in Children. 299
Clinical Picture 300
Mode of Infection in Children 300
X-ray Findings 301
Management 301
Nontuberculous Infections in Adults 301
Clinical Picture 301
X-ray Findings 302
Management 302
Disc Space Abscess 303
Tuberculosis of the Lumbar Spine 303
Signs and Symptoms 303
X-ray Findings 303
Management 304

14. Tumors of the Spine 306
Benign Tumors 307
Hemangiomas. 307
Pathology 307
X-ray Findings 307
Signs and Symptoms 307
Treatment 308
Osteomas 308
Malignant Tumors 309
Sarcomas 309
Multiple Myeloma 310
Metastatic Tumors 311
Symptoms 311
Physical Findings 312
X-ray Diagnosis 313
Management 314
Intradural Tumors 314
Neurilemmomas (Schwannoma Neurofibroma) 314
Meningiomas 315
Surgery of Spinal Cord Tumors 315

15. Uncommon Causes of Low Back Pain and Sciatica 321
Pelvic Disease 323
Low Back Pain and Pregnancy 323
Intra-abdominal Vascular Disease 324
Sciatic Neuritis. 325
Entrapment Neuropathy 325
Trauma 325
Primary Sciatica 325
Tumors Involving the Sciatic Nerve 326
Entrapment Neuropathies 326
Obturator Neuropathy. 326
Technique of Obturator Nerve Block 326

Iliohypogastric and Ilioinguinal Neuritis (Inguinal Neuritis) 327
    Anatomy 328
    Mechanism of Injury 328
    Technique of Block 330
    Management 330
Meralgia Paresthetica 330
    Pathophysiology 330
    Signs and Symptoms 330
    Diagnosis 330
    Treatment 331
Adhesive Arachnoditis 332
Arthritis of the Hips 332
Ilium-Transverse Process Pseudoarthrosis 333
    Treatment 333
Ankylosing Spondylitis 333
    Symptoms 333
    Examination 336
    Laboratory 336
    X-ray 336
    Treatment 336
    Confusion with Lumbar Disc Disease 336
Charcot's Disease of the Spine (Vertebral Osteoarthropathy) 336
Sacral Cysts 337

16. Lumbar Spinal Fusion 343
    Surgical Techniques 344
        Posterior Fusion 344
        Vertebral Body Fusion 345
    Complications of Anterior Interabdominal Lumbar Fusion 345
    Indications for Lumbar Spinal Fusion 345

17. Experimental and Unorthodox Treatments for Low Back and Sciatic Pain 348
    Evaluating Treatment 349
    Intervertebral Discolysis 350
        Chymopapain Injection 350
        Collagenase Injection 352
    Intradiscal Hydrocortisone Injection 352
    Prolotherapy 353
        Proliferating Solutions 353
        Injection Technique 353
        Site of Injection 354
        Complications 354
        Present Status of "Prolotherapy" 356
    Facet Rhizotomy 356
        Principle of Facet Rhizotomy 356
        Technique of Facet Rhizotomy 356
    Dorsal Column Stimulation 359
        Indications 360
        Surgical Technique 361
    Index 367

Low Back Pain

1
Basic Science

ANATOMY OF THE LOW BACK

Development of the Low Back

Embryology
Degenerative Effects of Living
Spinal Curves

Lumbar Vertebrae

Vertebral Foramina and the "Lateral
Bony Recess"

Sacrum and Coccyx

Articulations and Ligaments of the Lumbar Spine

Vertebral Body Articulation
Vertebral Arch Articulation

Pelvic Articulations and Ligaments

Pelvic-vertebral Articulation
Sacroiliac Articulation
Sacrococcygeal Articulation
Symphysis Pubis

Blood Supply of the Lumbar Spine

Blood Supply of the Intervertebral Disc

Nerve Supply of the Lumbar Spine

Low Back Musculature

Extensors of the Lumbar Spine
Flexors of the Lumbar Spine
Abductors of the Lumbar Spine

BIOMECHANICS OF THE LUMBAR SPINE

Mobility of the Lumbar Spine

Biochemical Changes in the Intervertebral Disc

Biomechanics of the Intervertebral Disc

The Skeleton as a Structural Unit

Stress Studies of the Lumbar Spine

Axial Compression
Torsion
Clinical Verification of Stress Studies

Extrinsic Spinal Support

Pressure Measurements in Lumbar Discs

1
Basic Science

ANATOMY OF THE LOW BACK

DEVELOPMENT OF THE LOW BACK

Embryology

A week after fertilization the embryo comes into direct contact with the uterine mucosa and adheres to it. By digesting the uterine tissue it embeds itself in the endometrium.[15]

After the second week the embryo has become completely buried and the endometrial defect has been closed over by the uterine epithelium.

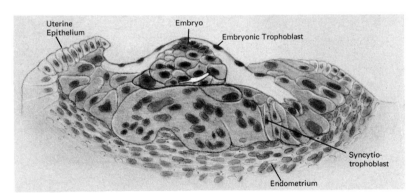

Fig. 1-1. A 1-week-old embryo in process of embedding into the uterine mucosa.

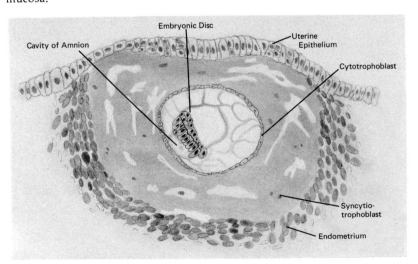

Fig. 1-2. After the second week the embryo has become completely buried and the endometrial defect has been closed over by the uterine epithelium.

Demarcation of the embryo begins with formation of the flat oval embryonic disc formed from the thickened layers of the germ disc.

The primitive groove occupies the midline in the caudal portion of the embryonic disc. The primitive node, or Hensen's node, is a clump of cells located at the cephalic end of the primitive groove. This node forms a special column of cells in the midline, which becomes the notochord.

Parallel to the long axis of the embryo, the thickened lateral ectoderm rises into rounded ridges on each side of the notochord forming the neural groove.

By the third week the column of mesoderm, which lies along both sides of the notochord, becomes organized into regularly arranged somites or primitive segments which are the precursors of body segmentation for the skeletal, muscular and nervous systems.

The primitive segments are separated by direct arterial branches of the aorta (intersegmental arteries) and each vertebral seg-

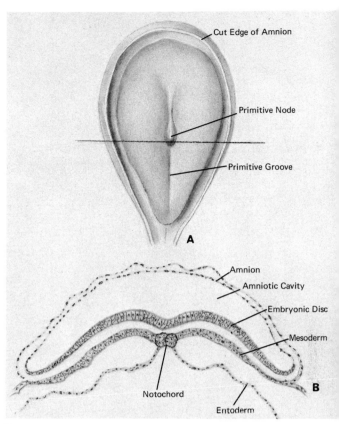

Fig. 1-3. Two views of 16-day-old presomite human embryo. A, Embryonic disc with amnion excised; B, Cross-section of embryo.

Fig. 1-4. Eighteen-day-old embryo.

Fig. 1-5. The somites or primitive segments are clearly seen by three weeks.

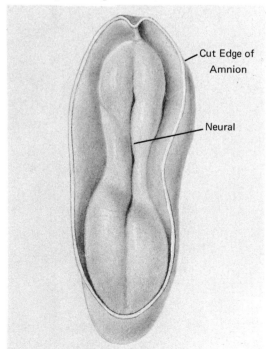

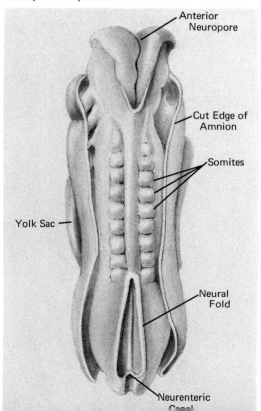

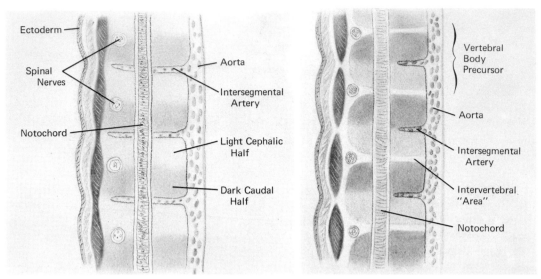

Fig. 1-6. Diagramatic representation of the primitive segments and surrounding structures.

Fig. 1-8. The cell mass closest to the nutrition afforded by the intersegmental arteries from precursors of the vertebral bodies.

Fig. 1-7. At 3 or 4 weeks the surface landmarks become recognizable.

Fig. 1-9. By 8 or 9 weeks the human embryo is externally well developed.

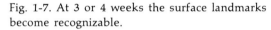

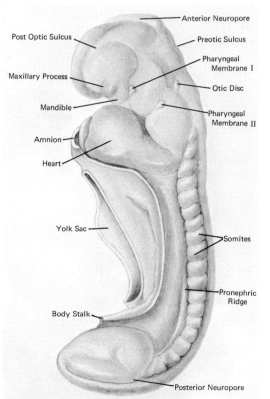

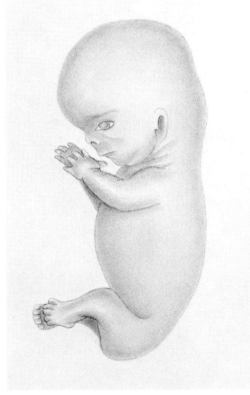

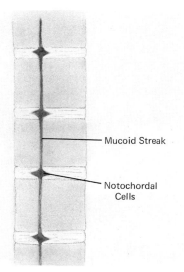

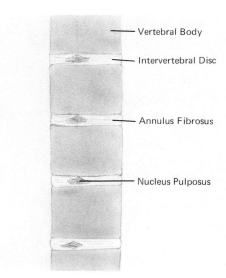

Fig. 1-10. A mucoid streak running through the vertebral body marks site of obliterated notochord.

Fig. 1-11. Development of annulus and nucleus pulposus.

ment or protovertebra consists of a condensed or dark caudal half and a lighter cephalic half.

The cells nearer the intersegmental arteries receive more nutrition than those farther removed and are more rapid in their differentiation to fuse and form the precursor of the vertebral bodies.

The cranial portion of the condensed caudal mass, being the farthest removed from the nutrition provided by the artery, remains undifferentiated as the precursor of the intervertebral disc. It is significant that the embryologically avascular development of the intervertebral disc is carried through into adult life with the limited nutritional demands of this tissue fulfilled by diffusion of lymph.

With the rapid addition of cytoplasm to the cells of the vertebral region and fusion of the cephalic and caudal masses to form the vertebral body, the cells of the notochord in this region are obliterated. Some embryologists theorize that there is an actual pressure gradient, with the notochordal cells being extruded or "squeezed" into the intervertebral region where the pressure is less. In any event, the notochordal cells become

Fig. 1-12. Twelve-week fetus.

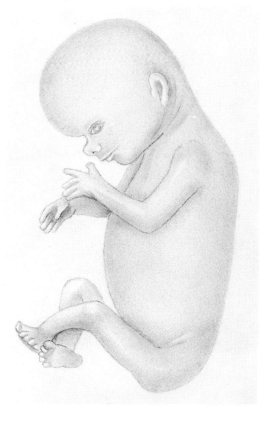

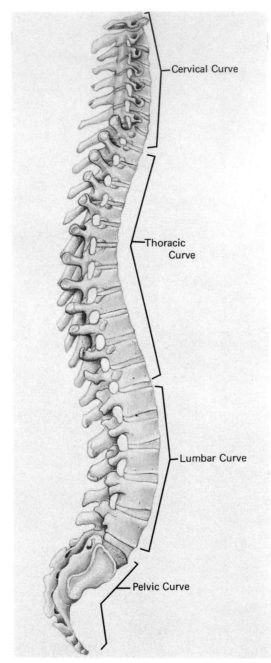

Fig. 1-13. Lateral view of the vertebral column.

attaching above and below to the vertebral bodies. These cells are formed from the cranial portion of the dark caudal masses and develop into the annulus fibrosis. Thus, the adult intervertebral disc has a double origin, the central nucleus pulposus derived from the notochord, the annulus from the fibroblastic extensions of the vertebral bodies.

Degenerative Effects of Living

The intervertebral disc undergoes progressive changes throughout life, so that its normal biologic state is specifically age-related.[8]

At birth the original notochordal cells are present within the nucleus pulposus with fine strands of fibrocartilage interlacing the mucoid center.

By the age of 4 years notochordal cells may be present but are increasingly difficult to find. The fibrous element and cartilage cells are increasingly prominent.

By the age of 12 years the notochordal cells have been completely replaced by loose fibrocartilage with abundant gelatinous matrix. With the passage of time, the fibrocartilage continues to replace the gelatinous mucoid material of the nucleus pulposus. This process is associated with progressive decrease in resiliency until old age, with the intervertebral disc composed almost entirely of dense irregularly arranged fibrocartilage. The water content of the nucleus pulposus decreases progressively with age.[18]

Spinal Curves

The vertebral column is formed by a series of 33 vertebrae—7 cervical, 12 thoracic, 5 lumbar, 5 sacral, and 4 coccygeal. The cervical, thoracic, and lumbar vertebrae remain distinct and separate from each other throughout life and may be considered "true" vertebrae. The adult sacral and coccygeal vertebrae are fused or united with each other to form 2 bones, the sacrum and the coccyx, and can be considered pseudo vertebrae. The bodies of the true or movable vertebrae are separated from each other by

obliterated within the vertebral body and migrate to the intervertebral region.

After 10 weeks, the cells around the periphery of the intervertebral region begin to differentiate into an elongated fibroblastic type and are arranged along a vertical axis intervertebral discs with the exception of the first and second cervical vertebrae.

A lateral view of the vertebral column reveals several curves which are identified by the predominant region in which the curve occurs.

The cervical curve, the least marked of all the curves, is convex anteriorly and extends from the first cervical to the second thoracic vertebra.

The thoracic curve extends from the second thoracic vertebra to the twelfth thoracic vertebra and is concave anteriorly.

The lumbar curve extends from the twelfth thoracic vertebra to the lumbosacral articulation and is convex anteriorly.

The pelvic curve begins at the lumbosacral joint and ends at the termination of the coccyx. It is concave anteriorly and is inclined in a somewhat downward direction.

The thoracic and pelvic curves are termed primary curves because they are present during fetal life.

The cervical curve becomes well established at the age of 4 months when the infant is able to hold up its head; the lumbar curve at 12 months when the infant begins to walk. The cervical and lumbar curves are termed compensatory or secondary curves.

The early fetal spine, which is completely concave anteriorly, embodies both the thoracic and pelvic curves. These primary curves are shaped by the configuration of the vertebral bodies which are wider posteriorly. The secondary cervical and lumbar curves are formed by the intervertebral discs which are wider anteriorly.

LUMBAR VERTEBRAE

The lumbar vertebrae are more massive and heavier than the other vertebrae, consistent with their primary role of weight bearing. The somewhat kidney-shaped bodies are wider in the transverse than in the anteroposterior diameter.

Fig. 1-14. A, The early fetal spine, which is completely concave, embodies both the thoracic and pelvic curves; B, the secondary cervical and lumbar curves are superimposed.

Fig. 1-15. Cephalad view of fourth lumbar vertebra.

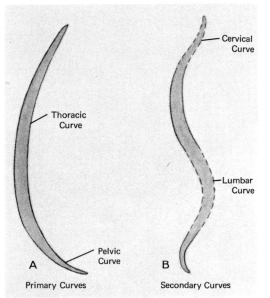

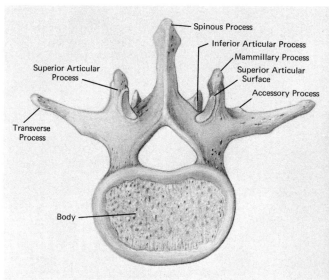

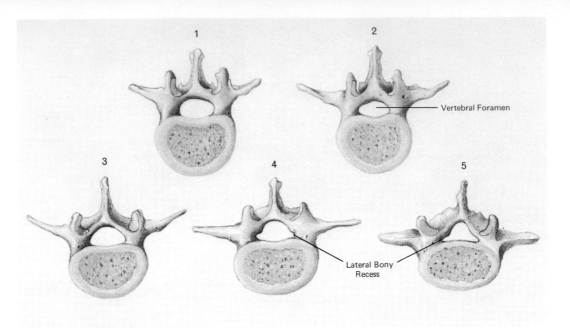

Fig. 1-16. The 5 lumbar vertebrae. Note the lateral bony recess formed by the last 2 vertebrae.

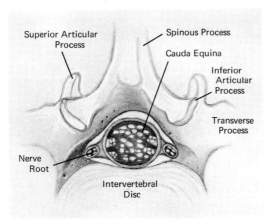

Fig. 1-17. Prior to exiting from the intervertebral foramina, the nerve root lies at the lateral-most portion of the vertebral foramen.

Vertebral Foramina and the "Lateral Bony Recess"

Changes in configuration of the lumbar vertebral foramina are of considerable clinical and surgical significance. The lumbar vertebral foramina are basically small and triangular in shape; but of prime importance is the progressive pinching of the lateral angles in the fourth and fifth lumbar vertebrae.

Prior to exiting from the intervertebral foramina, the nerve root lies snugly within this lateral bony recess.

The L5 and S1 nerve roots lying within this lateral recess are more vulnerable to compression from a protruding intervertebral

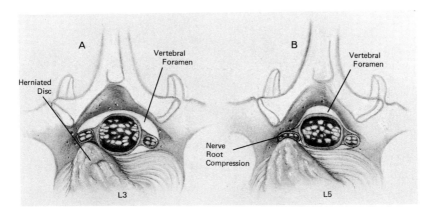

Fig. 1-18. A, A relatively small intervertebral disc protrusion may not produce significant nerve root compression when the vertebral foramen is oval permitting elevation of the root. B, When the nerve root lies within a lateral bony recess, even a small disc protrusion may produce severe root compression.

8

disc than the higher lumbar roots lying within a "rounder" vertebral foramen.[13,29]

The minute anatomy of the vertebral foramina exhibits considerable variation and it is not surprising to find a well-developed lateral bony recess as high as the third and occasionally even the second lumbar vertebra.

SACRUM AND COCCYX

The sacrum is a large triangular bone inserted like a wedge between the two hip bones.

The base of the sacrum articulates with the fifth lumbar vertebra, producing the rather acute lumbosacral angle which is formed by increased anterior width of both the fifth lumbar vertebral body and the L5-S1 intervertebral disc.

The sacral canal (vertebral canal) encloses the sacral nerves which pass out of the sacrum through the anterior and posterior sacral foramina.

The coccyx is usually a solid bone formed by the fusion of 4 rudimentary vertebrae. Occasionally the first coccygeal vertebra exists as a separate segment. The coccygeal cornua project upward and articulate with the sacral cornua to form a foramen through which the first coccygeal nerve passes. No vertebral canal exists within the coccyx itself.

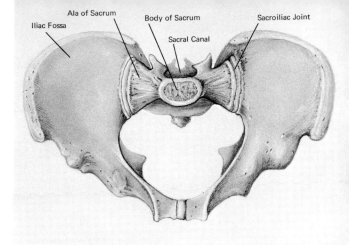

Fig. 1-19. The pelvis from above.

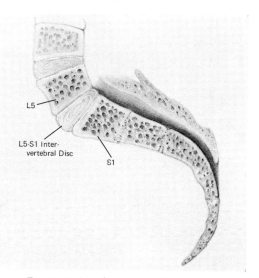

Fig. 1-20. Lumbosacral articulation.

Fig. 1-21. Sacrum and coccyx.

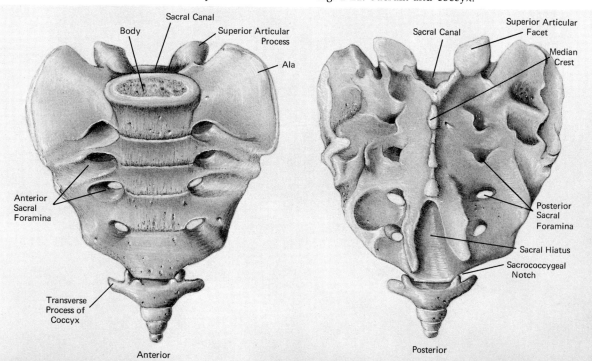

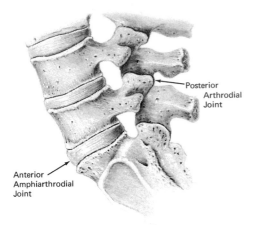

Fig. 1-22. Amphiarthrodial and arthrodial joints.

ARTICULATIONS AND LIGAMENTS OF THE LUMBAR SPINE

The articulations of the vertebral column consist of 2 types of joints. The joints between the vertebral bodies (amphiarthrodial) and the joints between the vertebral arches (arthrodial).

Vertebral Body Articulation

The joint between the vertebral bodies is called an amphiarthrodial joint, a joint in which the contiguous bony surfaces are either connected by discs of fibrocartilage or by an interosseous ligament. This type of joint, of course, permits only very limited movements but when this slight degree of movement takes place in all of the lumbar vertebrae, the total range of movement is considerable.

There are 4 ligaments involved in the amphiarthrodial vertebral body articulation:

1. intervertebral discs
2. anterior longitudinal ligament
3. posterior longitudinal ligament
4. lateral vertebral ligaments

Intervertebral Discs. The intervertebral discs contribute approximately one third of the overall length of the lumbar spine, while in the remainder of the vertebral column they contribute just a bit more than one fifth of the overall length.

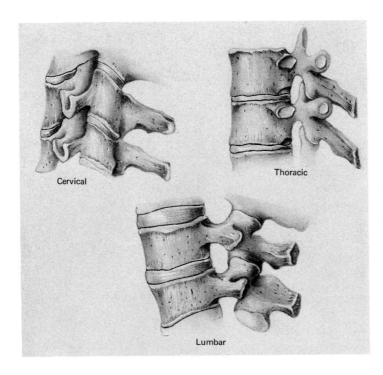

Fig. 1-23. Note the striking difference in bone-disc ratio in the cervical, thoracic, and lumbar spines. The lumbar intervertebral disc contributes about one third of the overall length of the lumbar spine while in the remainder of the vertebral column the intervertebral discs contribute just a bit more than one fifth of the overall length.

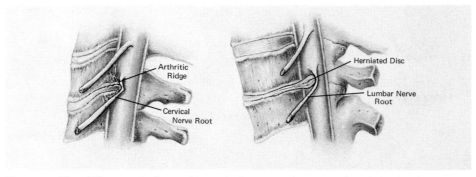

Fig. 1-24. The difference in bone-disc ratio between the cervical and the lumbar spines accounts for the different types of root compression lesions found in these two different areas. Most lumbar disc lesions are "soft tissue" in nature in contrast to the primarily bony lesions seen in the cervical spine.

This striking difference in bone-disc ratio in conjunction with the primary weight-bearing role of the lumbar spine accounts for the unique characteristics of lumbar disc disease. Most lumbar disc lesions are "soft tissue" in nature resulting from protrusion of the bulky lumbar intervertebral disc, causing nerve root pressure. This is in contrast to cervical nerve root compression syndromes, which are either exclusively bony lesions resulting from hypertrophic osteoarthritic ridging or a combination of bony spurs in association with some soft disc protrusion.

Structure. The vertebral surface adjacent to the lumbar disc is composed of a thin layer of cortical bone, which is most compact centrally and somewhat more porous at the periphery. A cartilaginous plate composed of hyaline cartilage overlies the cortical bone. This hyaline cartilage ends abruptly in the anterior and lateral regions, when it abuts on the outer raised bony rim of the vertebral body called the epiphyseal ring. Posteriorly the cartilaginous plate extends to the margin of the vertebral body. Blended intimately with the cartilaginous plate is a layer of fibrocartilage, which gives attachment to the fibers of the annulus fibrosus and nucleus pulposus. The annulus fibrosus forms a dense fibrocartilaginous retaining envelope for the fibrogelatinous nucleus pulposus. It is composed of approximately 12 concentric lamellae with the fibers of one layer running at an angle to those of the preceding layer.

The peripheral fibers of the annulus at the anterior and lateral margins of the vertebral body becomes very firmly attached to the outer raised bony rim of the vertebral body (epiphyseal ring).

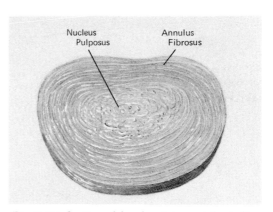

Fig. 1-25. Sectioned lumbar intervertebral disc.

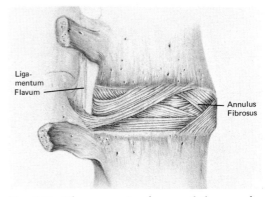

Fig. 1-26. The successive layers of the annulus fibrosus run in alternating oblique directions.

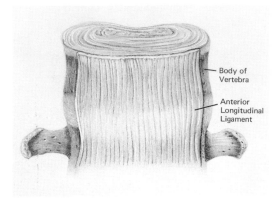

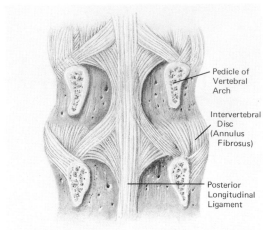

Fig. 1-27. The anterior fibers of the annulus fibrosus completely merged with the anterior longitudinal ligament fibers creating a powerful and virtually inseparable coupling of the lumbar spine.

Fig. 1-28. The fibers of the posterior longitudinal ligament are not as broad as the anterior longitudinal ligament and merge with the annulus fibrosus only in the posteromedial portion of the disc. This leaves the posterolateral portion relatively unsupported.

The anterior fibers of the annulus completely merge to form an intertexture with the anterior longitudinal ligament, creating a powerful and virtually inseparable coupling of the lumbar spine.

The posterior juncture is less secure. The annulus fibers are not as dense and firm posteriorly and the posterior longitudinal ligament is much thinner and less powerful than its anterior counterpart.

The centrally situated nucleus pulposus is composed of a loose network of fibrous tissue within a mucoprotein gel. In its normal state it has a gelatinous consistency and is semitransparent. The degenerated nucleus is denser, more fibrous and completely opaque.

Anterior Longitudinal Ligament. The anterior longitudinal ligament is a broad strong band of fibers, extending along the anterior surfaces of the vertebral bodies, from the body of the axis to the upper portion of the anterior sacrum.

It consists of 3 layers of dense fibers all running in a longitudinal direction. The most superficial fibers are the longest and extend over 4 or 5 vertebrae. The middle layer extends between 2 or 3 vertebrae. The innermost layer extends from one vertebra to the next, adhering intimately to the intervertebral discs and the outer raised bony rim of the vertebral body (epiphyseal ring)

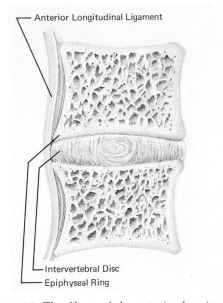

Fig. 1-29. The fibers of the anterior longitudinal ligament increase in thickness as they pass over the concave anterior surface of the vertebral bodies and fill in the concavities.

but not to the midportion of the vertebral bodies. The fibers increase in thickness as they pass over the concave anterior surface of the vertebral bodies and fill in the concavities.

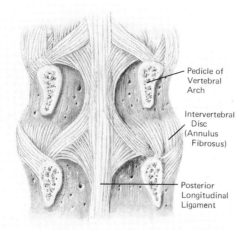

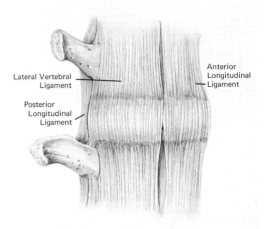

Fig. 1-30. The posterior longitudinal ligament is narrow and thick over the centers of the vertebral bodies where it is only loosely adherent, but at each intervertebral disc and at the raised bony rims of the vertebral body it is densely adherent.

Fig. 1-31. The lateral vertebral ligaments consist of short fibers firmly adherent to the intervertebral discs and passing over the vertebral body to the adjacent intervertebral disc.

Posterior Longitudinal Ligament. The posterior longitudinal ligament lies within the vertebral canal, extending along the posterior surfaces of the vertebral bodies from the axis to the sacrum. This ligament consists of 2 layers, the superficial layer extending over 3 or 4 vertebrae, and a deep layer extending between adjacent vertebrae. The ligament is narrow and thick over the centers of the vertebral bodies where it is only loosely adherent; but at each intervertebral disc it forms a thin lateral extension which is densely adherent to the annulus fibrosis of the intervertebral disc and the raised bony rim of the vertebral body.

Lateral Vertebral Ligaments. The lateral vertebral ligaments are situated between the anterior and posterior longitudinal ligaments. They consist of short fibers firmly adherent to the intervertebral discs and passing over the vertebral body to the adjacent intervertebral disc.

Vertebral Arch Articulation

The joint between the vertebral arches is called an arthrodial joint, one permitting only a gliding movement.

The articular facets which arise from the vertebral arches form the joint. The superior

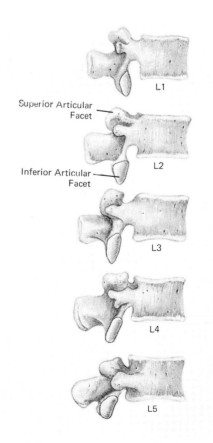

Fig. 1-32. The lumbar superior and inferior articular facets from the lumbar arthrodial joints.

facet is slightly concave and the inferior facet slightly convex. The lumbar facets lie generally in a sagittal plane, but the lumbosacral facets incline toward the coronal plane.

The gliding nature of the arthrodial joint permits flexion and extension of the lumbar spine. It is widely held that because of the shape and plane of these facets, rotation is not possible. However, the facets are only

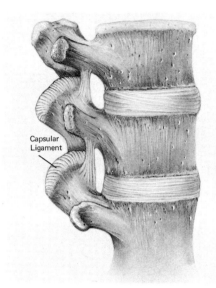

Fig. 1-33. The lumbar articular facets are enveloped by joint capsules which are lined with synovial membranes. The capsular ligaments are rather thin and loose to permit joint mobility.

loosely bound to each other, so that opposing articular facets are usually not in close opposition at the same time. This limited play allows for slight rotation of the lumbar spine. These joints are enveloped by capsules lined with synovial membranes.

The following ligaments are involved in the vertebral arch articulation:

1. capsular
2. yellow
3. supraspinal
4. interspinal
5. intertransverse

Capsular Ligament. The capsular ligaments are composed partly of yellow elastic tissue and partly of white fibrous tissue. They encapsulate the synovial joints between the superior and inferior articular processes of adjacent vertebrae. They are rather thin and loose to permit joint mobility.

Yellow Ligaments. The yellow ligaments connecting the laminae of adjacent vertebrae are composed of yellow elastic tissue. The

Fig. 1-34. A, The yellow ligaments are composed of thick, strong fibers attached to the anterior surface of the lamina above extending to the posterior surface and upper margin of the lamina below, producing a "shingle-like" configuration; B, they extend laterally to the medial and posterior edge of the intervertebral foramen forming a portion of the foraminal roof.

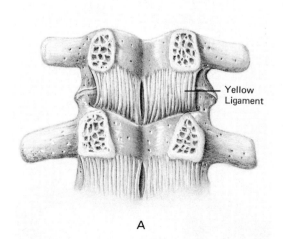

A

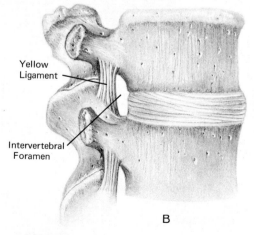

B

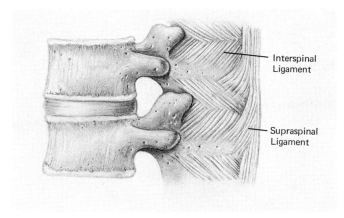

Fig. 1-35. Supraspinal and interspinal ligaments.

thick, strong fibers are attached to the anterior surface of the lamina above and to the posterior surface and upper margin of the lamina below. They extend laterally to the medial and posterior edge of the intervertebral foramen, forming a portion of the foraminal roof.

Supraspinal Ligament. The supraspinal ligament is a strong fibrous cord which extends without interruption along the tips of the spinous processes from the seventh cervical to end at the median sacral crest. Between the spinous processes it is continuous with the interspinal ligaments.

Interspinal Ligaments. The interspinal ligaments are fibers which decussate as they pass from the root of one spine to the tip of the next. Although they are thin and membranous in the cervical and thoracic spine, they are thick and well developed in the lumbar region.

Intertransverse Ligaments. The intertransverse ligaments are flat membranous bands passing between the apices of the transverse processes. They are relatively weak and unimportant as bonds of union.

PELVIC ARTICULATIONS AND LIGAMENTS

Pelvic-vertebral Articulation

Articulation of the pelvis with the vertebral column occurs at the interspace between the fifth lumbar vertebra and the sacrum. It is similar in almost all respects to those articulations which connect the vertebrae with

Fig. 1-36. Intertransverse ligament.

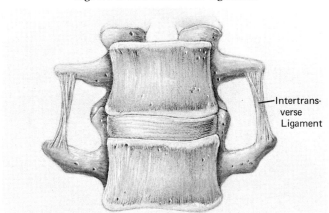

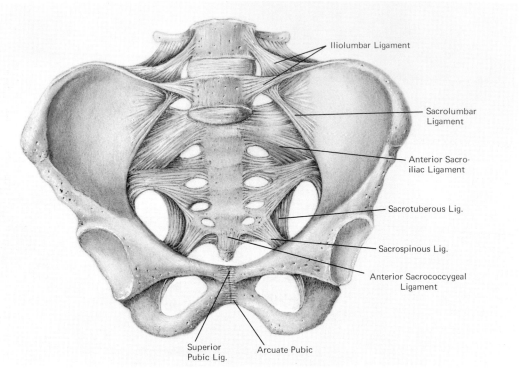

Iliolumbar Ligament

Sacrolumbar Ligament

Anterior Sacro-iliac Ligament

Sacrotuberous Lig.

Sacrospinous Lig.

Anterior Sacrococcygeal Ligament

Superior Pubic Lig.

Arcuate Pubic

Fig. 1-37. Pelvic joints and ligaments, anterior aspect.

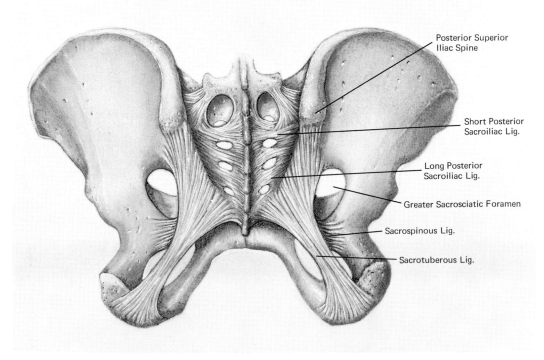

Posterior Superior Iliac Spine

Short Posterior Sacroiliac Lig.

Long Posterior Sacroiliac Lig.

Greater Sacrosciatic Foramen

Sacrospinous Lig.

Sacrotuberous Lig.

Fig. 1-38. Pelvic joints and ligaments, posterior aspect.

each other. In addition, the iliolumbar ligament connects the pelvis with the vertebral column on either side.

Sacroiliac Articulation

The sacroiliac articulation is an amphiarthrodial or slightly movable joint. The articular surfaces of the sacrum and ilium are covered with cartilaginous plates in close contact with each other and bound together by fibrous strands.

The ligaments of the sacroiliac articulation are the anterior sacroiliac, posterior sacroiliac, and interosseous.

Sacrococcygeal Articulation

The sacrococcygeal articulation is a joint similar to the articulations between vertebral bodies.

The ligaments of this symphysis are anterior sacrococcygeal, posterior sacrococcygeal, lateral sacrococcygeal and interarticular.

Symphysis Pubis

The pubic symphysis is an amphiarthrodial joint formed between the 2 oval symphyseal surfaces of the pubic bones.

The ligaments of this articulation are superior pubic, arcuate pubic and interpubic fibrocartilaginous lamina.

BLOOD SUPPLY OF THE LUMBAR SPINE

The 4 lumbar arteries arise in pairs from the posterior aspect of the aorta in front of the bodies of the first 4 lumbar vertebrae. In front of the fifth lumbar vertebra a fifth pair of arteries may arise from the middle sacral artery, and will appear in approximately 50 percent of all dissections. This fifth lumbar artery is always smaller than the first 4 arteries and is frequently unpaired and more often seen on the left side. The right arteries are longer than the left to compensate for the left paramedian position of the aorta. These arteries curve posteriorly around the bodies of the vertebrae to the interspaces between the transverse processes where a posterior ramus is given off, which in turn furnishes the vertebral (spinal) branch supplying the bodies of the vertebrae and their ligaments.

The spinal rami accompany the spinal nerves through the intervertebral foramina, traverse the dura mater and arachnoid and divide into radicular branches which supply each nerve root.

Blood Supply of the Intervertebral Disc

It should be recalled that the developmental precursor of the disc is that con-

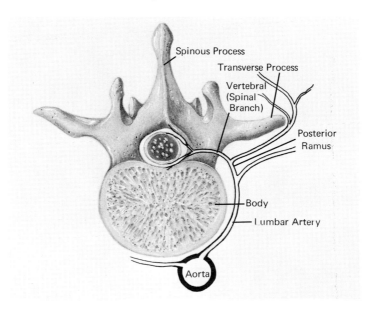

Fig. 1-39. The spinal branch of the lumbar artery accompanies the spinal nerves through the intervertebral foramina, traverses the dura mater and arachnoid and divides into radicular branches which supply each nerve root.

Spinous Process

Transverse Process

Vertebral (Spinal Branch)

Posterior Ramus

Body

Lumbar Artery

Aorta

densed mass most removed from the nutrition provided by the artery. In children and young adults one can find small vessels within the periphery of the cartilaginous end-plates. These vessels gradually become obliterated so that by the age of 20 or 30 years the intervertebral disc is found to be completely avascular in common with most cartilaginous or fibrous tissues subjected to weight bearing.

The disc's limited nutritional demands are probably fulfilled by the diffusion of lymph through minute perforations from the marrow cavity to the cartilaginous end-plates, which permits a scanty lumph supply to diffuse through the intervertebral disc.

NERVE SUPPLY OF THE LUMBAR SPINE

In 1949 as a neurology resident I assisted in my first neurosurgical procedure, a hemilaminectomy for excision of a herniated lumbar disc. The operation remains keen in my memory, because it was performed with the patient under local anesthesia, since, in addition to excising the offending lesion, the surgeon hoped to demonstrate the structures of the lumbar spine which were pain producing. This was to be accomplished by subjecting the various structures and tissues to noxious stimuli prior to anesthetizing them with procaine. He used a hemostat to pinch structures, such as the yellow ligament or the annulus fibrosis, and also exerted pressure upon these tissues. Other methods can be used such as injections of minute amounts of hypertonic saline into the various tissues and a variety of electrical stimuli. These varied noxious stimuli techniques furnish results that are far from conclusive because of the inherent difficulties in working with a partially sedated, intimidated, apprehensive patient undergoing an uncomfortable experience and who is often not especially receptive to the imposed demands of "clinical research." Of equal importance is the artificial nature of the stimuli, which cannot exactly reduplicate the physiological conditions producing pain.

A number of painstaking anatomical–histologic studies have been carried out in attempting to trace the nerve supply of the lumbar spine subserving low back pain.[26] It has been demonstrated that nerve strands originate beyond the dorsal root ganglia of the posterior primary division of the root and pass back through the intervertebral foramen, reentering the vertebral canal. This recurrent sinuvertebral nerve curves around

Fig. 1-40. Branches of the recurrent sinuvertebral nerve.

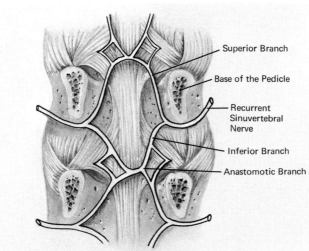

the base of the pedicle and gives off branches extending to the intervertebral discs above and below. Filaments of this nerve supply the posterior longitudinal ligament, periosteum, epidural blood vessels and dura mater. The posterior rami of the posterior primary divisions of the spinal nerve roots supply sensory fibers to the skin, muscle, fascia, ligaments and the posterior arthrodial joints.

LOW BACK MUSCULATURE

Determining the exact function of each of the various muscles involved in the low back is difficult. Anatomical studies, the construction of mechanical models and electrical stimulation of individual muscles are all valuable in investigating this problem. However, the interrelationship of these associated muscles so increases the complexities that we can only approximate the primary function of the individual low back muscles.

Extensors of the Lumbar Spine

Quadratus Lumborum. The quadratus lumborum derives its name from its irregularly quadrilateral shape, broader at the base than above. It arises from the iliac crest and iliolumbar ligament and inserts into the lower border of the last rib and to the transverse process of the first 4 lumbar vertebrae.

Sacrospinalis. The sacroscpinalis muscle, also called the erector spinae, is a long strong band of muscle running from the sacrum to the occipital portion of the skull and serving as a very powerful extensor of the spine.

It originates from a broad and strong aponeurosis which is attached to the sacrum, iliac crest, the spinous processes of all the lumbar vertebrae and the last 2 thoracic vertebrae. The muscle fibers divide in the upper lumbar region into 3 separate columns. The most lateral slip, the iliocostalis, is inserted into the angles of the ribs. The intermediate slip, the longissimus, is inserted into the tips of the transverse processes of all the thoracic and cervical vertebrae. The medial slip, the spinalis, is inserted into the spinous processes of the thoracic and cervical vertebrae.

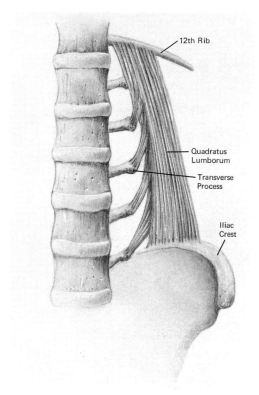

Fig. 1-41. Quadratus lumborum.

Fig. 1-42. The sacrospinalis muscle runs from the sacrum to the occipital portion of the skull and is a very powerful extensor of the spine.

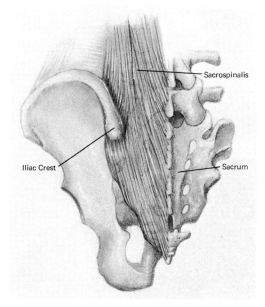

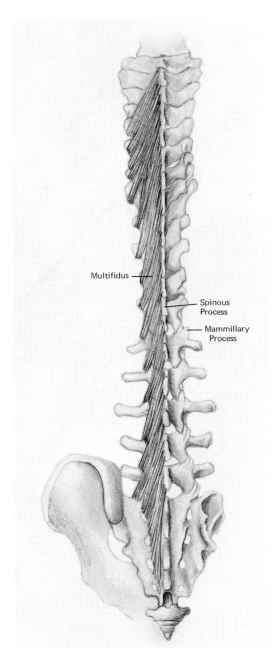

Multifidus —

Spinous
Process

Mammillary
Process

Fig. 1-43. The multifidus muscles consist of numerous small muscular slips arising from a small bony prominence on the articular facet called the mammillary process and ascending obliquely toward the midline and inserting into the spinous process of the vertebra 2 to 4 segments above. These muscles which are best developed in the lumbar spine act as extensors and can also abduct and slightly rotate the vertebral column.

Multifidus. The multifidus muscles extend from the sacrum to the cervical vertebrae but are best developed in the lumbar spine. They consist of numerous small muscular slips or fasciculi arising from the mammillary process, a small bony prominence on the dorsal margin of each superior articular process, and ascending obliquely toward the midline and inserting into the spinous process of a vertebra 2 to 4 segments above.

Although categorized as extensors of the lumbar spine, these muscles acting unilaterally will abduct and slightly rotate the vertebral column.

Intertransversarii. The intertransversarii are small muscles between the transverse processes of the vertebrae. In the lumbar region there are 3 muscle groupings: medial, dorsal lateral and ventral lateral. They lie between the psoas and sacrospinalis muscles.

The medial intertransverse muscle arises from the accessory process (a minute bony eminence arising at the angle between the superior articular process and the transverse process) of the superior vertebra and is inserted into the mamillary process of the inferior vertebra.

The dorsal lateral slip arises from the accessory process of the superior vertebra and is inserted in the transverse process of the inferior vertebra.

The ventral lateral slip connects the inferior border of one transverse process with the superior border of the next.

Interspinalis. The interspinalis muscles consist of short muscular fasciculi that extend from the superior surface of the spinous process below to the inferior surface of the above. They occur in pairs on either side of the interspinous ligament.

Flexors of the Lumbar Spine

Abdominal Muscles. *External oblique.* This broad, thin, irregular quadrilateral muscle is the largest and most superficial of the 3 flat abdominal muscles. It originates from 8 fleshy digitations from the lower 8 ribs and inserts into a broad, strong abdominal aponeurosis that extends over the rectus

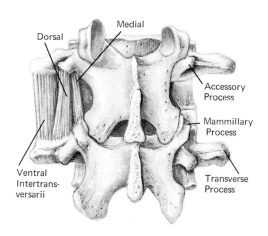

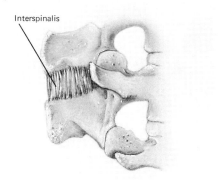

Fig. 1-44. The intertransversarii.

Fig. 1-45. Interspinalis muscle.

to the linea alba where the more superficial fibers originating from the last 2 ribs insert into the anterior wall of the iliac crest.

Internal oblique. The internal oblique lies under the external oblique and is smaller and thinner. It originates from the lumbodorsal fascia, the anterior two thirds of the iliac crest, and the lateral half of the inguinal ligament. The fibers, which run perpendicular to the external oblique fibers, pass upward in a vertical direction and insert into the lower 3 ribs and the remainder extend toward the lateral margin of the rectus muscle and terminate in its sheath.

Transversalis. The transversalis muscle is the innermost of the flat abdominal muscles and takes its name from the direction of its fibers. It originates from the lateral third of the inguinal ligament, the anterior three fourths of the iliac crest, the lumbodorsal fascia, and from the inner surface of the cartilages of the lower 6 ribs. The fibers take a nearly transverse course across the abdominal wall inserting either at the midline in the linea alba or in the lower attachments,

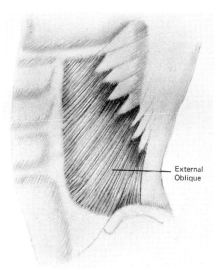

Fig. 1-46. External oblique.

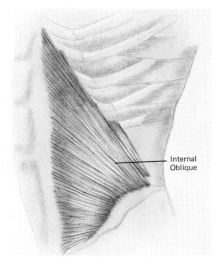

Fig. 1-47. Internal oblique.

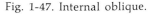

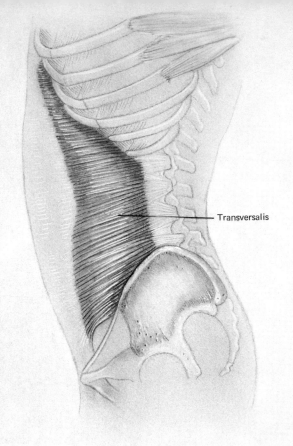

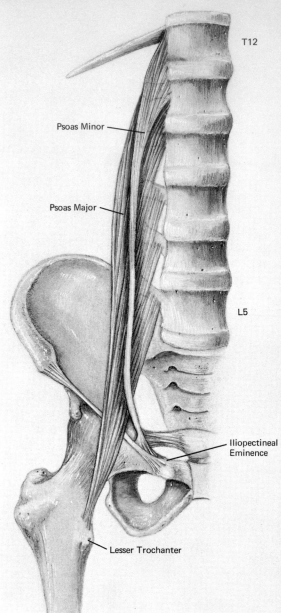

Fig. 1-48. Transversalis.

Fig. 1-49. Rectus abdominus.

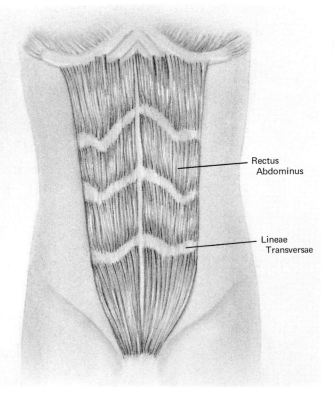

Fig. 1-50. Psoas major and minor.

curving behind the spermatic cord and attaching to the lacunar ligament and pectineal fascia.

The chief function of this muscle is to act as a living girdle in supporting the abdominal viscera. It is such support that helps maintain fixation of the lumbar spine.

Rectus abdominis. The rectus abdominis is a long, flat, bandlike muscle which extends along the length of the anterior abdominal wall. It originates as a short thick tendon which divides into two. The thicker lateral tendon is attached to the crest of the pubis. The muscle inserts into the cartilages of the fifth, sixth, and seventh ribs. The muscle is crossed by 3 fibrous bands (lineae transversae) passing transversely or obliquely across the muscle.

Psoas Major. The psoas major is a long fusiform muscle originating as a series of thick fasciculi attached to the fifth lumbar vertebra and the transverse processes of the lumbar vertebrae. The muscle extends downward across the brim of the minor pelvis and ends in a tendon which is inserted into the lesser trochanter of the femur.

Psoas Minor. The psoas minor is a long slender muscle lying anterior to the psoas major. It originates from the twelfth thoracic and first lumbar vertebrae and the interven-

ing disc. The muscle fibers end in a long flat tendon which inserts into the iliopectineal eminence.

Abductors of the Lumbar Spine

Identifying a muscle as either a flexor or extensor of the lumbar spine implies bilaterally simultaneous muscle action. Unilateral action will produce abduction or lateral bending of the spine. For example contraction of the right quadratus lumborum or right psoas major will produce right lumbar abduction.

Abductors of the Lumbar Spine
  Quadratus lumborum
  Psoas major and minor
  Abdominal muscles
  Intertransversarii

Fig. 1-51. Cross-section of body musculature and fascia through third lumbar vertebra.

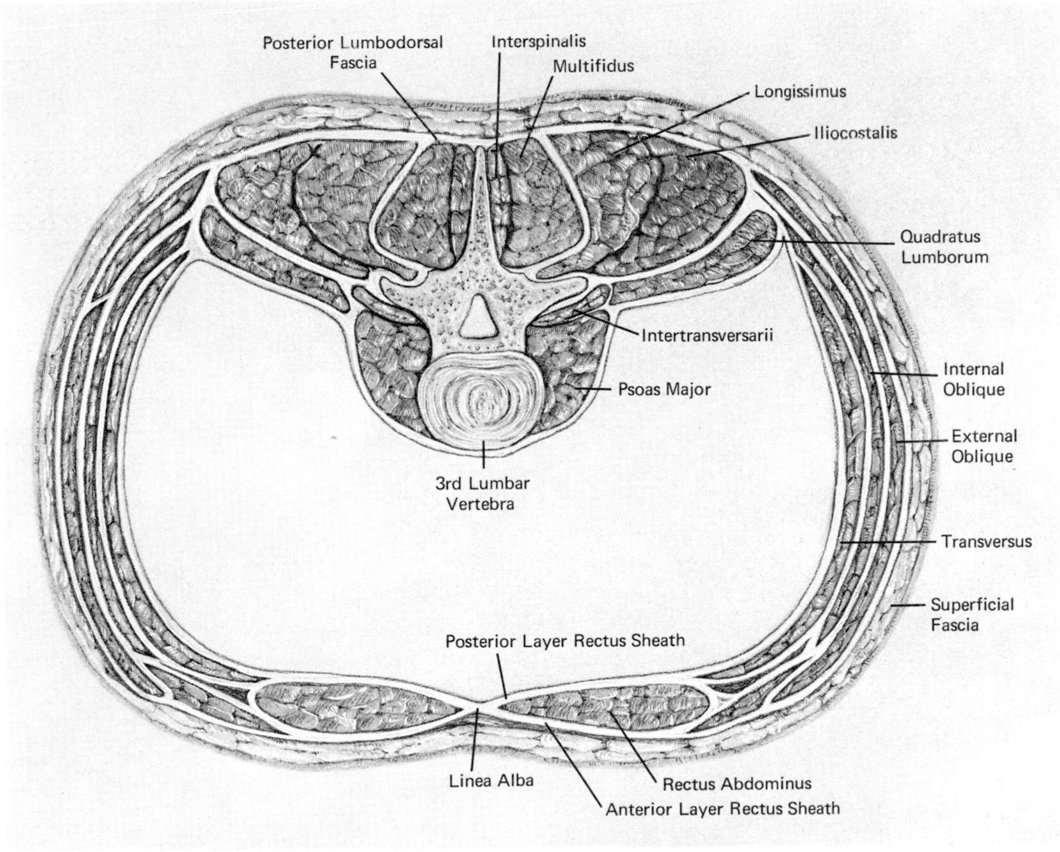

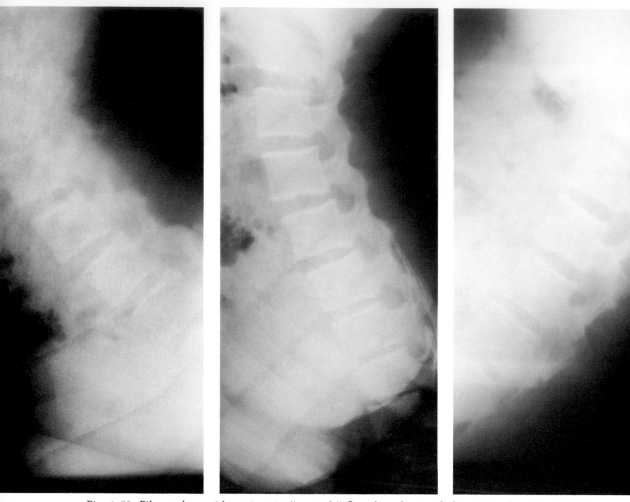

Fig. 1-52. Films taken with patient in "neutral," flexed, and extended position (see Fig. 1-53B).

BIOMECHANICS OF THE LUMBAR SPINE

MOBILITY OF THE
LUMBAR SPINE

In 1950 a patient with low back dysfunction who had been previously evaluated in another area was seen in consultation by me. Included in his original x-ray folder were several "mobility films" of the lumbar spine. This was the first time I had ever carefully examined such films, and to my inexpert eye they appeared to indicate markedly decreased mobility. Since the clinical examination revealed excellent mobility of the lumbar spine, I presumed that improvement had occurred in the interim. To demonstrate x-ray evidence of this improvement, I ordered a second set of mobilization films which, to my surprise, were identical to the originals. This experience impressed upon

my mind the striking difference between the rather limited range of lumbar mobility as viewed radiographically and what we think we see when examining the patient.

Rotation of the pelvis on the femoral heads during flexion is difficult to differentiate from lumbar flexion and may obscure a relatively nonmobile lumbar spine. Since relatively little rotation of the pelvis occurs during extension, the extension films of the lumbar spine more closely approximate what we clinically visualize.

David Allbrook[1] carried out a study in which lateral lumbar spine films were obtained in full flexion, the erect position and full extension. He then traced the vertebral bodies and sacrum on transparent paper while superimposing the sacrum in all 3 positions; thus, giving a fixed point for measur-

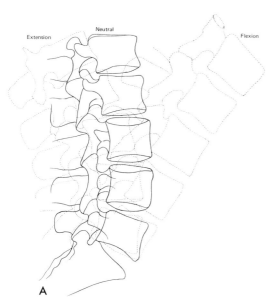

A

Fig. 1-53A. Tracing of x-ray films of patient in "neutral," flexed, and extended positions.

ing movement of each lumbar vertebra between the position of full flexion and full extension. Using these tracings, individual vertebral movement was measured.

Shelby J. Clayson and coworkers[7] also carried out measurements of lumbar mobility using x-rays and found an angulation of 115° from the "relaxed standing position" with flexion and 11° angulation with extension. They report the greatest movement to be between the fifth lumbar vertebra and the sacrum while Allbrook found the greatest movement to be between the fourth and fifth lumbar vertebrae. Both studies indicated a progressive decrease in the degree of motion from each vertebra to the next up the lumbar spine. Clayson placed the subjects in the knee to chest position for maximal flexion in contrast to forward bending with knees straight in Allbrook's report. These modifications may account for the minor differences in measurements.

In addition to flexion, extension and lateral movements of the lumbar spine, rotation or torsion of the lumbar vertebrae occurs during walking and many other activities of daily living. The degree and nature of this torsion primarily depends upon the position of the facets. When walking, the greatest rotation

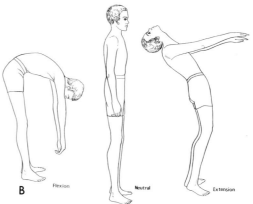

B

Fig. 1-53B. "Neutral," flexed, and extended positions.

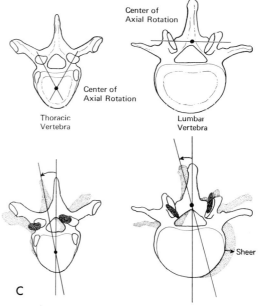

C

Fig. 1-53C. Because of the arrangement of facet joints, the axis of rotation of the thoracic vertebrae is near the center of the vertebral body in comparison to the lumbar vertebrae where the center of axial rotation is posterior to the body. This subjects the lumbar discs to considerably more sheer stress during rotation.

occurs in the midthoracic spine. The axis of rotation in the thoracic vertebrae is through the center of the disc. In comparison, because of the arrangement of the facet joints, the lumbar vertebrae rotate around an axis posterior to the disc, subjecting the lumbar discs to much more sheer stress.[16]

BIOCHEMICAL CHANGES IN THE INTERVERTEBRAL DISC

The biochemical structure of the intervertebral disc is specialized to fulfill its function of absorbing and redistributing the forces applied to the vertebral column. The 2 principal macromolecules of which the disc is composed are collagen and mucopolysaccharide. Many of the chemical details of the various processes relating to the synthesis and deterioration of these constituents have yet to be worked out.

In 1930 Püschel[28] published a paper indicating that with advancing age, the water content of the intervertebral disc progressively decreased. This was followed 5 years later by DePukey's[10] observation that the average person is 1 percent shorter at the end of the day when compared to body length in the morning on first arising. This report was based on measurements of 1,216 persons of various ages. In harmony with Püschel's paper was the finding that the average daily oscillation in body length is 2 percent in the first decade and only 0.5 percent in the eighth decade. The difference was attributed to decreasing water content of the intervertebral disc with advancing age.

Following these early works are many articles describing changes in the disc constituents including the collagen and mucopolysaccharide ratio plus the changes in water content resulting from both age and protrusion.[3,11,17] With the development of improved investigative techniques, the more recent articles utilize increasingly sophisticated means of measuring the constituents of the intervertebral disc including x-ray crystallographic, biochemical and electron microscopic studies.

Since the protruded disc in a younger man demonstrates a loss of water, an increase in collagen and protein and a decrease in mucopolysaccharides, which is consistent with what is found in nonprotruded discs from older individuals, it is felt by some that disc degeneration represents a premature aging process.[21]

On the other hand, Dr. Arthur Naylor, who has devoted many years to the analysis of the biochemical constituents of the intervertebral disc, suggests that neither age nor trauma is the sole factor; and some cause responsible for a basically spontaneous onset should be considered. He advances a tentative hypothesis considering an auto-immune phenomenon as the etiology for lumbar disc protrusion.[4,25] When I first read this hypothesis it seemed farfetched to me. However, the longer I deal with low back dysfunction the more I realize how scanty are the basic facts upon which we establish our working hypothesis. I now attempt to view this and other theories without prejudice in the realization that we remain only on the threshold of investigation into a very complex problem.

BIOMECHANICS OF THE INTERVERTEBRAL DISC

The unique construction and composition of the intervertebral disc enables this structure to withstand stresses varying in duration and magnitude. Both the annulus and the nucleus act to absorb forces that occur primarily in a vertical axis and redistribute them evenly in all directions. This is possible because the nucleus pulposus alters its shape freely under pressure, transmitting some of these forces radially to the annulus and the rest over the entire cartilaginous end-plate. It is the liquid property of the nucleus, rendering it almost incompressible, that is the basis of this shape-altering property.

The importance of the entire phenomenon of fluid exchange as it affects the intervertebral discs has been the subject of considerable investigation since the pioneer papers of Püschel and DePukey. It was originally postulated that fluid exchange was governed by osmotic pressure. The cartilaginous end-plates were thought to act as semipermeable membranes with the nucleus drawing water from the vertebral bodies.[5] It is presently thought that the hydrodynamics of the disc depends upon the nucleus pulposus possessing the properties of a gel rather

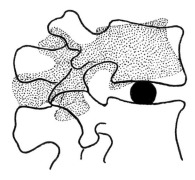

Fig. 1-54. The movement of contiguous lumbar vertebrae is partially dependent on a ball-bearing-like action of the nucleus pulposus.

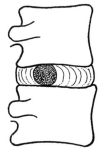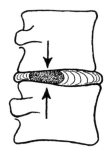

Fig. 1-55. Axial vertebral compression produces slight flattening of the nucleus and a compensatory "stretching" of the annular fibers.

than upon osmosis.[18] This gel contains some cartilaginous cells, fibroblasts, collagen framework and the ground substance, which is mostly mucopolysaccharide with varying amounts of salts and water. A high imbibition pressure is produced by the gel which can bind almost 9 times its volume of water. This water content is not chemically bonded, as demonstrated by the tendency to express significant quantities of water from the nucleus by prolonged mechanical pressure. The daily oscillation in body length (with the average person 1 percent shorter at the end of the day when compared to body length upon arising in the morning) is the most striking example of this phenomenon.

The normal nucleus, occupying about half of the disc surface area bears most of the vertical load while the annulus, bears the tangential load. When there is degeneration

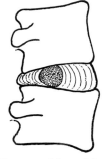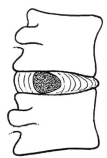

Fig. 1-56. Normal lumbar spinal movement produces a slight protrusion of the annulus fibrosus.

of the nucleus resulting in impairment of the gel's imbibition pressure, a marked change occurs in the transmission of forces occurring along the vertical axis of the spine. The degenerated nucleus is unable to redistribute

Fig. 1-57. A, The normal nucleus bears about half the vertical load while the annulus bears the other half tangentially. B, The degenerated nucleus is unable to redistribute much of the load radially causing the annulus to sustain much of the vertical load.

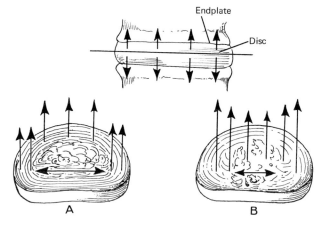

much of the load radially, causing the annulus to sustain most of the vertical load and little tangential load.

THE SKELETON AS A STRUCTURAL UNIT

Using engineering principals, one may consider the skeleton as a structural unit and theoretically estimate the forces brought to bear on the lumbar spine. All of these theoretical calculations employ the fulcrum-lever concept utilizing the nucleus pulposus of the L5-S1 or the L4-5 intervertebral disc as the fulcrum. When lifting a heavy weight, the hands, arms and trunk are considered to be like a long anterior lever which is counterbalanced by a much shorter lever comprising the distance from the nucleus pulposus (ful-

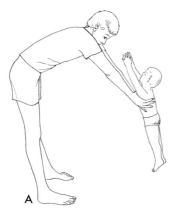

A

Fig. 1-58A. A most common and dangerously inefficient lifting position.

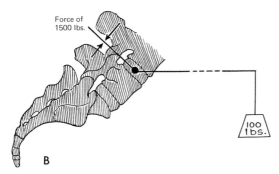

B

Fig. 1-58B. The fulcrum-lever concept of estimating stress on the spine.

crum) to the spinous process. This mechanical concept was originally advanced by Bradford and Spurling, and they estimated the ratio between the anterior and posterior levers at about 15 to 1. Thus, it follows that if a 100-pound weight were lifted, the posterior lever is activated by a 1,500-pound muscle contraction, subjecting the nucleus pulposus to a total pressure of 1,600 pounds.

A more complex series of calculations was employed by Morris, Lucas and Bresler[22] utilizing similar principles. The conditions they assumed are that a 170-pound man lifts a 200-pound weight; the weight being lifted at a distance of 14 inches from the L5-S1 intervertebral disc and that flexion of the spine at the pelvis is 40°. They calculated that the head, neck and upper limbs weigh 30 pounds (17.7% of the body weight) and that the portion of the trunk above the L5-S1 disc weighs 51 pounds (30% of body weight). The weight of the head, neck and upper limbs act at a distance of 18 inches from the L4-S1 disc and the weight of the trunk 7 inches from the disc. Employing these measurements in their calculations, a force of 2,071 pounds is exerted on the L5-S1 intervertebral disc.

STRESS STUDIES OF THE LUMBAR SPINE

The previous calculations are based on the skeletal spine functioning as an isolated unit being acted upon by the forces of the weight lifted, the body weight and the contraction of the deep muscles of the back.

Stress studies, however, of the isolated skeletal lumbar spine, both as a unit and segmentally, clearly demonstrate its inability to tolerate such tremendous forces. Lucus and Bresler[20] conducted studies in which they fixed the isolated ligamentous spine at the base and produced progressively increasing compression in a vertical plane. The critical load valve above which point the spine would buckle was found to be approximately 4½ pounds, or much less than the weight of the body above the pelvis.

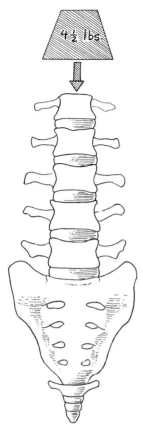

Fig. 1-59. The isolated spine will buckle under 4½ pounds of pressure.

Axial Compression

Compression tests have been carried out on segments consisting of two vertebral bodies with their intervening disc. This testing segment or unit demonstrates a hydrostatic pressure within the disc which is 30 to 50 percent higher than the pressure applied to the entire segment. Because of the hydrostatic nature of the nucleus pulposus, an axially compressive load upon the testing segment produces compressive stress upon the nucleus, which in turn causes a different type of stress on the fibers of the annulus fibrosus, a tensile stress.

For example, consider a wooden barrel filled with water, the weight of which is producing pressure upon the staves. In order to restrain these staves from flying outward it is necessary to place steel rings or hoops around them. This so called "hoop stress" occurs whenever there is a chamber full of fluid under hydrostatic pressure.

In this fashion compressive loading in an axial direction produces a hydrostatic pressure, which in turn causes a circumferential tensile stress around the periphery of the disc. This circumferential stress upon the

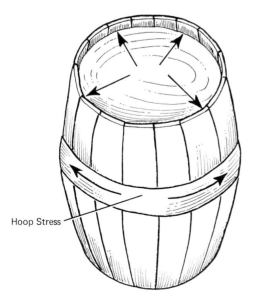

Fig. 1-60. The integrity of this water-filled barrel is maintained by "hoop stress."

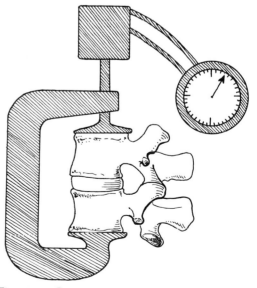

Fig. 1-61. Compression tests on autopsy specimens.

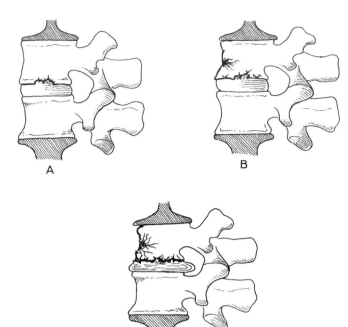

Fig. 1-62. A, The cartilaginous end-plates are most susceptible to spinal compression. B, The vertebral body is the second most susceptible unit of the spine. C, The normal nucleus pulposus and annulus fibrosus are least susceptible to pressure.

annulus fibrosis is 3 to 5 times higher than the compressive stress applied to the testing segment.

Compression tests performed on autopsy specimens from the 20- to 30-year-old age group demonstrated structural damage at loads in excess of 600 Kg. In specimens from the over-60 age group structural failure was produced at 260 Kg., which is a decrease of more than 50 percent.

Such studies indicate a decrease in the lumbar spine's resistance to axially compressive loading of approximately 20 percent per decade over the age of 30. This is significantly higher than the decrease in functioning capacity of other anatomical structures and systems.[9,14,27]

In these compression tests it was found that when the annulus was complete, its elastic limits could not be exceeded without vertebral fracture. The cartilaginous endplates are the most susceptible to compression of the spine and will crack or sometimes collapse as the first evidence of structural failure. The vertebral body itself is the second most susceptible unit of the spine and usually collapses and disintegrates. The nor-

mal nucleus pulposus and annulus fibrosis are the portion of the unit least susceptible to pressure.

Most experimental spinal stress studies have been performed on isolated segments of the lumbar spine involving two vertebrae with the intervening intervertebral disc. King and Vulcan carried out experiments using entire adult male cadavers.[19] In this study, all abdominal organs were eviscerated and the abdominal cavity was filled with tightly crumpled newspaper. The cadavers were then seated in an accelerator sled housed in an eight-story elevator shaft of the School of Medicine, at Wayne State University. Fractures of the lower thoracic and upper lumbar vertebrae were produced by rapid caudocephalad acceleration with this sled. This study and others of a similar nature were carried out to obtain data relative to the mechanisms of vertebral compression fractures sustained by pilots ejecting from disabled aircraft.

Torsion

In addition to axially compressive stress, the lumbar spine is subjected to rotation or torsion. The ability of the lumbar spine to sustain torsional loads depends upon 3 structures. The intervertebral disc provides between 35 and 45 percent of the mechanical resistance to torsion. The articular processes provide an equal or slightly greater amount accounting for approximately 80 to 90 percent of the total strength of the vertebral structure in rotation. The remaining 10 percent comes from ligamentous or capsular attachments. These percentages remain valid at almost every vertebral level so that we have a spinal system in which the disc is responsible for a large share of the torsional strength.

We can measure torque load by removing the posterior elements of a lumbar vertebral testing segment and subjecting it to torsion. Abnormalities in the disc reduce its capacity to aid in supporting torsional loads of the spine by about 40 percent.

In a normal disc the first 2 or 3 degrees of rotation require more force than is necessary to obtain the next few degrees. In a degenerated disc the first 2 or 3 degrees are almost free and occur with the application of minimal force.

In the lumbar vertebral testing segment with posterior elements removed, rotation may approach 30 degrees. If the testing segment is intact, a 12- to 16-degree rotation capability is present.

Under torsional load the stresses are not uniformly distributed throughout the disc. The stress is zero in the center of axial rotation and this increases as it goes outward. Since the disc is not a uniform circle, the stresses at the periphery are not uniformly distributed. In the lumbar spine with the center of axial rotation posteriorly, the greatest sheer stress occurs at the posterolateral angle of the disc. It is in this region that we would expect to see torsional load failures with separation and tearing of the annular fibers.

Clinical Verification of Stress Studies

Correlation of the information we derive from in vitro stress testing with the clinical situation is based on similar loads producing similar types of tissue failure. If we have an in vitro test loading that produces a compression fracture of a vertebra and we see the same type of compression fracture clinically, which is produced by an axially compressive stress, we can reasonably assume that similar loads were in effect.

Compression fractures of the lumbar spine are often seen in certain types of injuries. A fall on ice or on a slippery floor when the lower extremities slip forward causing the patient to land directly on the buttocks may result in wedging of the midlumbar vertebrae. The high incidence of lumbar compression fractures resulting from snowmobile injuries occurs when the buttocks are momentarily raised from the seat and then smash down again when speeding over a crest or embankment.

The forces involved in the above types of injuries are difficult to estimate because of the several variables involved. One frequent cause of lumbar compression fracture, in which the forces involved can be studied, is the seat ejection injury.[6][12] Jet pilots are seat ejected by means of a catapult mechanism when a crash is imminent, since, at the high speeds they are moving, it would be impossible for them to "bail out" of a plane by climbing out of the cockpit. Although the development of such escape systems was initiated by the German Luftwaffe over thirty years ago, frequent and persistent design improvements have not yet resulted in the elimination of compression fractures. Some pilots suffer vertebral fractures when the ejection force approximates 1,000 Kg. Since these men are usually young and healthy, their vertebral load compression tolerance should be extremely high.

EXTRINSIC SPINAL SUPPORT

A large discrepancy exists between the theoretical calculations indicating the great load brought to bear on the lumbar spine when weight-lifting in forward flexion and the limited ability of the lumbar vertebrae

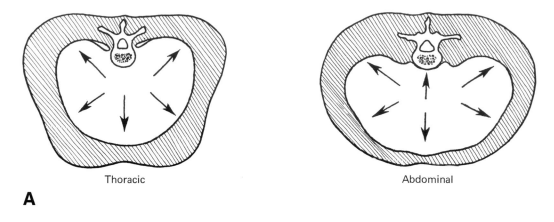

Thoracic   Abdominal

A

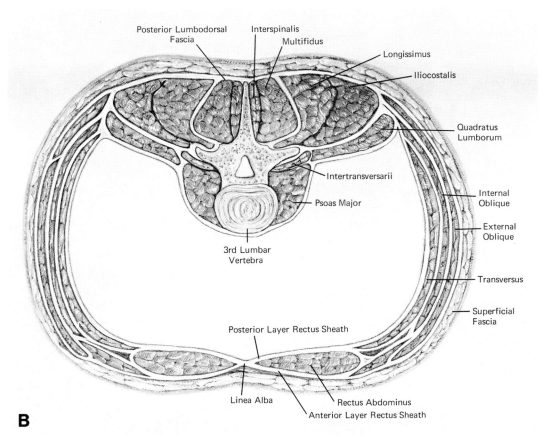

B

Fig. 1-63. A, The spine is enclosed within the thoracic and abdominal cavities which can be converted into almost rigid-walled cylinders by the trunk muscles. This mechanism diminishes the direct load on the spine. B, Cross-section of body musculature and fascia through third lumbar vertebra.

to tolerate great loads as demonstrated by both experimental stress studies and clinical experience. If both the theoretical calculations and experimental stress studies are accepted as valid, it must be presumed that the support and stability of the spine depends, to a considerable degree, upon extrinsic forces. That the mechanism of such additional support for the spine can be provided by the musculature and compartments of the trunk was advanced first by Bartelink[2] and further developed by Morris, Lucas and Bresler[22] in what has since become a classic and often referred to paper.

They consider the spine to be a segmented elastic rod or column supported by the paraspinal musculature. This column is within 2 chambers, the thoracic and abdominal cavities, separated by the diaphragm. The thoracic cavity is filled largely with air and the abdominal cavity with a semifluid mass. The action of the trunk muscles converts these chambers into almost rigid-walled cylinders which are capable of resisting a part of the stress imposed in the trunk and in this way diminishing the load on the spine itself.

To test this hypothesis, the intrathoracic and intra-abdominal pressures and the electrical activity of the trunk muscles were recorded simultaneously while subjects lifted weights or pulled against a measurable fixed resistance (strain ring). Lifting weights is referred to as dynamic loading and pulling on the strain ring as static loading.

It was found that when lifting weights of 100 to 200 pounds, there is generalized contraction of the trunk muscles including the intercostals, the muscles of the abdominal wall and the diaphragm.

The shoulder girdle and paraspinal muscles are, of course, active during lifting, just as the muscles of the thigh help maintain body balance an the erect position.

When inspiration and the action of the intercostal muscles, which stabilize the rib cage, increase intrathoracic pressure the thoracic cage and spine become a solid sturdy unit capable of supporting a considerable load.

Diaphragmatic contraction and contraction of the abdominal musculature, especially the transversus abdominis, compresses the abdominal cavity into a semirigid cylinder also capable of supporting a large load.

The important fact to bear in mind is that these thoracic and abdominal changes are involuntary and reflex mechanisms brought to bear whenever heavy loads make it necessary to increase the intracavitary pressures to aid in support of the spine.

It is of considerable interest to note that an air pressure corset increased the recorded abdominal pressure while at rest. However, when lifting weights with a corset, the recorded abdominal pressure was equal to that recorded when lifting the same weight without a corset. The electrical activity of the abdominal muscles is markedly decreased when an inflatable corset is worn. This indicates that when compression or restraint is accomplished by external apparatus there is decreased need for contraction of the abdominal muscles.

The contribution of the trunk compartments to the support of the spine reduces the load on the lumbar spine by about 30 percent and on the lower thoracic portion of the spine by 50 percent.

PRESSURE MEASUREMENTS IN LUMBAR DISCS

Dr. A. Nachemson and his associates have published a number of important reports[23,24] utilizing a direct method to measure the intradiscal pressure. They constructed a spinal needle with an opening on its side which was covered by a pressure sensitive polyethylene membrane and was connected to a pressure transducer.

Using this apparatus on autopsy material, the hydrostatic properties of the nucleus pulposus was determined. It was demonstrated on cadaver specimens that the pressure in the nucleus pulposus is 50 percent higher than the externally applied load. For example, a load of 10 Kg. per square cm. will

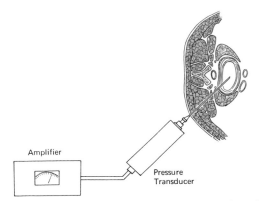

Fig. 1-64. Schematic drawing of the method used in intravital disc pressure measurements (discometry). (*After* Nachemson, A.: In vivo discometry in lumbar discs with irregular nucleograms. Acta Orthop. Scand., *36:*422, 1965.)

give a pressure of 15 Kg. per square cm. within the disc.

When measurements are performed in the living man, the needle is inserted from behind at a 45° angle into the L2, L3 or L4 intervertebral discs using x-ray guidance.

The load or pressure in an intervertebral disc in the unsupported upright sitting position is related directly to the body weight above that disc. A man weighing 70 Kg. places a 140 Kg. load in the L3 disc. When he stands up the intradiscal pressure unexpectedly falls to 100 Kg. The probable reason for this decrease is the alteration in lumbar curvature. In standing position with a lumbar lordosis, the line of gravity falls closer to the nucleus pulposus of the middle lumbar discs; in a sitting position, the lor-

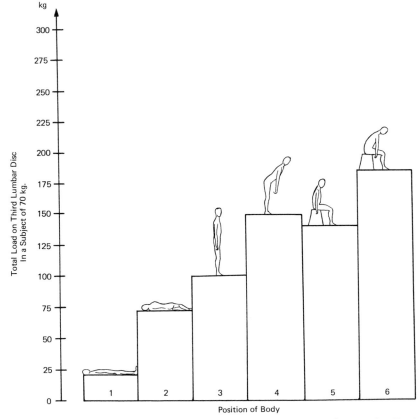

Fig. 1-65. Total load on the L-3 disc in different positions in a subject weighing 70 kg. Positions shown are (1) reclining (relaxed, supine), (2) reclining (lateral decubitus), (3) standing upright, (4) standing and 20° forward leaning, (5) sitting upright, arms and back unsupported, (6) sitting and 20° forward leaning. (*After* Nachemson, A.: Acta Orthop. Scand., *36:*426, 1965.)

dotic curve becomes flattened, decreasing the anterior height of the annulus fibrosis and increasing the pressure within the disc. Compatible with this line of reasoning, when the sitting subject leans forward 20°, this increases the position of lumbar flexion and raises the intradiscal pressure to 190 Kg. Lying on his side produces 70 Kg. and supine 20 Kg. intradiscal pressure.

While in the sitting or erect position, if the subject holds weights, the intradiscal pressures are increased appropriately.

Disc pressure measurements were obtained in some subjects wearing tightly fitting inflatable corsets and in all cases so studied there was a considerable decrease in the total load on the disc. These findings are compatible with the theoretical calculations of Morris, Lucas and Bresler.

The intradiscal pressure in discs spanned by a posterior fusion was approximately 30 percent less.

REFERENCES

1. Allbrook, D.: Movements of the lumbar spinal column J. Bone Joint Surg., *39B*:339, 1957.
2. Bartelink, D. L.: The role of abdominal pressure in relieving the pressure on the lumbar intervertebral discs. J. Bone Joint Surg., *39B*:718, 1957.
3. Blakey, P. R., Happey, F., Naylor, A., and Turner, R. L.: Protein in the nucleus pulposus of the intervertebral disc. Nature (London) *195*:73, 1962.
4. Bobechko, W. P., and Hirsch, C.: Autoimmune response to nucleus pulposus in the rabbit. J. Bone Joint Surg., *47B*:574, 1965.
5. Charmley, J.: Imbibition of fluid as a cause of herniation of the nucleus pulposus. Lancet, *1*:124, 1952.
6. Chubb, R. M., Detrick, W. R., and Shauven, R. H.: Compression fractures of the spine during U.S.A.F. ejections. Aerospace Med., *36*:968, 1965.
7. Clayson, S. J., *et al.*: Evaluation of mobility of hip and lumbar vertebrae of normal young women. Arch. Phys. Med. Rehabil., *43*:1, 1962.
8. Comfort, A.: The Biology of Senescence. New York, Rinehart, 1956.
9. Crocker, J. F., and Higgins, L. S.: Phase IV. Investigation of Strength of Isolated Vertebrae. Final Technical Report T I 1313-66-4 Contract No. MASW-1313, Technology, Inc., 1966.
10. DePukey, P.: The physiological oscillation of the length of the body. Acta Orthop. Scand., *6*:338, 1935.
11. Dickson, I. R., Happey, F., Naylor, A., Pearson, C. H., and Turner, R. L.: Decrease in hydrothermal stability of collagen on aging in the human intervertebral disk. Nature, *215*:50, 1967.
12. Eiving, C. L.: Vertebral fractures in jet aircraft accidents: A statistical analysis of the period 1959 through 1963, U. S. Navy Aerosp. Med., *37*:505, 1966.
13. Epstein, J. A., Epstein, B. S., Rosenthal, A. D., Carra, R., and Levine, L. S.: Sciatica caused by nerve root entrapment in the lateral recess: the superior facet syndrome. J. Neurosurg., *36*:584, 1972.
14. Evans, F. G., and Lissner, H. R.: Biomechanical studies on the lumbar spine and pelvis. J. Bone Joint Surg., *41A*:278, 1959.
15. Gray, H.: Anatomy of the Human Body. ed. 27. Philadelphia, Lea & Febiger, 1966.
16. Gregersen, G. G., and Lucas, D. B.: An in vivo study of the axial rotation of the human thoraco-lumbar spine, J. Bone Joint Surg., *49A*:259, 1967.
17. Happey, F., Pearson, C. H., Polframan, J., Render, R., Naylor, A., and Turner, R. L.: Proteoglycans and glycoproteins associated with collagen in the human intervertebral disc. Z. Klin. Chem., *9*(1):79, 1971.
18. Hendry, N. G. C.: The hydration of the nucleus pulposus and its relation to intervertebral disc derangement, J. Bone Joint Surg., *40B*:132, 1958.
19. King, A. I., and Vulcan, A. P.: Experimental studies on stresses in the lumbar vertebrae caused by caudocephalad acceleration. Neckache and backache: Proceedings of a workshop sponsored by the American Association of Neurological Surgeons in cooperation with the National Institutes of Health, Bethesda, Maryland.
20. Lucas, D. B., and Bresler, B.: Stability of the ligamentous spine, Biomechanic Laboratory, Technical Report No. 40, University of California, San Francisco, 1960.
21. Lyons, H., Jones, E., Quinn, F. K., and Sprunt, D. H.: Changes in the protein-polysaccharide fractions of nucleus pulposus from human intervertebral disc with age and disc herniation. J. Lab. Clin. Med., *68*:930, 1966.
22. Morris, J. M., Lucas, D. B., and Bresler, B.:

Role of the trunk in stability of the spine J. Bone Joint Surg., *43A*:327, 1961.

23. Nachemson, A.: The load on lumbar disks in different positions of the body. Clin. Orthop., *45*:107, 1966.

24. Nachemson, A., and Morris, J. M. In vivo measurements of intradiscal pressure. J. Bone Joint Surg., *46A*:1077, 1964.

25. Naylor, A.: (1) The structure and function of the human intervertebral disc (2) Pathogenesis of disc prolapse and degeneration. Oxfordian, *3*:7, 1970.

26. Pederson, H. E., Blunck, C. F. V., and Gardner, E.: The anatomy of the lumbosacral posterior rami and meningeal branches of spinal nerves (sinu-vertebral nerves). J. Bone Joint Surg., *38A*:377, 1956.

27. Perey, O.: Fracture of the vertebral end plate in the lumbar spine. Acta. Orthop. Scand., suppl. 25, 1957.

28. Puschel, J.: Der Wassergehalt normaler and degenerieter Zuracken werbelscheben. Beitr. Pathol., *84*:123, 1930.

29. Schlesinger, P. T.: Incarceration of the first sacral nerve in a lateral bony recess of the spinal canal as a cause of sciatica: Anatomy—two case reports. J. Bone Joint Surg., *37A*:115, 1955.

2
Evaluation

EXAMINATION OF THE PATIENT

History

Sit Back and Listen
Low Back Pain
Sciatica
Motor Impairment
Sensory Impairment
Sphincter Impairment

True Sciatica Versus Musculoligamentous
  Pain
Past Medical History

Examination

Systematic Approach

X-RAY LUMBOSACRAL SPINE

Retrograde Reasoning

Equivocal Diagnosis

Common Radiographic Abnormalities

X-RAY CONTRAST STUDIES

Myelogram

History
Patient Apprehension
Principle of Myelography
Myelogram Controversy
Indications for Myelography
Preparation of Patient
Positioning
Myelogram Technique
Postmyelogram

Myelogram Tracing

Discogram

Basic Principles
History of Discography
Technique of Midline Lumbar Discography
Interpretation of Discogram
Lateral Approach
Advantages and Disadvantages of Discog-
  raphy
Postmortem Discography
Role of Discography

2
Evaluation

EXAMINATION OF THE PATIENT

HISTORY

When Thomas Carlyle, the Scottish author, wrote in 1845 "histories are as perfect as the historian is wise and is gifted with an eye and a soul," he assuredly did not have low back dysfunction in mind. However, the quotation is quite apt and appropriate when applied to this clinical problem.

Sit Back and Listen

In evaluating a patient with low back pain, a most searching and deliberative history is required to properly appraise the problem. In dealing with any pain syndrome, the examiner should keep in mind the importance of allowing the patient to freely express himself, since pain is such a subjective entity and so often the patient's statements are misinterpreted by a preoccupied physician. The examiner should maintain an open mind and not prejudge every patient with back and sciatic pain as having a "disc problem," and although lumbar disc disease is a fairly common cause for back and sciatic pain, many other entities need to be considered.

Low Back Pain

In eliciting a history from a patient who is being seen for low back pain, one commonly finds that the patient is most eager to speak about the specific most recent episode of pain for which treatment is being sought. The present painful condition may so dominate the history that it obscures previous episodes of similar, but possibly less severe, attacks. For this reason, even when previous episodes of low back pain are denied, it may be advisable to pursue this point a bit farther with leading questions asking if long auto trips, heavy lifting, extended periods of stooping had ever previously produced low back dysfunction.

How the symptoms developed is of interest. We tend to think of the spontaneous onset of low back pain as caused by an entity such as tumor and expect the onset of a herniated disc to be associated with an injury. Attributing too much importance to mode of onset, however, may be misleading. Many patients with low back pain can, in hindsight, recall some injury to the low back that may conceivably have been responsible for the symptoms; it may have been a direct fall, lifting heavy weights or merely leaning forward to pick up something of negligible weight from the floor. In reviewing a recent series of 14 patients presenting with low back pain as the initial symptom caused by unsuspected metastatic neoplasm, 5 attributed the onset of their symptoms to trauma. A history of injury or trauma is of interest but must be considered in its proper perspective.

Are the low back symptoms intermittent? Between episodes of back pain is the patient completely free of any discomfort? Is it a pain of gradual onset and unremitting progression? Certainly, the latter history should alert one to the possibility of neoplasm.

What is the relationship of the pain to mechanical factors? Is the pain eased by bed rest and made worse with physical activities, or is the pain worse at night while lying supine in bed, which is true of many tumors? What type of activity aggravates the pain most? Is standing worse than sitting? Does forward bending or stooping aggravate the pain? It is usually necessary to ask specific and sometimes leading questions to elicit such details. Recently, a medical student noted on the chart that a patient under my care for very severe lumbar disc pain was not adversely affected by heavy lifting or stooping. On reviewing the chart and seeing this unexpected allegation, I went back to the patient's room and asked if such strenuous activities increased his pain. The patient denied such aggravation and when I expressed surprise at this answer, he explained that he never did heavy lifting or stooping because of his low back pain.

It is important to find out what relieves the pain. Is it eased when sitting or standing? Is there any specific body position that relieves the pain? What medications are helpful? Does aspirin help or is it necessary to take more powerful analgesics? Learning the type of medication required helps the physician assess the intensity of pain.

What previous treatment has been carried out? Low back manipulation? Was it helpful or did it seem to aggravate the symptoms? Have low back supports or girdles been of help?

Does the patient have a spinal list or scoliosis? Is it always to the same side or does it alternate? Does one leg seem longer than the other?

Sciatica

Sciatica can occur with or without back pain. Where is the sciatic radiation? Is the symptom exclusively one of pain, or is it associated with numbness and tingling? The distribution of the sciatic radiation may be helpful in diagnosing the level of the lesion. Did the back and leg pain occur simultaneously or did the back pain occur first and the leg pain occur subsequently? Did sciatica occur without a previous history of low back pain?

To determine the aggravating effect of increased intraspinal pressure, the examiner asks if coughing, sneezing or straining at stool causes increased pain in either the back or sciatic distribution of the pain. One must

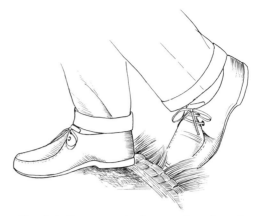

Fig. 2-1. Frequent tripping on the edge of a rug with the painfully affected limb may indicate a partial foot drop.

be cautious in attributing the effects of increased intraspinal pressure to a cough or sneeze, since a vigorous cough or sneeze can produce a sudden body movement which might aggravate pain of any sort. For example, a sneeze might aggravate the pain of a fractured limb, which would have nothing to do with increased intraspinal pressure. Straining at stool or a Valsalva maneuver is not likely to cause any sudden body movement and if this phenomenon causes pain, one is more likely to consider increased intraspinal pressure as the aggravating factor.

Motor Impairment

It is sometimes difficult to differentiate weakness from pain. The patient may state: "I'm paralyzed and can't move my legs," and examination will disclose no actual motor dysfunction but such severe muscle spasm and pain that it is almost impossible for the patient to move. Oftentimes, the patient is not aware of any specific weakness, and the examiner must search for subtle clues to decide whether a motor deficit does exist. For example, if a patient has a partial foot drop, an increased unilateral shoe slap may be heard when walking on hard surfaces. Another clue to a partial foot drop is the tendency to trip over small surface elevations such as curbs, rocks or even the edge of rugs

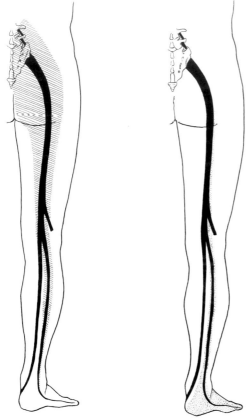

Fig. 2-2. Predominant site reversal of nerve root pain and sensory symptoms. Pain is most severe proximally and numbness is most severe distally.

Oftentimes, the patient will complain "My leg gives out from under me unexpectedly."

Sensory Impairment

As a rule, sciatic pain is most severe proximally, since it begins in the hip and decreases in intensity as it progresses distally. Although sensory symptoms may follow a similar course, the predominant site of symptoms is usually the reverse of pain. Oftentimes, numbness is primarily appreciated distally, and the patient will be aware of what is described as a "pins and needles feeling" in the foot or lower leg.

The subjective sensory symptoms distally are of much greater diagnostic help than those more proximal. It is almost impossible to clinically differentiate the L5 from the S1 roots in the posterior thigh; but when these dermatomes extend down to the foot, they assume a relatively consistent distribution. Sometimes no objective sensory changes can be elicited by examination, and we have only the subjective sensation of numbness to help us localize a lesion.

The number of dermatomes affected is of great importance. Whenever more than one root is involved, either unilaterally with a major portion of one lower extremity affected or when there is bilateral sciatica, one is alerted to the possibility of neoplasm.

Sphincter Impairment

Sphincter changes are usually elicited in the history only by direct questions. The patient is not apt to volunteer inadequacy of sphincter mechanisms, particularly if these are not severe, since there may be incomprehension of any relationship between back pain and increased difficulty in voiding. A recent onset of constipation is of interest and may be the initial evidence of sphincter impairment.

True Sciatica Versus Musculoligamentous Pain

It is important to differentiate the pain of true sciatica from hip disease which is associated with an ill-defined, diffuse, deep, dull,

and carpets. The patient has habitually cleared these obstacles in the past without using any special precautions and, not realizing that the extensors are a bit weaker as a result of a partial foot drop, the tip of the shoe will abut against rugs or curbs.

Once aware of this phenomenon, some patients habitually overcorrect by elevating the affected foot a bit higher with each step to avoid tripping, producing a characteristic gait abnormality.

Weakness of the quadriceps is often first noted on climbing stairs, when it is necessary to elevate the weight of the body using the quadriceps and gluteus muscles primarily.

aching discomfort extending into the buttock or posterior thigh due to ligamentous, periosteal and joint capsule dysfunction. In the case of hip joint pain, internal and external rotation of the hip is productive of pain. As a rule, the radiating pain of sciatic neuralgia is readily distinguished from the musculoligamentous pain of hip disease. However, nerve root compression may produce reflex spasm of those muscles innervated by the irritated root making differentiation of these two entities an occasional problem.

Past Medical History

In addition to questions relating specifically to low back dysfunction, additional information must be elicited before the problem can be properly evaluated. The past medical history must include a review of previous hospitalizations. Such information may furnish special insight into the patient's personal characteristics as well as rounding out the general, overall medical picture. For example, was the patient hospitalized for vague gastrointestinal complaints on one occasion and again for vague chest pains and were the studies performed during both of these hospital stays negative? A past history of multiple surgical procedures performed for obscure indications should ring a warning bell in the mind of the examiner. Is litigation anticipated or is the amount of compensation to be received likely to be an issue? Potential secondary gain may be a factor in prolongation of symptoms.

EXAMINATION

Systematic Approach

Examination of the patient with low back pain should take no more than 15 minutes, and yet, if properly done, can be most comprehensive. An orderly and systematic approach is more than a time-saver. It develops into an aid in proper evaluation. When the examining physician becomes accustomed to a somewhat fixed and specific examining routine, each positive or negative finding falls into a pattern as he moves along in the

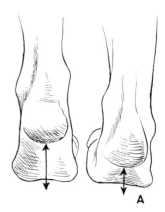

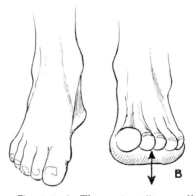

Fig. 2-3. A, The patient "toe walks" away from the examiner for determination of plantar flexion weakness; B, "heel walks" back toward the examiner for determination of foot extensor weakness.

examination, so that by the end of the examination he will find that it is easy to reach a diagnostic opinion. In contrast, if the examination is done in a haphazard fashion, instead of having a group of patterned findings he has a mixed jumble of facts to mentally sort out and try to piece together.

The following 12-point examination is quite comprehensive and can easily be performed in 15 minutes.

1. Inspection. Examination begins when the patient enters the office. Often a great deal can be learned by observing the patient walking the short distance to a chair and sitting down while he is not overly self-conscious about being scrutinized. During the taking of the history it is well to note

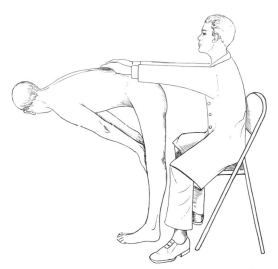

Fig. 2-4. Lumbar mobility can be assessed visually and by palpation.

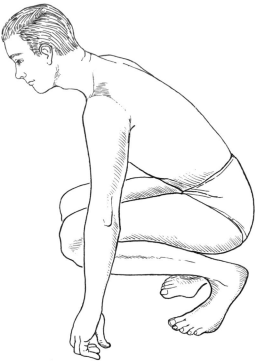

Fig. 2-5. If hip and knee dysfunction are present, squatting is usually pain producing at the pathologic joint.

external manifestations of pain and any unusual features of stance or carriage.

Exposure of the patient should enable the examiner to visualize the entire spine and both buttocks. Inspect the back for any evidence of midline congenital defect such as a tuft of hair or a scar indicating a spina bifida occulta. If the patient is having severe discomfort at the time of examination, the lumbar spine may be splinted by severe paraspinal muscle spasm. This produces a flattening of the normal lumbar lordotic curvature which may be associated with slight flexion of both the thoracic and cervical spines. With a thoracolumbar scoliosis, the hip on the side of the convexity protrudes laterally.

2. Gait. Observe the patient walking back and forth. Even moderately severe back pain is usually associated with decreased mobility of the lumbar spine, producing restriction of normal spinal movement. When lumbar paraspinal muscle spasm is so severe that a "poker spine" or "frozen spine" is present, both lumbar flexion and extension may be completely absent. Even in the presence of severe muscle spasm, a certain degree of lateral flexion and rotation of the spine is usually retained so that the patient often walks in a stiff, guarded fashion depending mainly on hip movement and lateral spine flexion to ambulate rather than using the normal gait which involves a more complete range of active spinal movement.

After observing the patient's gait, the patient is requested to walk on his toes away from the physician. The examiner observes and compares the height of the heels and notes any tendency for one heel to consistently drop closer to the floor with weight-bearing, which is indicative of some weakness of the gastrocnemius, soleus and plantaris muscles. Weakness of this muscle grouping is compatible with S1 nerve root compression. The patient then walks back toward the physician on the heels, permitting the physician to determine whether one foot consistently drops a bit with weight bearing in comparison to the other foot. This is indicative of weakness of the tibialis anterior, the

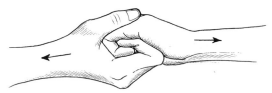

Fig. 2-6. Opposing hand pull for reinforcement of deep tendon reflexes.

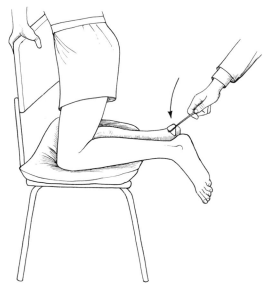

Fig. 2-7. Comparison of Achilles reflexes is best done with patient kneeling on a cushioned chair.

extensor digitorum longus and the extensor hallucis longus muscles. Weakness of this muscle grouping is compatible with L5 nerve root compression.

3. Mobility. When examining the patient for mobility of the lumbar spine, the examiner is seated with the patient standing in front of him. The examiner's hand is placed on the patient's lumbar spine, and the patient is asked to bend forward, backward and to either side. During these movements, the palpation of the examiner's hand determines whether increased paraspinal muscle spasm develops with any specific movement. The degree of lumbar mobility can be assessed visually and by palpation.

Total spinal mobility is of lesser importance than the specific extent of lumbar spine mobility. Some individuals with a surgically fused lumbar spine can bend forward and actually touch their toes by compensating for the lack of lumbar mobility with hip movement and hypermobility of the remaining vertebrae. For this reason, during flexion, one should very carefully observe any changes in the lumbar spine. By placing the thumb and third fingertips over the second and fifth lumbar spinous processes during flexion, one will normally see approximately a one-inch spread of these fingertips when the patient demonstrates an adequate reversal of the normal lumbar lordosis in the presence of good spinal mobility. If mobility of the lumbar spine is poor, little or no apparent separation of the fingertips occurs.

Limited flexion may occur with any lumbar spine dysfunction associated with paraspinal muscle spasm, such as lumbar disc protrusions or hypertrophic spurring. Occasionally,

flexion can be performed quite freely without limitation or discomfort; but on attempting to "straighten up" and resume the erect position, the patient may appreciate increased discomfort. If in association with this finding, hyperextension of the spine produces increased pain, the differential diagnosis should include stenotic lumbar spinal canal, midline lumbar disc herniation or lumbar neoplasm.

Rotation and lateral flexion are not specifically affected by any of the more common lesions causing low back or sciatic pain. Such movements may be limited as a result of extensive paraspinal muscle spasm, which would tend to limit any mobility of the lumbar spine and are a specific finding in iliac-transverse process pseudoarthrosis.

When a specific movement produces pain either in the back or sciatic radiation, determine as accurately as possible the exact location and nature of the pain so produced.

The range of mobility of the lumbar spine is not usually recorded in degrees but as normal, or slightly, moderately or markedly limited.

4. Squatting. The patient is asked to squat

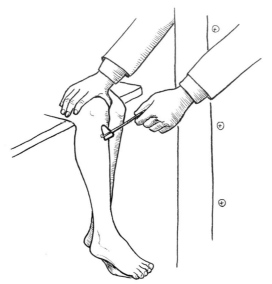

Fig. 2-8. Comparison of patellar reflexes is best done with the legs hanging freely over the edge of an examining table or bed.

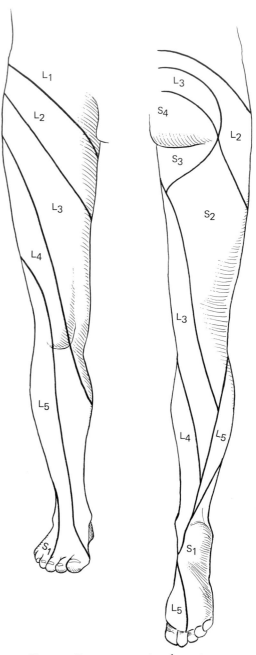

Fig. 2-9. Lower extremity dermatomes.

with complete flexion of the knees and hips. Does this action cause pain in the low back or does it cause pain in hip or knee joints? If dysfunction is present involving the knee or hip, this movement is usually pain-producing at the site of the pathology.

5. Reflexes. Reflex examination can be carried out with the patient in a sitting position. If the deep tendon reflexes are difficult to elicit, they can sometimes be brought out by various forms of reinforcement. Most commonly, this consists of an opposing hand pull, but almost any muscular activity can be used which will direct the patient's concentration away from the area to be tested.

If the ankle jerks cannot be elicited or if there is difficulty in doing so, kneeling the patient on a cushioned chair using reinforcement is usually helpful.

A diminished or absent patellar jerk usually implicates the L3 or L4 nerve root while a diminished or absent ankle jerk implicates the S1 nerve root.

6. Leg Length. Measure leg length from the anteriorsuperior iliac spine to the medial malleolus. Occasionally, a patient with low back pain derives relief with a shoe lift on the short side.

7. Sensation. Sensation is tested with the application of a wisp of cotton for light touch, and the gently applied sharp end of a pin for pain. If the patient has no subjective appreciation of paresthesia, the examiner is less likely to elicit a dermatomal sensory impairment. Occasionally, even when one of

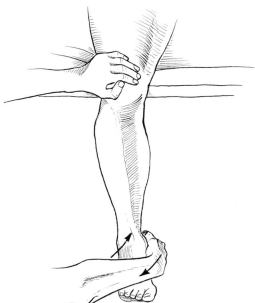

Fig. 2-11. Testing knee joint flexor strength.

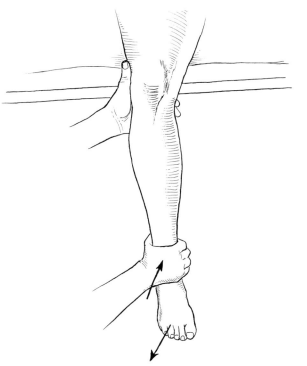

Fig. 2-10. Testing knee joint extensor strength.

the primary complaints is annoying paresthesia extending into a specific dermatomal distribution, a most careful examination will frustratingly not demonstrate any objective change. When mapping out a sensory dermatome, it is useful to go from the zone of numbness toward the area of sensitivity.

Because of the considerable variation in dermatomal patterns, there are no charts of the dermatomes that can be considered "absolute." It is generally agreed that the lateral portion of the foot is subserved by the S1 root; the dorsum of the foot extending toward the great toe is subserved by the L5 root, after which the variability increases and the dermatomal charts become more disparate.

8. Motor Strength. Loss of lower extremity muscle tone is determined by palpating the quadriceps and calf muscles to elicit any significant differences in muscle mass or tone with the patient in the erect position.

Measurement of thigh and calf circumference is carried out with the patient lying

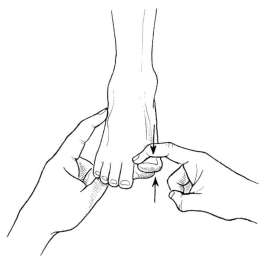

Fig. 2-12. Testing dorsiflexion strength of the great toe.

supine and the muscles relaxed. The thigh circumference is measured at a specific distance above the upper pole of the patella and compared with similar measurements on the opposite leg. The calf circumference is measured in one leg at the level of estimated greatest circumference. Then, using the same

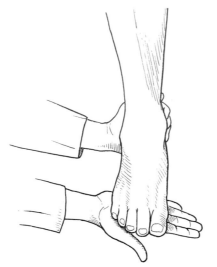

Fig. 2-13. Testing plantar flexion strength of the ankle.

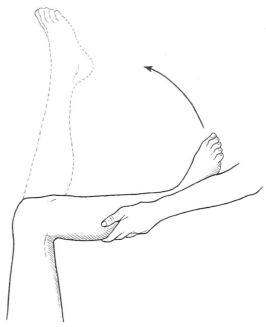

Fig. 2-14. The Lasègue test.

distance from that point to the tibial tuberosity, the opposite calf is measured.

To determine flexion and extension power of the knee joint, the patient grasps the back of a chair or tabletop to maintain balance and attempts squatting and elevating the body first with the presumed normal thigh and then the suspected one.

Flexion and extension strength of the knee joint can also be tested with the patient in a sitting position with both feet free of the floor. The examiner grasps one ankle at a time and asks the patient to flex and extend the knee joint against resistance.

Test dorsiflexion strength of the great toe and foot.

Normally the average patient should be able to dorsiflex the foot despite moderate opposition of the examiner. Weakness of these muscles implicates the fifth and sometimes the fourth lumbar nerve roots.

Plantar flexion of the ankle also can usually be maintained by the average patient despite moderate resistance. The muscles involved in this movement are primarily subserved by the first sacral nerve root.

Larger muscles are usually subserved by more than one nerve root so that the quadri-

ceps which is innervated by the L3, L4 and L5 roots would be less affected by a single root lesion than the extensor hallucis longus, which is primarily innervated by the L5 root. The gastrocnemius, also a larger muscle, is innervated by the S1 and S2 roots so that although some weakness may be caused by S1 root involvement it is not as apparent as the extensor hallucis longus. Gluteal muscle weakness may be present and is usually apparent by comparitive inspection and palpation of the buttocks while the patient is in a standing position.

9. Straight Leg Raising. The straight leg raising test is often mistakingly identified as the Lasègue sign. Ernest Charles Lasègue, who wrote a paper in 1864,[14] commenting upon the physical signs of patients with sciatic neuritis, described the following test: With the patient supine he flexed both the knee and hip; after the hip had been flexed to 90°, he slowly extended the knee producing severe pain in the patient suffering from sciatica. The Lasègue is less valuable than the straight leg raising test, since the movements

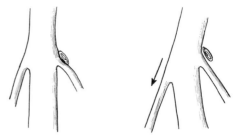

Fig. 2-16. Mechanism of pain relief with straight leg raising of the unaffected leg.

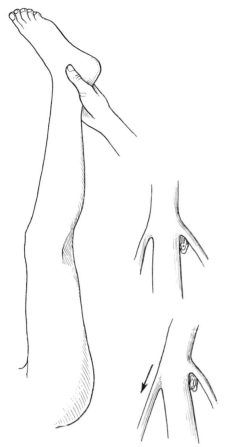

Fig. 2-15. The well leg raising test of Fajerstajn.

of 2 joints are involved, causing increased difficulty in interpretation.

The more valuable straight leg raising test was first described by J. J. Forst, a pupil of Lasègue, 17 years later. This test is done with the patient lying supine, the examiner elevating the straight leg to approximately 90°, which would normally cause no discomfort other than a feeling of tightness behind the knees and in the hamstrings. Straight leg raising performed in the presence of sciatica caused by nerve root pressure will produce severe pain either in the back or the sciatic distribution of the affected leg or in both. As a rule, with unilateral root involvement, straight leg raising is diminished on the affected side. In some cases where the root pressure is extensive, as a result of a sizable disc protrusion within the "axilla" between the spinal dura and the exiting root sleeve, straight leg raising of the unaffected leg may aggravate pain in the involved leg. The mechanism of this phenomenon is that elevating one leg causes a tug on the cauda equina and may impinge the already compromised root against the protruding disc.[25]

When sciatic pain is caused by a laterally placed disc protrusion, straight leg raising of the unaffected leg may act to relieve root compression and so reduce sciatic pain.

If the straight leg raising test appears to be positive, sciatica can be confirmed by lowering the raised leg an inch or two until the pain is no longer present, at which point the foot is dorsiflexed, producing a recurrence of pain. In carrying out this confirmation test, pain produced by ligamentous or muscle pull is ruled out, since it is presumed that dorsiflexion of the ankle will stretch the sciatic nerve by means of tightening the posterior tibial branch of this nerve.

When performing the straight leg raising test, each leg should be tested separately, since when both legs are raised together, an upward tilt of the pelvis occurs, diminishing the desired angulation of straight leg raising.

The straight leg raising test is recorded in degrees, 90° being considered normal. In addition, one should record the location and intensity of pain produced by this maneuver.

10. Hip Rotation. Internal and external rotation of the hip is performed to rule out hip

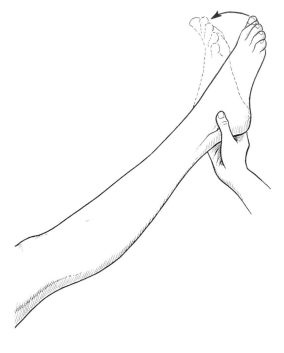

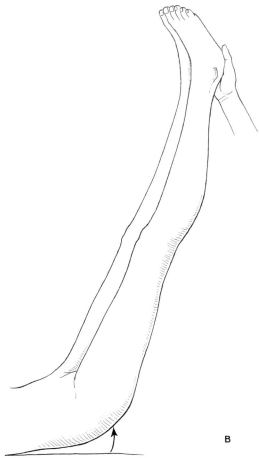

A

Fig. 2-17A. Confirmation of sciatica.

B

Fig. 2-17B. Raising both legs together produces an upward tilt of the pelvis which diminishes the desired angulation of straight leg raising.

disease. External rotation was originally described by Hugh Talbot Patrick, a Chicago neurologist, and is carried out with the patient supine. The thigh and knee are flexed, and the external malleolus is placed over the patella of the opposite leg and the knee forcibly depressed. If pain is produced by this maneuver, hip disease is indicated. Doctor Patrick originally called this test, the "fabere sign," from the initial letters of movements necessary to elicit it; namely, flexion, abduction, external rotation and extension.

Internal rotation of the hip produces distraction of the sacroiliac joint and if painful may be compatible with sacroiliac dysfunction.

11. Spinal Pressure. With the patient in the prone position, pressure over the spinous processes of the lumbar spine and sacrum is performed. No tenderness should be elicited over the sacrum, unless neoplasm involving

the sacrum or nonorganic disease is present. In the presence of nerve root pressure and irritation, paraspinal pressure on the side of involvement at the affected interspace may cause a twinge of sciatic pain.

12. Arterial Pulses. Every patient who is suspected of having sciatica should have careful examination of the arterial pulses in the inguinal, popliteal and dorsalis pedis sites. It is rarely difficult to differentiate vascular occlusive disease from sciatica, but confusion in this regard can occur and may not only be embarrassing to the physician but of considerable detriment to the patient.

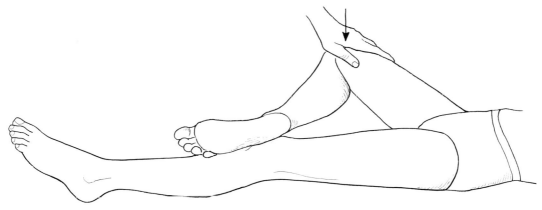

Fig. 2-18. Patrick's sign (external rotation of hip).

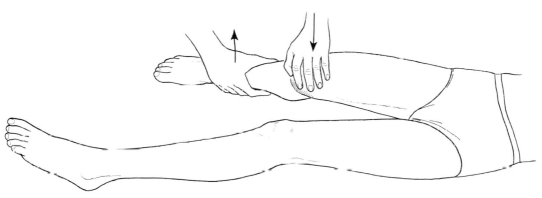

Fig. 2-19. Internal rotation of hip.

X-RAY LUMBOSACRAL SPINE

Careful study of plain lumbosacral spine x-rays is important in clinically evaluating the patient with low back pain and sciatica. Certain conditions such as fractures, dislocations, infections, tumors and certain metabolic diseases are clearly seen on x-ray and will enable the clinician to demonstrate radiographically the specific cause of back pain. These entities comprise a small portion of the backache patients encountered in a general hospital population. In the vast majority of patients, the specific cause of low back symptomatology is not clearly demonstrated by x-rays.

Retrograde Reasoning

A patient manifesting symptoms of low back symptomatology with anatomical variations of the lumbar spine demonstrated by x-ray induces the physician, who is trained to document symptomatology with objective evidence relating to the etiology of the symptoms, into a form of retrograde reasoning in which he seizes upon this anatomical variant and designates it as the cause of the patient's problems. Opportunities to compare spine films of patients with and without back pain are limited because persons without low back dysfunction rarely have x-rays of the spine. One of the first papers to bring this to our attention was written by Dr. C. A. Splitoff[20]; since that time, a number of other investigators[8,11,12] have demonstrated a discrepancy between factual knowledge and the physician's inclination to attribute low back symptoms to a number of anatomical variations demonstrated radiologically.

EQUIVOCAL DIAGNOSIS

Although many patients are labeled with a diagnosis of lumbosacral strain, the diagnosis is eventually found to be a completely different entity. They may have early lumbar disc disease prior to the onset of obvious nerve root signs or symptoms; occult malignancies have occasionally been so misdiagnosed before the true nature of the disease process became evident; and a host of medical, genitourinary, and gynecological conditions can give rise to low back dysfunction as the presenting symptom. Because of frequent indistinguishable symptoms in the early stages of these other entities, lumbosacral strain is considered by some as a sort of wastebasket diagnosis into which any low back dysfunction which is not readily identified may be placed. Though our factual knowledge of this disease is wanting, and we are not even sure what causes the pain in strain, this condition does exist as a specific entity with special characteristics and findings. It is classified as acute lumbosacral strain and chronic lumbosacral strain.

Common Radiographic Abnormalities

A review of some of the common radiographic abnormalities noted on lumbar spine x-rays and discussion of their clinical significance follows.

Transitional Vertebrae. By transitional vertebrae we mean either a sacralized lumbar vertebra or lumbarized sacral vertebra. This anatomical variant occurs in 5 to 7 percent of the population as a whole.[4] Some physicians give considerable importance to this x-ray finding and believe it is associated with an increased incidence of low back dysfunction. One industrial physician actually considers this finding sufficient grounds to prevent an employee applicant from carrying out heavy duties. There are no statistics to demonstrate a significantly increased incidence of low back dysfunction with transitional vertebrae; and based on my own personal experience, I feel that there is no direct relationship.

Spina Bifida. With the posterior elements either partially or incompletely absent, one might anticipate some loss of stability, which would normally be furnished by the muscle and tendinous attachments to these missing posterior elements. Available statistics, however, do not indicate an increased incidence of back pain, a finding compatible with my personal experience.

Increased Lumbar Lordosis. The patient with chronic lumbosacral strain traditionally has been noted to have an increased lumbar lordosis. What statistics we do have in the population as a whole are equivocal but may indicate that this is possibly more than an incidental finding that could conceivably be a factor relating to low back pain.

Scoliosis. When a physician sees a patient with low back pain and upon reviewing the x-rays notes a scoliosis in the lumbodorsal area, he cannot help considering a direct relationship between what is seen on the films and the presenting symptoms. However, a significant discrepancy in this line of reasoning is demonstrated by the fact that scoliosis clinics, where patients of all ages are seen, have a rather remarkable infrequency of low back complaints in their patients. There is no question that the intervertebral disc at the apex of the scoliosis has an increased tendency toward degeneration, since it is at the site of greatest stress. Despite this fact, statistics indicate surprisingly little increase in the incidence of back pain in long-range studies of scoliotic patients. Further-

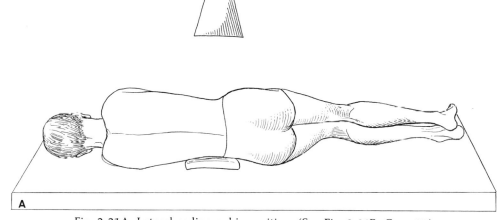

Fig. 2-20A. A-P radiographic position. (See Fig. 2-20B, C, p. 53.)

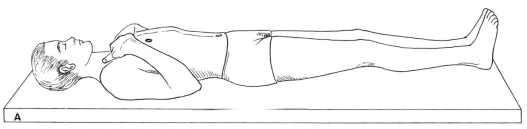

Fig. 2-21A. Lateral radiographic position. (See Fig. 2-21B, C, p. 55.)

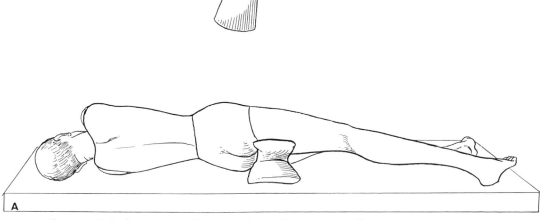

Fig. 2-22A. Left posterior oblique radiographic position. (See Fig. 2-22B, C, p. 57.)

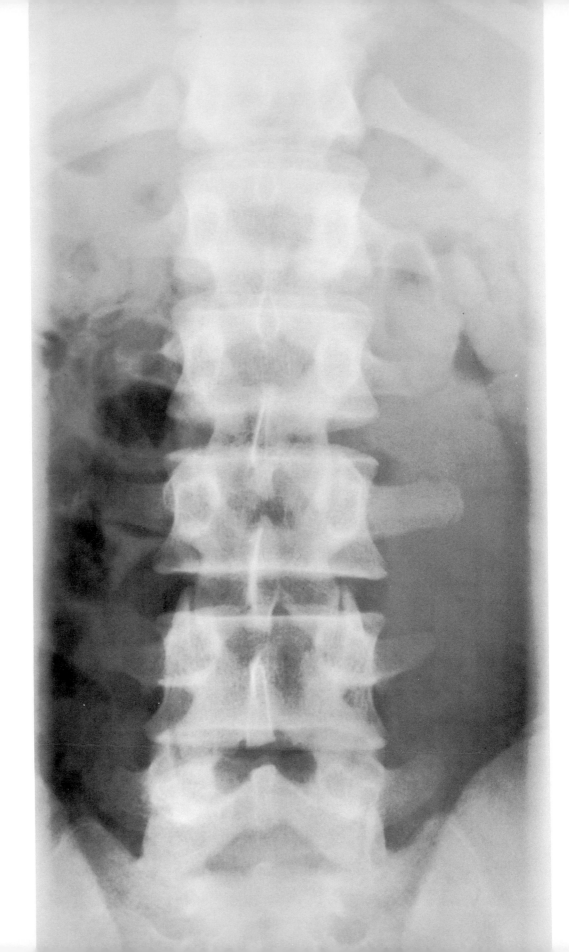

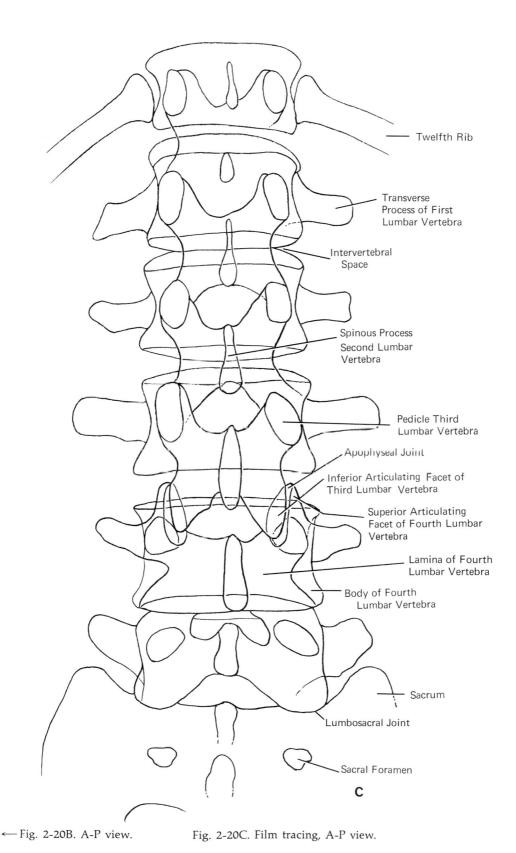

Twelfth Rib

Transverse
Process of First
Lumbar Vertebra

Intervertebral
Space

Spinous Process
Second Lumbar
Vertebra

Pedicle Third
Lumbar Vertebra

Apophyseal Joint

Inferior Articulating Facet of
Third Lumbar Vertebra

Superior Articulating
Facet of Fourth Lumbar
Vertebra

Lamina of Fourth
Lumbar Vertebra

Body of Fourth
Lumbar Vertebra

Sacrum

Lumbosacral Joint

Sacral Foramen

C

←Fig. 2-20B. A-P view.   Fig. 2-20C. Film tracing, A-P view.

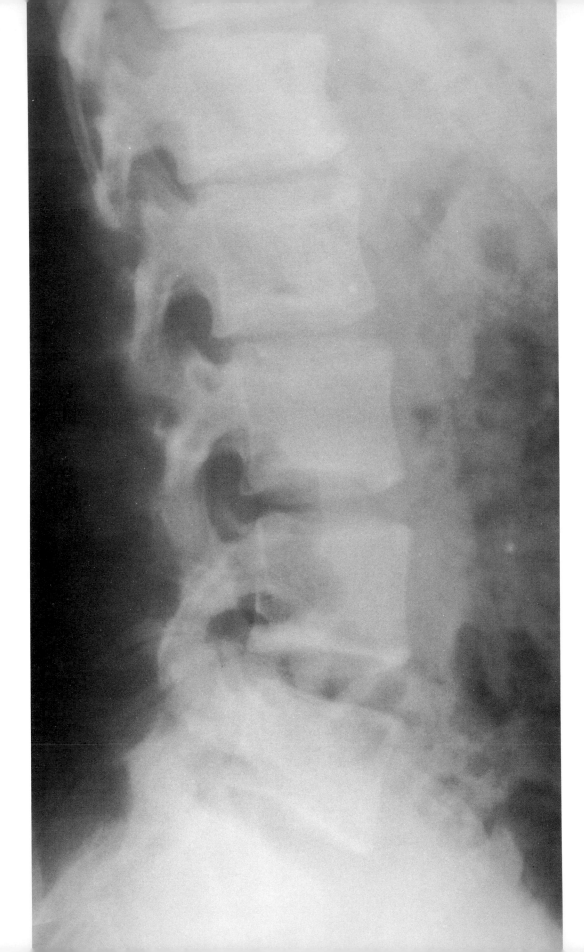

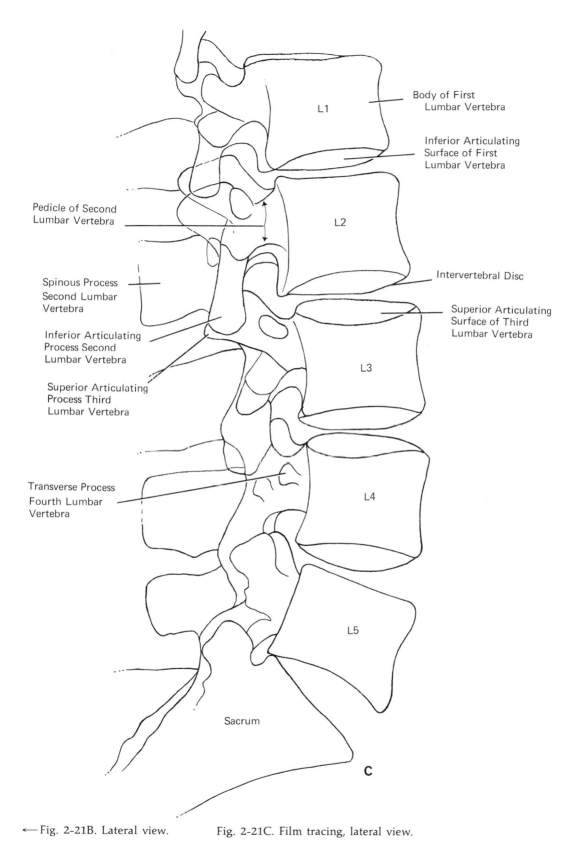

Body of First
Lumbar Vertebra

Inferior Articulating
Surface of First
Lumbar Vertebra

Pedicle of Second
Lumbar Vertebra

Intervertebral Disc

Spinous Process
Second Lumbar
Vertebra

Superior Articulating
Surface of Third
Lumbar Vertebra

Inferior Articulating
Process Second
Lumbar Vertebra

Superior Articulating
Process Third
Lumbar Vertebra

Transverse Process
Fourth Lumbar
Vertebra

L1

L2

L3

L4

L5

Sacrum

C

←—Fig. 2-21B. Lateral view.   Fig. 2-21C. Film tracing, lateral view.

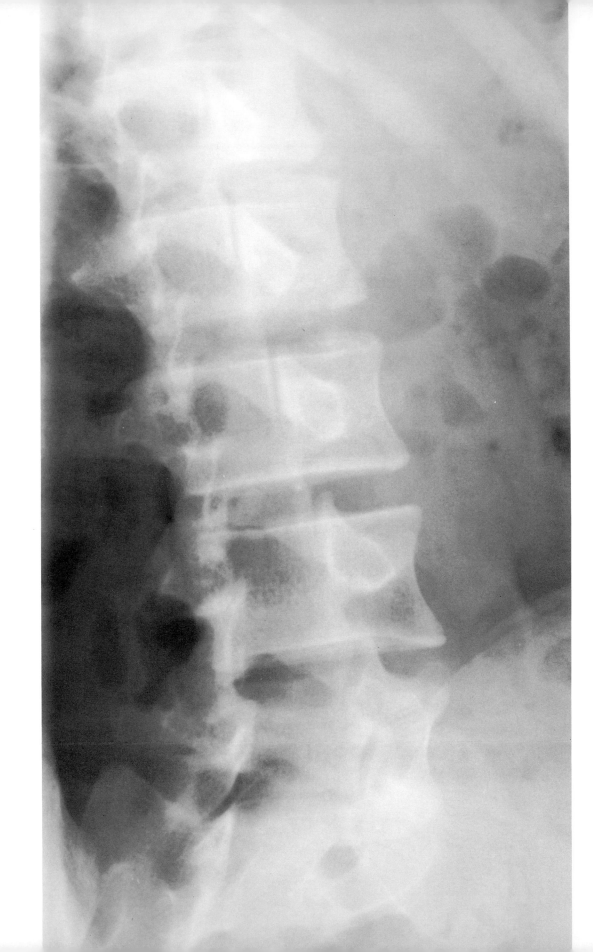

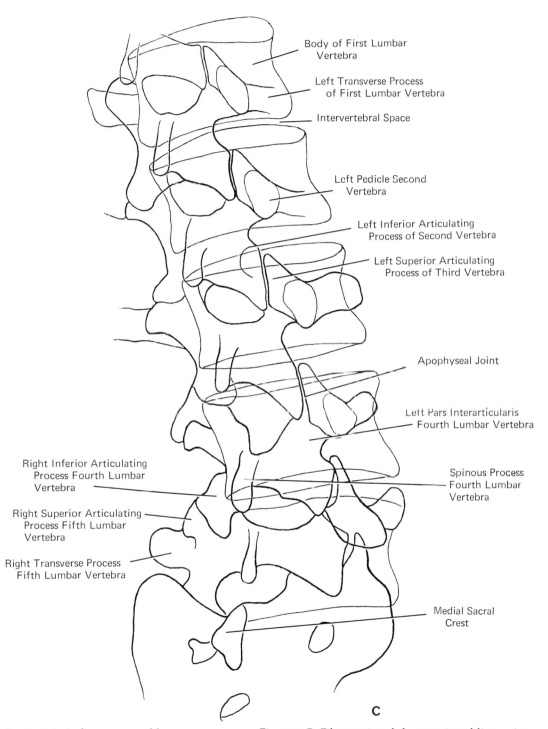

Body of First Lumbar
Vertebra

Left Transverse Process
of First Lumbar Vertebra

Intervertebral Space

Left Pedicle Second
Vertebra

Left Inferior Articulating
Process of Second Vertebra

Left Superior Articulating
Process of Third Vertebra

Apophyseal Joint

Left Pars Interarticularis
Fourth Lumbar Vertebra

Right Inferior Articulating
Process Fourth Lumbar
Vertebra

Spinous Process
Fourth Lumbar
Vertebra

Right Superior Articulating
Process Fifth Lumbar
Vertebra

Right Transverse Process
Fifth Lumbar Vertebra

Medial Sacral
Crest

C

←Fig. 2-22B. Left posterior oblique view.   Fig. 2-22C. Film tracing, left posterior oblique view.

more, despite the fairly high incidence of scoliosis, this condition does not seem to be overwhelmingly predominant in patients with low back dysfunction.

Intervertebral Disc Narrowing. Narrowing at the L5 to S1 interspace is a relatively common finding in patients over the age of 50. There is certainly a very direct relationship to such narrowing and age. Degenerative changes at the disc interspace are also associated with this finding. Less commonly, one sees x-ray evidence of disc degeneration and narrowing at the L4-5 interspace, and this is seen less frequently above that level. There does seem to be a definite relationship between such findings and an increased tendency toward low back pain. However, one must keep in mind the fact that a large number of patients with these incidental findings do not have low back dysfunction.

Pars Defects. Defects in the pars interarticularis is associated with an increased incidence of low back pain. This condition increases the mechanical stress upon the intervertebral disc and may be followed by disc degeneration, producing increased stress upon the annulus fibrosis with a greater tendency toward low back dysfunction.

Asymmetrical Lumbosacral Facets. This condition has been called tropism, which term derives from the Greek word tropē, meaning "turning." When one of the lumbosacral facets is in a more coronal plane than the other, an abnormal rotary motion acts on the annulus in addition to the normal flexion and extension movements. The torque stress on the annulus is increased and is probably associated with an earlier breakdown, since rotational stresses are not as well tolerated by the lumbar discs as are flexion and extension.

Osteoarthritis. Hypertrophic osteoarthritis of the lumbar spine is associated with an increased incidence of low back pain.[10] However, it must be emphasized that many people with osteoarthritis do not have a great deal of pain. The vast majority of elderly patients in "rest homes" or "nursing homes" will reveal on spine x-rays rather advanced hypertrophic osteoarthritic changes, and most of these patients do not have low back pain.

X-RAY CONTRAST STUDIES

MYELOGRAM

History

In the early 1900's when greater attention was directed to the surgery of spinal lesions, the limitations of plain roentgenography of the spine became increasingly clear. In 1919, Dr. Walter Dandy[3] described the use of air injected into the lumbar subarachnoid space to delineate the cerebral ventricles, pointing out its use as a contrast agent in the spinal canal. Within two years, Bingel[1] in Germany, Jacobaeus[13] and Wideroe[23] in Norway, unaware of Dandy's work, independently carried out air myelography to demonstrate tumors of the spinal cord. However, air myelography never became universally popular, because the contrast was not great and the air shadow often indistinct.

The introduction of lipiodol myelography by Sicard and Forestier[19] in 1922 gave such satisfactory visualization of the spinal canal that air was largely neglected as a spinal contrast medium. Adversely, this compound of iodine and poppy-seed oil produced meningeal irritation when allowed to remain in the subarachnoid space; and because of its high viscosity, removal of this substance was difficult and often painful.

In 1944 Pantopaque, a medium containing iodine in organic combination, was introduced by the University of Rochester group.[21] Because of its lower viscosity, it outlined the finer structures of the spinal canal, such as the root sleeves, and was more easily removed by gentle aspiration. This material has received widespread and general acceptance in America. In Europe, especially the Scandinavian countries, Pantopaque myelography has not gained universal acceptance and many clinics prefer water soluble contrast agents.

Patient Apprehension

Most patients with a prolonged history of low back dysfunction have heard the term myelogram, and some of them view the test with fear and apprehension because of the horror stories they have been told, which are usually pure fantasy. Occasionally, someone does suffer an unfortunate experience, but with few exceptions this study can be performed in a relatively painless fashion.

Principle of Myelography

The type of myelography used primarily in the United States utilizes Pantopaque, a radiopaque oil substance, heavier than spinal fluid which is introduced into the subarachnoid space. By tilting the patient up and down under fluoroscopic guidance, one can follow the column of dye along the length of the spine to be investigated.

Myelogram Controversy

The question as to whether myelography should be utilized on a "routine" basis prior to surgery is a source of some lively discussion and a difference of opinion. A number of specialists feel that lumbar disc surgery can be carried out after the careful evaluation of the presenting signs and symptoms. They reserve the use of myelography for situations in which the clinical picture is not clear or when neoplasm may be suspected. The following considerations can be cited to vindicate this latter position:

1. Pain during the performance of the myelogram, which usually relates to nerve root irritation either from direct trauma of the lumbar puncture needle or, more frequently, from removal of the radiocontrast material when the root is aspirated against the needle bevel.

2. Postmyelogram radiculitis resulting from nerve root trauma, which may be the cause of persisting pain for a variable period of time.

3. Postspinal headache, which may produce considerable discomfort and be quite disabling to some patients.

4. Meningeal irritation, in reaction to introduction of a foreign material into the subarachnoid space. Infrequently, this may take the form of an aseptic meningitis with nuchal rigidity, severe headache and increased white cells in the cerebrospinal fluid.

5. Rarely, bacterial meningitis which may result from faulty technique.

6. The irritative effects of the Pantopaque, which may produce adhesive arachnoiditis years after the myelogram has been performed. This complication is more likely to occur if a traumatic lumbar puncture produces subarachnoid bleeding and inadequate withdrawal of Pantopaque results in a blood-Pantopaque mixture remaining in the subarachnoid space. When complete removal of this material is not achieved, serial x-rays taken at yearly intervals will usually demonstrate gradual diminution in the quantity of visible radiopaque material. The rate of absorption of this material is estimated to be approximately 1 cc. per year. The absorption rate varies, and some patients have very little absorption over a period of many years, while in others it may be absorbed more rapidly.

7. Dye retained in the subarachnoid space which, when the patient lies in such a position that the head is lower than the lumbar spine, may flow into the basilar cisterns and cerebral ventricles and produce a basilar adhesive arachnoiditis, and which in turn may lead to obstructive hydrocephalus with all the potential complications of this condition.

8. Faulty lumbar puncture technique used in performing the myelogram, which may deposit Pantopaque outside the subarachnoid space making removal much more difficult and at times impossible. This may create a localized tissue reaction at the site of the deposited radiopaque material.

9. The incidence of a 10 percent error due to inability to visualize laterally placed discs

where they may impinge against the root within the lateral recess and would have no contact with the dural sac. This 1 to 10 incidence of error may cause the surgeon to withhold indicated surgery.

10. Pantopaque sensitivity.[4,6,9] Spinal fluid examination 1 or 2 days following Pantopaque myelography, will usually demonstrate from 10 to 20 white blood cells per cubic centimeter, associated with a moderate increase in the spinal fluid protein. Symptoms resulting from these spinal fluid changes are not commonly apparent, but occasionally a patient will develop nuchal rigidity, headache, low-grade temperature elevation and malaise. Spinal fluid culture will reveal no organisms, and the clinical course is self-limiting, responding to bed rest and analgesics within a week or two.

Several reports of more severe and even fatal reactions attributed to a unique hyper-sensitivity to Pantopaque have appeared in the literature. As a result of the increased sensitivity to this radiopaque material, a widespread aseptic leptomeningitis may occur, involving not only the spine but extending into the brain, particularly the posterior fossa. This may produce an obstructive hydrocephalus with some cases terminating in death.

The rarity of these tragedies makes it impossible to establish reasonable criteria to prevent similar future complications. Intradermal Pantopaque skin tests have been used but have proven to be unreliable. Until satisfactory guidelines can be developed, patients with a severe allergic background, including a specific allergy to iodine, should probably not have Pantopaque myelography.

Reviewing the rather formidable list of objections to myelography, one should rightly pause before considering the use of this test. The physician must be cognizant of every objection to the use of myelography, because it is not totally innocuous and carries with it a number of potential risks to the patient. The alternative to myelography is, however, even more formidable; namely, exploratory surgery of the spine.

The potential complications of exploring an extra interspace needlessly, removing one protruding disc when two are present, operating for lumbar disc disease when the symptoms are produced by a stenotic lumbar spinal canal, or not being aware of the pres-

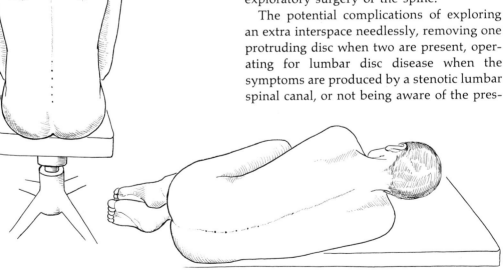

Fig. 2-23. Accurate midline placement of the lumbar puncture needle is best done with the patient in the sitting position or prone position. The distortion of spinal alignment with the patient in the lateral decubitus position creates increased difficulty in midline needle placement.

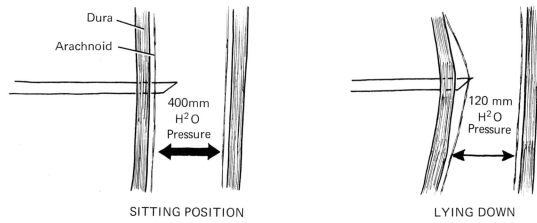

SITTING POSITION   LYING DOWN

Fig. 2-24. Meningeal distension of the caudal sac, produced by increased subarachnoid pressure when the patient is in the sitting position, allows the lumbar puncture needle to cleanly penetrate the dura and arachnoid with less tenting of these membranes, decreasing the possibility of epidural or subdural Pantopaque injection.

ence of a neoplasm are all so serious that they far outweigh the recognizably serious potential, but rarely occurring, complications of myelography. Exploring a "negative" interspace and retracting a root "ever so gently" medially to determine whether a disc is, indeed, protruded is far more likely to produce persisting symptoms than is myelography.

Indications for Myelography

1. Patients with clinical evidence of a protruding lumbar disc who fail to respond to conservative treatment and on the basis of this failure are being considered for surgery.
2. Significant motor weakness resulting from nerve root compression.
3. A long-standing history of low back pain which has not responded to conservative management.
4. Diagnostic possibility of a neoplasm.

Preparation of Patient

No premedication is ordinarily given unless the patient is suffering from severe pain and is receiving large amounts of medication for pain during bed rest. If this be the case, a dose of the same medication is administered prior to being sent to x-ray. Meals are not routinely withheld.

Positioning

The lumbar puncture should be performed with the patient either in the sitting position or in a prone position on the x-ray table. The needle should not be introduced with the patient in the lateral decubitus position, because the distortion of spinal alignment in this position creates increased difficulty in accurate midline needle placement.

Sitting Position. Advantages of the sitting position are:

1. In the sitting position the dura and arachnoid are distended from hydrostatic pressure produced by the upright spinal subarachnoid canal. When penetrating this distended dura with a spinal needle, the myelographer is more likely to be alerted to the puncture by a "dural ping."
2. As a result of increased compression of the arachnoid against the dura, the needle is less likely to tent the arachnoid and create a subdural injection.
3. Increased spinal fluid pressure in the sitting position produces a free flow of spinal fluid with proper placement of the needle tip. When the spinal fluid flow is noted to be less than copious and escapes drop by drop, this is a warning of partial obstruction at the

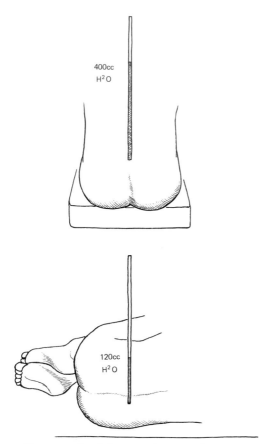

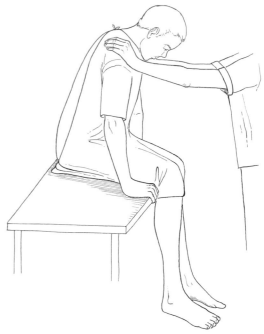

Fig. 2-26. To prevent a serious fall resulting from syncope, a nurse or x-ray technician must remain in front of the sitting patient during a lumbar puncture.

Fig. 2-25. Caudal sac gradients in the sitting and recumbent positions recorded by the spinal manometer.

needle bevel, which can often be cleared by replacing the stylet and rotating the needle or advancing the needle a millimeter.

Prone Position. An alternative to the sitting position is the prone position which has its own advantages which are:

1. In the sitting position the patient may become apprehensive and syncopal during the lumbar puncture. Because of this possibility, it is necessary to have either a nurse or an x-ray technician standing in front of the patient for reassurance and, if necessary, physical support.

2. In the sitting position, the spinal needle cannot be introduced under fluoroscopic guidance, with image intensification television monitoring, as can be done in the prone position. Utilization of this technique is quite

helpful; particularly in instances when the physician finds it difficult to introduce a lumbar puncture needle into the subarachnoid space either in a very obese person or someone who has marked scoliosis.

3. Although one can usually approximate the interspace using the iliac crest as a landmark, with fluoroscopic control the lumbar puncture can be performed at the desired interspace with a high degree of certainty. When a lumbar puncture is performed in the prone position, a large triangular sponge is placed under the abdomen to maintain a slight degree of lumbar flexion.

4. It is possible to tilt the x-ray table to a 45° "head up" position to increase spinal fluid pressure within the caudal sac. This will provide some of the advantages of dural-arachnoid distension associated with the sitting position.

Myelogram Technique

Because technical deficiencies so often thwart the proper interpretation of myelograms, the technique will be discussed in some detail.

Needle Placement. The site at which the lumbar puncture is performed is determined in accordance with the level of the suspected lesion. As a rule, the L3-4 interspace is the preferred needle placement site since both the L4-5 and L5-S1 interspaces comprise 90 percent of all lumbar disc lesions.

The interlaminar space becomes smaller as we go higher, so that the lumbar puncture becomes a bit more difficult above the L3-4 level. Also, above the L3-4 level it is more difficult to remove the Pantopaque, since the column begins to "break up" at the L2 to 3 level. When there is clinical evidence that the lesion is in the middle or upper lumbar levels, the injection site can electively be the L4-5 or L5-S1 interspaces.

Occasionally, it is necessary to introduce the dye from above, in which case 2 methods are suitable:

1. Cisternal tap. A cisternal tap can be done with the patient in the sitting position and dye introduced through this needle will drop down to the lumbar region. After the dye has been injected, the needle is withdrawn. At the termination of the myelogram, the dye can be removed by means of a lumbar puncture; or if small amounts of dye are used, some physicians make no effort to remove the dye and allow it to remain in the subarachnoid space.

Technique of cisternal puncture. The spinous process of C2 can usually be palpated by having the patient gently flex and extend the neck. The C1 spinous process can be palpated only in extremely thin individuals. A small area of the suboccipital and upper cervical area is shaved and cleansed with alcohol. With the patient in the sitting position, the head is firmly held in a slightly flexed position by an assistant. Using 1 percent Xylocaine, a skin wheal is placed exactly in the midline, one half inch above the C2 process, after which the syringe is removed and the hypodermic needle left in place to mark the site. An 18-gauge spinal needle is introduced through the skin wheal and aimed toward the supraorbital ridge. The

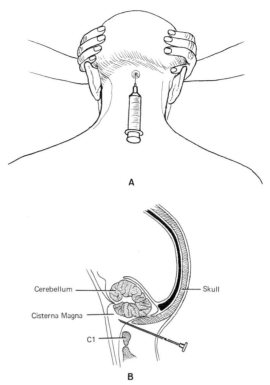

Cerebellum

Cisterna Magna

Skull

C1

B

Fig. 2-27. Cisternal puncture.

needle is advanced slowly and carefully until the characteristic snap or "ping" indicates penetration of the posterior atlantooccipital ligament. At the time of ligamentous penetration, the immediately adjacent dura may also be penetrated or it may be necessary to carefully advance the needle further and a second "ping" may be appreciated, signaling dural penetration.

It should be noted that the cerebrospinal fluid pressure, at the level of the cisterna magna, in the erect position may be zero so that occasionally CSF will flow sluggishly from the needle. For this reason it is advisable to remove the stylet at regular intervals and gently aspirate, using a 1 or 2 cc. syringe. Occasionally, I am surprised at aspirating spinal fluid without having appreciated penetration of either the atlantooccipital ligament or the dura. Depending upon the thickness of the neck and angulation of the spinal needle, the cisterna magna may vary from 3 to 6 cm. beneath the skin.

2. High cervical lateral puncture. The lumbar

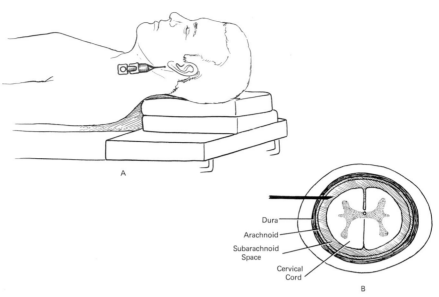

Fig. 2-28. A, Site of Xylocaine wheal for high cervical lateral puncture;
B, diagrammatic cross-section of high cervical lateral puncture.

puncture needle can also be introduced laterally between the first and second cervical vertebrae, employing a technique originally devised for percutaneous cordotomy.

Technique of high cervical lateral puncture. With the patient lying supine on the biplane x-ray table, a 25-gauge hypodermic needle is inserted 1 cm. below and behind the tip of the mastoid process and 1 percent Xylocaine is used to infiltrate the skin and subcutaneous tissue. An 18-gauge, short beveled lumbar puncture needle is introduced through the anesthetized skin and slowly advanced medially as 1 percent Xylocaine is infiltrated along the needle pathway. After some experience, the surgeon is able to appreciate the various layers penetrated; but it is well to check the position of the needle at various levels of penetration by A-P and lateral films of the high cervical spine using Polaroid film. Penetration of the dura is signaled by the typical sensation of resistance and then perforation of a parchmentlike membrane. Once the dura is penetrated, cerebrospinal fluid will flow freely from the needle when the stylet is withdrawn. An A-P and lateral film is obtained to check the position of the needle. Optimal placement of the

needle tip is approximately 10 mm. behind the posterior border of the body of C2 and 10 to 12 mm. from the midline.

After satisfactory needle position has been established, a short plastic connector tube is attached to the needle and allowed to fill with cerebrospinal fluid. The head of the x-ray table is then elevated approximately 35°; and under TV-image intensification, Pantopaque is injected into the subarachnoid space.

This method has the advantage of allowing the injection to be carried out with the patient lying supine. In this position the Pantopaque can be injected under fluoroscopic guidance until a sufficient quantity has been introduced to establish an adequate contrast column. As with cisternal tap, the spinal needle is removed after injection of the Pantopaque; if contrast material recovery is carried out, it must be done by means of a standard lumbar puncture at the termination of the myelogram. The disadvantage of this technique is the possibility of injury to the high cervical cord. It is best performed by a physician familiar with the technique of high cervical percutaneous cordotomy.

Lumbar Puncture Technique. The optimal position of the needle tip in lumbar punctures should not be directly over the interspace but preferably over the upper third of the vertebral body, because there may be constriction and narrowing directly over the interspace, resulting from a combination of a bulging annulus and thickened yellow ligament. Introducing a needle into this narrowed space may cause the needle point to penetrate the anterior floor of the dural canal and provoke bleeding or a subdural spinal fluid extravasation, which may lead to injection of the Pantopaque into the subdural rather than the desired subarachnoid space.

Since the interspace is, as a rule, a bit higher than the body of the vertebrae, which in most cases are somewhat concave on their posterior surfaces, removal of the Pantopaque through a needle directly over the interspace may become a problem. When the bevel of the needle is optimally placed over the vertebral body, the tip can be dropped quite low below the level of the roots in withdrawing the contrast material; and the dye can be pooled and siphoned out without difficulty.

In most patients the first interspace above the iliac crest is the L3-4 interspace.

Disposable needle. A disposable lumbar puncture needle is used to be assured of using a needle with no burs or one which has been blunted by previous use. A dull or burred needle may impinge the dura, pushing it forward and reducing the A-P (anteroposterior) diameter of the subarachnoid space to a width sometimes less than the length of the bevel; or after perforating the dura, it may tent the arachnoid away from the dura, creating a false subdural space. Most myelographers prefer an 18-gauge needle for facilitation of Pantopaque retrieval; some advocate the finer 20-gauge needle, citing a reduced incidence of postspinal headaches.

Site of puncture. The skin overlying the interspace to be injected can be marked using the thumbnail to indent a cross at that site. It may be helpful to indent the midspinous processes 2 and 3 interspaces above the puncture site and use these 3 marks in conjunction with the buttock crease to determine

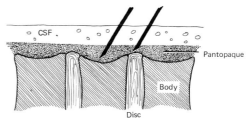

Fig. 2-29. For Pantopaque removal, the optimal position for the needle tip is over the vertebral body rather than over the intervertebral disc.

whether there is a significant scoliosis of the spine.

Allergy to local anesthesia. The patient is questioned about previous dental surgery carried out under local anesthesia and whether any untoward reaction resulted from this or other local anesthetic blocks. If a hypersensitivity or allergic history is elicited, no local anesthetic is used. In the absence of local anesthesia, one can usually pinch the skin overlying the proposed puncture site and then very quickly introduce the point of the lumbar puncture needle employing "vocal" anesthesia in the form of reassurance. Once the needle is beneath the skin, there is usually no significant discomfort.

Needle technique. Wearing sterile gloves, cleanse the skin of the low back with an antiseptic solution and then 1 or 2 cc. of 1 percent Xylocaine is injected to make a cutaneous wheal with a 25-gauge hypodermic needle.

When the lumbar puncture is performed in the prone position, fluoroscopic guidance is used. The skin is marked with a metal-tipped ballpoint pen held in a lead-gloved hand at the site of the desired interspace precisely over the midline. Since the ballpoint ink probably will be washed off by the prep solution, one should take care to indent the skin as well as mark it, so that this little indentation can be visualized.

The needle is then carefully introduced as close to the midline as possible and in a slightly cephalic direction, advancing the needle slowly. When the yellow ligament is

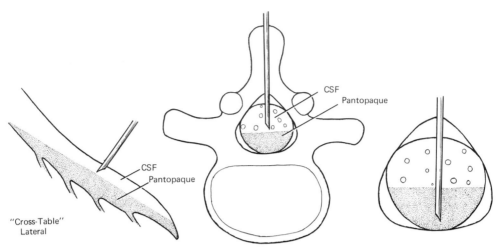

Fig. 2-30. When the lateral film reveals the needle tip to be a distance from the floor of the subarachnoid space, it can be depressed if the needle is in good midline position.

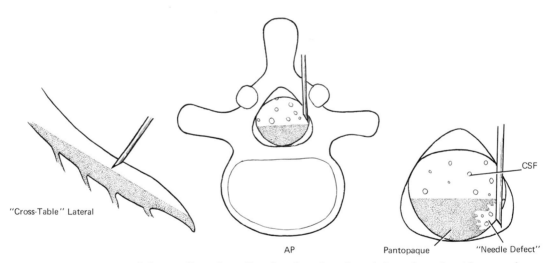

Fig. 2-31. If the tip of the needle is laterally placed at the edge of the subarachnoid space, do not make the mistake of attempting to depress the tip to the level of the floor of the canal as visualized on the cross-table lateral film, since this will result in a "needle defect."

perforated, this is appreciated by the physician as a slight dull resistance. At this point the stylet is removed and, if no spinal fluid escapes, it is replaced and the needle is advanced slowly until a "dural ping" is appreciated. The stylet is removed to assure free escape of cerebrospinal fluid and then replaced to advance the needle one millimeter. The stylet is removed again. Several cubic centimeters of cerebrospinal fluid are collected for analysis.

Pantopaque Injection. Using a plain-tipped syringe, introduce 9 cc. of Pantopaque into the subarachnoid space taking care not to change the position of the needle while injecting the dye. Prior to use it is important to test ease of movement of the 10 cc. syringe used to inject the Pantopaque. If the syringe

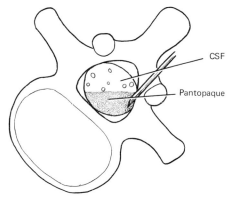

Fig. 2-32. When the tip of the needle is laterally placed, place the patient in an oblique position so that the Pantopaque is pooled beneath the needle bevel.

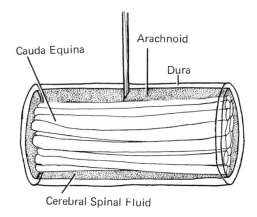

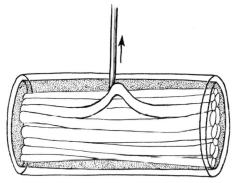

Fig. 2-33. Rapid aspiration will produce a convection current which may cause a root to float up against and to be aspirated into the needle bevel, producing pain.

is sticky and requires more than gentle pressure during the injection, movement of the needle may occur or the sticky syringe barrel may create a false impression that the Pantopaque is being injected under increased pressure. The myelographer thus may show undue concern that his needle may have moved and is not in the proper location. A sticky syringe is often caused by glove powder between the barrel and the plunger.

To avoid any movement of the needle during injection, it may be necessary to utilize a short flexible connector tube between the needle and the syringe. If this is done, the connector tube should be allowed to fill with cerebrospinal fluid before carrying out the Pantopaque injection, so that air will not be introduced into the subarachnoid space. The lumbar puncture needle is allowed to remain in place throughout the study.

Pantopaque Removal. After the spinal segment to be surveyed has been fluoroscopically visualized and documented with spot-films, including oblique views and the "cross table" lateral, it is helpful to examine the lateral film to visualize the tip of the needle in relationship to the floor of the canal. When the lateral film reveals the needle tip to be a distance from the floor of the subarachnoid space, it can be depressed if the needle is in good midline position.

If the tip of the needle is laterally placed at the edge of the subarachnoid space, do not make the mistake of attempting to depress the tip to the level of the floor of the canal as visualized on the cross table lateral film, since this will result in a needle defect.

In such instances allow the needle to remain undisturbed and place the patient in an oblique position so that the Pantopaque is pooled beneath the needle bevel.

Using a long plastic connector tube, very slowly and gently aspirate as the dye is pooled under the needle tip fluoroscopically. Rapid aspiration will produce a convection current which may cause a root to float up against and be aspirated into the needle bevel, producing pain.

It is important to use a syringe that will

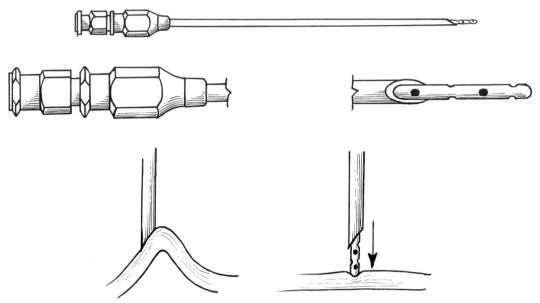

Fig. 2-34. The Cuatico myelography needle.

not stick, since an irregular, jerky withdrawal may aspirate a root against the needle bevel. After the tubing has been filled, it should no longer be necessary to aspirate, since the siphon effect of the tubing is usually sufficient for removal of the remaining Pantopaque. Aspiration of CSF is likely to float up a root against the needle bevel causing pain, which can be avoided by maintaining the dye pool beneath the needle at all times during the removal. The normal buoyant mobility of the cauda equina roots floating in cerebrospinal fluid is dampened by the oily Pantopaque.

Special Myelography Needle. To facilitate Pantopaque withdrawal, a needle* was designed for myelography.[2]

The needle set consists of an 18- or 17-gauge lumbar puncture needle with the usual solid, sharp-pointed stylet which conforms to the bevel of the needle which fits snugly into the needle shaft. This portion of the set is used to perform a lumbar puncture and injection of Pantopaque in the usual fashion.

At the completion of the myelogram, re-

*Cuatico myelography needle (Becton-Dickinson Company).

moval of the contrast material is attempted in the ordinary manner. If difficulty is encountered, either because of nerve root or arachnoid adherence at the bevel, then a hollow blunt-end aspiration cannula, which fits into the inner bore of the needle, is used. This aspiration cannula is 19-gauge, with multiple openings spaced within the first 5 mm. of the distal end. By using this cannula, whatever is adherent to the bevel is pushed aside. Gentle aspiration using a plastic venatube easily removes the Pantopaque through the holes at the tip of the cannula.

I have used the Cuatico needle in approximately 100 myelograms and found it particularly helpful in patients with stenotic lumbar spinal canals or adhesive arachnoiditis, which causes the nerve roots to be closely adherent making even gentle aspiration with an ordinary lumbar puncture needle either difficult or painful.

Technical Problems. If in the performance of the lumbar puncture a traumatic tap causes bleeding, discontinue the procedure and wait a week before rescheduling the myelogram. A mixture of blood and Pantopaque is thought to increase the likelihood of adhesive arachnoiditis.

If a lumbar puncture is performed but the

cerebrospinal fluid flow does not seem satisfactory, attempt a second lumbar puncture at the interspace above or below the original needle. However, do not remove the first needle, since this may cause a spinal fluid extravasation between the arachnoid and the dura, creating a false space, so that the second puncture will be technically unsuccessful.

If Pantopaque is inadvertently deposited in the subdural space, do not move the needle at all but very gently attempt to aspirate as much Pantopaque as possible. Occasionally, a surprising amount, sometimes all of it, can be removed in this fashion. However, in an attempt to remove more Pantopaque do not rotate the needle or do any manipulations with it, since the day may yet be saved and a second lumbar puncture should be performed above or below the original needle site. If a satisfactory flow of spinal fluid is obtained with the second lumbar puncture, inject 6 cc. of Pantopaque and proceed with the examination. This procedure may not be as technically satisfactory as desired, but oftentimes, a lesion can be clearly identified and the situation retrieved. Allow both needles to remain undisturbed until the study has been completed, after which the subarachnoid dye may be removed initially through the second needle. Following this, rotate or manipulate the original needle in the subdural space to remove the dye that could not be removed on the initial attempt. Both needles are to be removed only after no further dye can be removed.

If, during the aspiration of Pantopaque at the end of the myelogram procedure, severe pain occurs each time the aspiration occurs, replace the stylet and turn the needle. If this does not successfully relieve the pain with subsequent aspiration, allow the needle to remain in place and insert another needle above or below the original needle. It must be remembered that after the myelogram, once identification of the lesion has been made or a lesion ruled out, the needle can be placed into any interspace; and in fact, the myelogram should be helpful, since you now know the configuration of the subarachnoid space. For this reason, dropping a second

needle into a subarachnoid space filled with Pantopaque should be easy, since it can be completely visualized.

Postmyelogram

The introduction of 40 to 80 mm. of Depo-Medrol (methylprednisolone acetate) intrathecally following a myelogram reduces most postmyelographic discomfort, in addition to reducing the incidence of postspinal headaches. The patient is maintained in bed for 6 hours following a myelogram, after which bathroom privileges are permitted with instructions to remain as flat as possible within the limits of comfort and to force oral intake of fluids.

MYELOGRAM TRACING

When the myelogram is abnormal, it may be useful to have a graphic representation of the myelographic defect in the patient's office records. It serves as a helpful reminder of the lesion during follow-up visits. Occasionally, when a patient requires a second myelogram years later, the original films may be lost or destroyed by the radiology department to save storage space, so that it is impossible to compare the new and old films.

A practical and simple method of dealing with this problem was kindly demonstrated to me by Dr. William B. Scoville of Hartford, Connecticut. He routinely traces the myelographic defect on a sheet of tracing paper which he includes in the patient's office chart. I now follow this practice and find it profitable.

DISCOGRAM

Basic Principles

Discography involves introducing a needle under x-ray guidance into the nucleus of the intervertebral disc and injecting 2 cc. of a water soluble contrast material such as Diodrast, Hypaque or Conray. The roentgenologic configurations assumed by this injected material are studied to evaluate the pathology of the disc. In addition to the roentgenologic patterns, radicular symptoms produced

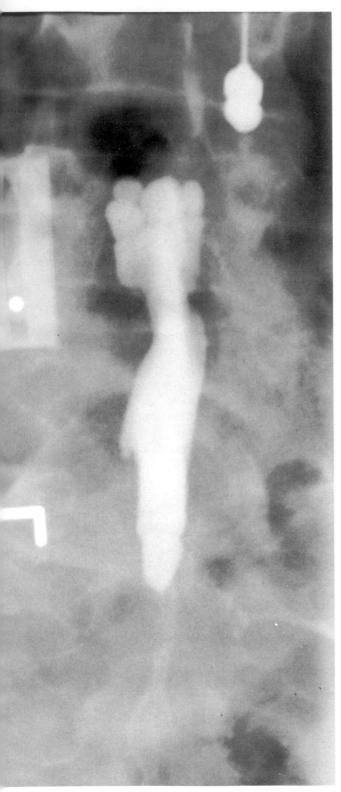

Fig. 2-35A. Myelogram.

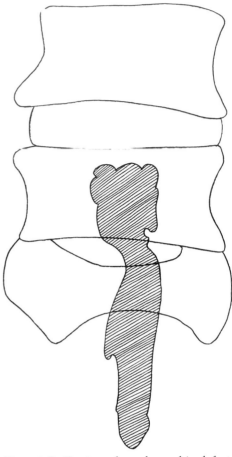

Fig. 2-35B. Tracing of myelographic defect.

by the injection are considered of diagnostic importance. The injection is normally followed by some low back discomfort, but if the injection is carried out into a pathologic disc which is the cause of radicular symptomatology, the injection will precipitate not only low back pain but also sciatic radiation. The pain produced by injection will reduplicate the patient's radicular complaints. A third diagnostic criterion is the injection pressure necessary to instill 1 cc. of contrast material into the nucleus and the amount of the material accepted by the disc. A normal disc will accept up to 1 cc. of dye with a fairly strong terminal pressure while injecting the last fraction of this dye. A degenerated disc will accept as much as 4 cc. of dye, and a ruptured disc will accept 6 cc. or more dye without severe pressure.

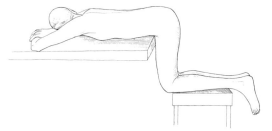

Fig. 2-36. Patient must be flexed over end of x-ray table.

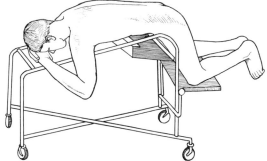

Fig. 2-37. Collis lumbar discography table.

History of Discography

The discography concept of evaluating the physical state of the intervertebral disc was initially developed by Schmorl as part of his elaborate and painstaking autopsy studies of the human spine. His technique involved postmortem injection of red lead into the intervertebral discs, followed by radiography of the spine, in order to differentiate normal from pathologic intervertebral discs.

Years later, Knut Lindblom, working in the famous Karolinska Institute of Stockholm, became involved in the physiologic aspects of disc disease and pursued this interest for many years. Working on cadaver material, he carried out anatomical studies on discs by injecting them anteriorly with red lead. This paint filled the central cavities of the nucleus pulposus. If the disc was herniated, the dye would pass through the rupture of the annulus fibrosis, spreading concentrally under the outermost layer of the annulus, or in some cases going outside the annulus, and spreading along the nerve roots and epidural tissues.[15] After carrying out these anatomic studies, Lindblom, who had originally intended to continue this type of investigation clinically, was discouraged from doing so by reports of disc lesions caused by lumbar punctures. However, his interest in clinical discography was revived in 1941 by Dr. E. Lindgren who read a paper before the Swedish Radiologic Society demonstrating x-rays of a patient whose normal disc he had injected with contrast material. It was later demonstrated by Dr. Karl Hirsch that intentionally performed disc puncture during surgery caused no immediate prolapses through

the puncture canal, and on subsequent follow-up no obvious dysfunction was noted. On the basis of these observations, Lindblom was encouraged to perform diagnostic disc punctures on patients. His original technique utilized the prone position with the needle inserted by means of the usual spinal puncture method, passing through the posterior and anterior dural walls and then into the disc itself. He utilized a 2-needle method, penetrating the posterior longitudinal ligament with a larger gauge outer needle through which a thinner needle was introduced, and this was used to penetrate the disc itself into the nucleus pulposus. Discography was first presented as a clinical diagnostic study by Lindblom in 1948.[16] This method was first done in the United States in 1950 by R. E. Wise and E. C. Weiford of the Cleveland Clinic.[24] They carried out discography on the 3 lower lumbar discs and reported a normal L3-4 disc and herniated L4-5 and L5-S1 discs, findings which were subsequently confirmed at surgery. Interestingly enough, although the procedure was initially developed in Sweden, its use in that country is on a less than routine, occasional basis. In the United States the study has received a more enthusiastic reception by a number of specialists and clinics which utilize this diagnostic method with great frequency. Some clinics utilize discography in the place of myelography, but most do prior myelograms after which discography is performed. In most instances, the lower 3 lumbar interspaces are done.

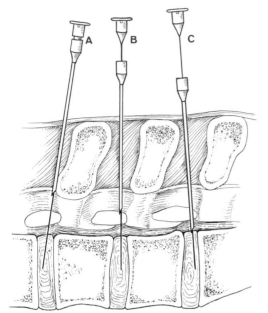

Fig. 2-38. The penetration depth of the 21-gauge needle is left to the discographer's choice. A, Through the interspinous ligament. B, Penetrating the posterior dura. C, Penetrating the anterior and posterior dura to the posterior longitudinal ligament.

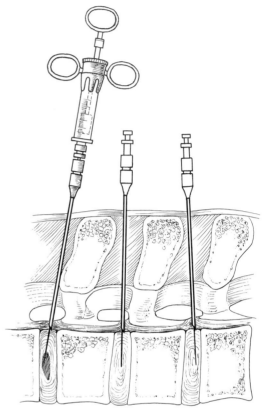

Fig. 2-39. Injection of contrast material into the nucleus pulposus.

Technique of Midline Lumbar Discography

Preparation of Patient. This procedure is a more painful one than myelography and the patient is sedated prior to the examination. However, he is not so heavily sedated that he is unable to cooperate during the examination and to report on the symptoms attendant to the procedure. Most patients are adequately sedated with 100 mg. of Nembutal and 100 mg. of Demerol given intramuscularly one hour before undergoing lumbar discography.

Positioning. The patient is placed in a kneeling-prone position on the x-ray table with both hips flexed over the end of the table and knees resting on a padded bench placed at the end of the table. Biplane x-ray positioning is important so that an A-P and lateral view of the lower lumbar spine can be obtained.

In clinics where discography is performed on a routine basis, a table specifically de-

signed for lumbar discography is commercially available. The knee rest of this table can be adjusted to the patient's size and comfort and thus facilitate the study.[17]

Positioning the patient prone on the x-ray table may provide inadequate reduction of the lumbar lordosis. Even with several pillows or pads under the abdomen, inadequate lumbar flexion may result, making lumbar discography difficult to perform.

Interspace Identification. The skin in the lumbar region is prepared in the usual fashion by shaving the hair and cleansing with antiseptic solution. A 25-gauge hypodermic needle is used to infiltrate the skin and subcutaneous tissues with 1 percent Xylocaine over what is judged to be the L4-5 interspinous space. The hypodermic needle is allowed to remain in place and radiologic verification of the needle placement site obtained. If the estimated L4-5 interspace is

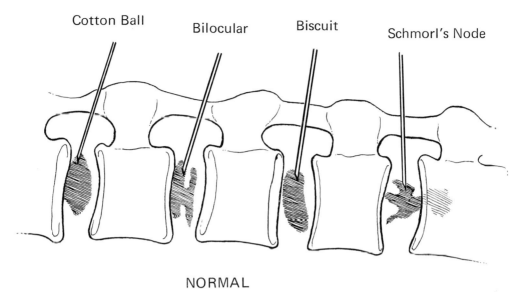

NORMAL

Fig. 2-40. Some normal discogram configurations. The Schmorl's node was included in the "normals" since it is not usually symptom productive.

found to be incorrect on x-ray check, the miscalculation will probably not be greater than one interspace. Since the proposed sites of injection are the L3-4, L4-5, and L5-S1 interspaces, the hypodermic needle will be radiographically visualized over one of these sites; and using this marker as a guide, the other 2 interspaces similarly will be infiltrated with Xylocaine leaving all 3 hypodermic needles in place. The 3 hypodermic needles can serve as a subsequent radiographic check, if deemed necessary, or to indicate the exact spot through which the 21-gauge spinal needles are to be introduced.

Needle Placement. Three 3-inch, 21-gauge spinal needles are inserted through the interspinous ligaments, to provide rigid support for the longer, thinner 26-gauge needles which, because of their increased flexibility, could not be accurately directed for more than a short distance. Some specialists prefer to advance the heavier, 21-gauge needle only through the interspinous ligaments and use the thinner needle to penetrate the ligamentum flavum, posterior dura, subarachnoid space and anterior dura in the belief that penetration of these important structures is best done with the finest needle possible. I prefer to penetrate all of the above structures

down to the posterior longitudinal ligament immediately over the intervertebral disc with the 21-gauge needle, because of the greater control afforded by a more rigid needle. As the needles are slowly advanced, biplane (A-P and lateral) radiologic guidance is necessary. The needle must be located in the center of the spinal canal to decrease nerve root trauma. The more laterally placed roots of the cauda equina are less apt to slip away from the needle tip, because they are more firmly fixed in their position as they are exiting laterally from the dural sac. The more medially positioned roots seem to have somewhat more "play," making them less vulnerable to needle impingement.

A-P and lateral films are obtained to confirm the correct position of the 21-gauge needles, either immediately over or directed toward the interspaces, depending on the preference of the physician. When satisfied with needle position, the 5-inch, 26-gauge spinal needles are passed through the 21-gauge needles into the intervertebral discs. As the needle penetrates the annulus fibrosus, slightly increased resistance is appreciated. If a firmer resistance is encountered, the tip of the needle is either impinging upon bone or the subchondral space and

Degenerated   Herniated   Extruded

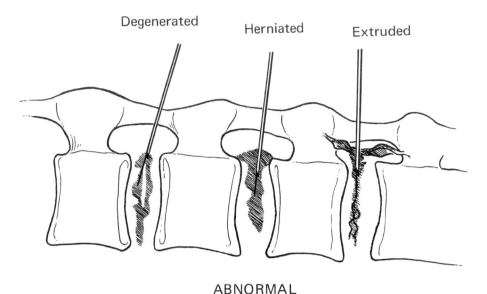

ABNORMAL
Fig. 2-41. Some abnormal discogram configurations.

must be repositioned. Before injection of contrast material, another A-P and lateral film is obtained. A properly placed needle tip is near the midline and not impinging upon the vertebral body or the cartilaginous plate.

Injection of Contrast Material. A 5 cc. "3-ring finger guard" syringe with a Luer-Lok tip is used to inject the 50-percent Hypaque or water soluble contrast material of preference into the intervertebral disc to the point of resistance. The "normal" disc will accept approximately 1 cc. of solution with some difficulty. In the absence of resistance, 3 cc. of contrast material is injected.

As a rule, the least suspected disc, which is usually the L3-4 disc, is first injected with dye. The disc most suspected is deferred until last so that if the L4-5 disc is clinically symptomatic, following the L3-4 disc, the next disc to be injected is the L5-S1 disc.

Immediately following each disc injection, a lateral x-ray is taken; and after injection of all 3 discs, a lateral and A-P film is obtained. Films taken 15 or 20 minutes after the last injection reveal absorption of most of the contrast material.

Interpretation of Discogram

The distribution and severity of pain produced by the injection is noted, along with the volume of dye accepted by the disc and the pressure required for injection.

The patient with a normal disc may experience some moderate discomfort during the injection unless excessive pressure is used, which may cause extravasation of solution anteriorly extending under the anterior longitudinal ligament or along the course of the needle tract. Such excessively applied pressure may be associated with severe back pain.

The x-ray appearance of the injected material is by far the most important single factor in discogram interpretation. In the face of a normal discogram, the injection pain response is disregarded. It is only in the presence of an abnormal discogram that pain response is interpreted as being of clinical significance. Then, if some reduplication of the patient's symptoms is produced by the injection with radiation into the clinically affected leg, the pain response is considered positive.

Lateral Approach

The advantage of performing a lumbar discogram by means of the lateral approach is that the spinal canal is not entered and the integrity of the dura remains intact. This method is particularly adaptable to the use

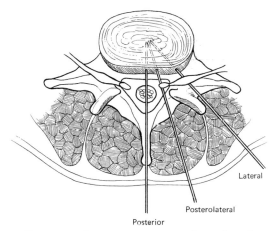

Fig. 2-42. The posterior, posterolateral, and lateral approaches.

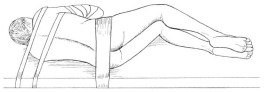

Fig. 2-43. Position for lateral approach.

of chymopapain for chemolysis of the nucleus pulposus. When using this chemolytic agent, great care must be taken to avoid introducing any of the material into the subarachnoid space, so a technique that completely skirts the spinal canal is advantageous.

A posterolateral extradural approach, which was first described by Erlacher in 1952, has been largely replaced by the lateral approach.[6]

Technique. The patient is positioned right side up on the x-ray table, and 6-inch, 18-gauge spinal needles are directed from a point 8 cm. lateral to the spinous process of the disc to be injected, with the needle maintained at an angle of 45° toward the disc. Injecting of the L5-S1 disc requires a 35° caudal angulation. Sometimes it is impossible to inject the L5-S1 disc using the lateral approach, and in such a case the posterior approach is required.

Advantages and Disadvantages of Discography

The advantages of discography are:

1. The only x-ray contrast study that examines the discs themselves.
2. Pain response associated with an abnormal discogram can be correlated with the clinical picture.

3. Avoids immediate or delayed reactions to contrast material injected into the subarachnoid space.

The disadvantages of discography are:

1. Invariably associated with some degree of pain.
2. Possible nerve root trauma.
3. Possibility that long-term untoward effects of injecting a needle into a normal disc may accelerate the normal degenerative changes of age and stress.
4. Possibility of infection following injection into an interspace.

Postmortem Discography

Dr. Jack L. Gresham and Dr. Roy Miller[9] carried out postmortem discography on 63 fresh autopsy specimens of patients from 14 to 80 years old with relatively asymptomatic "normal" backs. These were divided into 4 age groups with the following results:

Group I: 14–34 years of age—90% normal and 10% degenerated discs.

Group II: 35–45 years of age—25% normal discograms, majority at the L3-4 level.

Group III: 46–59 years of age—25% normal discograms, majority of normal discs at the L3-4 level and none normal at at the L5-S1 level.

Group IV: Over 60 years of age—5% normal discograms, none at L5-S1 level, one at L4-5 level, and two at L3-4 level out of 60 specimens.

The authors conclude that discography has its greatest clinical significance in the younger patient, with less weight given to this study if the patient is beyond the age of 35 years.

Role of Discography

Hazards and discomfort aside, the role assumed by any diagnostic test must be determined primarily by its clinical value in providing direction for proper management of the patient. This test, which is the only x-ray contrast study that actually examines the integrity of the discs, has provided us with important information on the degenerative effects of age upon the lower lumbar discs. The majority of symptom-free patients over the age of 35 reveal radiographic evidence of lumbar disc degeneration when subjected to this study.

As clinicians, we are principally concerned with the relationship between test findings and symptom-producing lesions. The discrepancy between radiographically demonstrated discogram lesions and clinical findings is controvertible. For this reason, universal acceptance of this study as a routine diagnostic measure is not general and widespread; although some advocates prefer this diagnostic procedure over myelography. I personally reserve its occasional use to unusual diagnostic problems.

REFERENCES

1. Bingel, A.: Intralumbale Lufteinblasung zur Hohendiagnose intraduraler extramedullarer Prozesse und zur Differential diagnose gegnuber intramedullarer Prozessen. Deutsche Ztochr. f. Nervenhlk. 72:359, 1921.
2. Cuatico, W.; Gannon, W.; Samoukos, E.: A needle designed for myelography J. Neurosurg., 28:87, 1968.
3. Dandy, W. E.: Roentgenography of the brain after the injection of air into the spinal canal. Ann. Surg. 70:397, 1919.
4. Epstein, B. S.: The Spine. A Radiological Test and Atlas. ed. 3, Philadelphia, Lea & Febiger, 1969.
5. Erickson, T. C., and Van Baaren, H. J.: Late meningeal reaction to ethyl iodophenylundecylate, used in myelography. Report of a case that terminated fatally. JAMA, 153:636, 1953.
6. Erlacher, P. R.: Nucleography, J. Bone & Joint Surg., 34B:204, 1952.
7. Finneson, B. E.: Diagnosis and Management of Pain Syndromes, ed. 2, Philadelphia, W. B. Saunders, 1969.
8. Ford, L., and Goodman, F. G.: X-ray studies of the lumbosacral spine. South. Med. J., 10:1123, 1966.
9. Gresham, J. L., and Miller, R.: Evaluation of the lumbar spine by diskography. Orthop. Clin., 67:29, 1969.
10. Hanraets, T. R. M. J.: The Degenerative Back and Its Differential Diagnosis. Amsterdam, Elsevier Publishing Company, 1959.
11. Horal, J.: The clinical appearance of low back disorders in the city of Gothenberg, Sweden Acta. Orthop. Scand., Supp. 118, 1969.
12. Hult, L.: The Munk Fors Investigation. Acta. Orthop. Scand., Supp. 16, 1954.
13. Jacobaeus, H. D.: On insufflation of air into the spinal canal for diagnostic purposes in cases of tumors in the spinal canal. Acta Med. Scand., 55:555, 1921.
14. Lasègue, C.: Considerations sur la sciatique. Arch. Gen. de Meil 2 4:558, 1864.
15. Lindblom, K.: Diagnostic puncture of intervertebral discs in sciatica. Acta Orthop. Scand., 17:231, 1948.
16. Lindblom, K.: Acta Radiol., 22:711, 1941.
17. Lumbar Discography Table, Orthopedic Equipment Company, Bourbon, Indiana, U.S.A.
18. Mason, M. S., and Raaf, J.: Complications of pantopaque myelography; case report and review. J. Neurosurg., 19:302, 1962.
19. Sicard, J. A., and Forestier, J.: Method radiographique d'exploration de la cavite epidurale par le lipiodol. Rev. Neurol., 37:1264, 1921.
20. Splitoff, C. A.: Roentgenographic comparison of patients with and without backache. JAMA, 152:1610, 1953.
21. Steinhausen, T. B., Dungan, C. E., Furst, J. B., Plati, J. T., Smith, S. W., Darling, A. P., Wolcott, E. C., Jr., Warren, S. L., and Strain, W. H.: Iodinated organic compounds as contrast medicine for radiographic diagnosis. III. Experimental and clinical myelography and ethyl iodophenylundecylate (Pantopaque). Radiology, 43:230, 1944.
22. Tarlov, I. M.: Pantopaque meningitis disclosed at operation. JAMA, 129:1014, 1945.
23. Wideroe, S.: On intraspinal luftinjektion og om dens diagnotiske betydning ved rygmervslidelser, saerlig ved svulster. Norsk. Mag. f. Laegevidensk, 32:491, 1921.
24. Wise, R. E., and Weiford, E. C.: X-ray visualization of intervertebral disc; report of case. Cleveland Clinic Quarterly. 18:127, 1951.
25. Woodhall, B., and Hayes, G. J.: The well-leg-raising test of Fajerstajn in the diagnosis of ruptured intervertebral disc. J. Bone Joint Surg., 32A:786, 1950.

3
Psychology of Low Back Dysfunction

PSYCHOLOGY OF PAIN

Organic Pain and "Imaginary" Pain

Pain and the Doctor-Patient Relationship

Reactions to Pain

Emotions
Adaptation
Socioeconomic and Cultural Factors
Athletics
Body Area
Psychosis

Absence of Pain

Pain and Sensory Deprivation

Evaluation of Pain

Difficulties in Diagnosis

Management of Pain

Overtreatment
Target Fixation

Secondary Loss and Secondary Gain

Prolongation of Symptoms and Secondary Gain

Placebos and the Placebo Effect

Double-blind Method
Mechanism of Action
"Placebo-Reactor Type": Fact or Fancy?

NONORGANIC BACKACHE

Apocryphal Diagnosis

Hypochondriac and Malingerer

Hypochondriac
Malingerer

Management

3
Psychology of Low Back Dysfunction

PSYCHOLOGY OF PAIN

Pain is a psychobiologic phenomenon with both physical and emotional components. This dual aspect of pain is linked to the distinction between its perception and reaction. Perception of pain may be evaluated in terms of quality and intensity, while reaction to pain is manifested by such symptoms as tachycardia, anxiety, fear, panic, and prostration.

ORGANIC PAIN AND "IMAGINARY" PAIN

In the practice of clinical medicine, emotional factors are often not considered part of a pain syndrome unless the pain is labeled "imaginary" or the patient is identified as a malingerer. Most patients complaining of pain usually have at least some physiological basis for their complaints, although neurotic mechanisms may greatly exaggerate their suffering. The very term "psychosomatic medicine" epitomizes the dual nature of the mind and body concept. The constant effort of physicians to separate the purely physiologic from the purely psychologic and label symptoms either as organic or functional has a certain futility about it.

The use of "organic phraseology" to depict an emotional or psychologic state is often encountered in the expressions used in daily conversations, such as "You are a pain in the neck," or "You make me sick" or "That job is a headache." That such symbolic uses of "organic expressions" are so completely understood and require no explanation indicates that the merging of mind and body is indeed a natural one; and it is only the so-called "trained" mind of the physician that often creates a somewhat false problem in attempting to separate the two when there is no actual division. For example, if an individual states that a certain job is a headache, no one would consider treating this condition medically. But when a patient with a backache of emotional etiology is seen in the office, it is much easier to treat him medically than to attempt to evaluate and to deal with the etiology of his backache. Thus, as physicians, we are always called on to make a "value judgment" regarding the organicity of pain.

If we do decide that the pain is actually organic, it is either because we can identify the etiology of the pain or because the characteristics of the pain fall into a known or readily classifiable pattern. When we are able to identify a pain successfully as organic in nature, we then carry out the appropriate therapeutic measures. If we are unable to diagnose the patient's pain as organic, we do not feel as comfortable in managing such a patient. Because of our own mental frame of reference with regard to nonorganic symptoms, this frame of reference in part resulting from our background and training, we are inclined to consider this painful response somewhat inappropriate. When we label a symptom as functional or psychogenic we are, in part, making light of it.

PAIN AND THE DOCTOR-PATIENT RELATIONSHIP

Whenever a physician is dealing with a pain problem, he must constantly bear in mind the relationship he has with the patient and the patient's attitude toward him. It is my experience that the vast majority of patients have a high regard for their physicians, and it gives them considerable regret if they are not significantly improved by treatment administered. As a rule, most patients rarely say that any particular method of treatment is completely ineffective. The physician is more likely to get the guarded response: "It's only a little better."

Because of the normal tendency to prefer praise to blame, we tend to become frustrated, and in some instances even antagonistic, and are apt to label the pain problem as functional when the patient does not improve. Most of us have had the experience of treating a symptom complex that we would ordinarily expect to improve with our method of therapy, and in not realizing the expected satisfactory result, develop a somewhat hostile attitude toward the patient. Although we are sometimes able to assess adequately our own feelings toward the patient, we must at the same time remain aware that the patient's feelings toward us often play a significant role in determining the success of therapy. In some instances, the patient may develop hostility toward the physician and announce with triumph at each visit that "Your medicine doesn't do a thing for me." The patient may not feel that he is able to complain overtly to his physician, but his continued suffering, despite treatment, is a form of covert criticism, which in fact renders the physician powerless to retaliate.

This example of hostility between doctor and patient is somewhat oversimplified, and, of course, persisting pain invariably has many more ramifications than described in this primitive psychological schema. But it is often with a sense of punishment or banishment that the patient is referred to a psychiatrist or other specialist. The patient feels that he has annoyed the physician, and in many cases he truly has. When this is in part true, the patient often feels somewhat rejected in being banished to a psychiatrist for symptoms he feels are certainly not imaginary. It is my own impression that probably 50 percent of all psychiatric referrals in a general hospital can be classified, at least in part, as pain syndromes.

REACTIONS TO PAIN

Emotions

There are no really satisfactory and universally accepted methods for gauging pain intensity, but studies based on the techniques currently available to us provide some information on individual "pain thresholds." The patient with a prefrontal lobotomy may have a normal threshold for pain but manifest a decreased reaction to a painful stimulus, although he may acknowledge it on direct inquiry.

A number of factors influence the reaction to pain. Conditioning experience and emotions may either increase or decrease the reaction to pain, as demonstrated by the howls of pain when a child who is ordered, against his will, to go upstairs to bed, barks his shin as he is sulking up the stairs. By contrast, an identical injury suffered by the same child while climbing to a stadium seat to see a ball game may go unnoticed. The pain of a superficial laceration is easily tolerated by most adults, but apprehension and inexperience will cause a child with the same wound to experience a much amplified reaction. Conversely, if an adult experiences a dull pain over the left anterior chest wall, this may provoke considerable apprehension and alarm. The child under identical stimulus will probably not interrupt his play.

The patient harboring malignant disease,

whose suffering is almost always most intense in the gloom of night after all routine activities have ceased and he is alone with his thoughts, illustrates the role of emotions in increasing the reaction to pain. Often cited to indicate the effect of emotions in decreasing appreciation of pain is the testimony of prize fighters who, during the course of a bout, may be cruelly battered about and yet not notice any pain. This experience, shared by soldiers in combat who often state that their wounds do not become painful until they are evacuated from the dangers of the combat area, is probably only partly due to emotional influences.

Initial absence of pain is a common phenomenon accompanying sudden trauma. For example, a bullet wound that shatters the tibia may be appreciated as a heavy but painless blow to the shin. The observation has been made during combat that if a man cries out noisily when wounded, it is likely that the wound is not a severe one. Although high-speed projectile wounds are more often mentioned in this connection, stab wounds are often first noticed when blood trickles down the skin, producing a sensation of wetness.

Adaptation

If a stimulus to a sensory receptor is maintained at a constant intensity, the frequency of discharge from this receptor gradually diminishes. This phenomenon is called adaptation, and the rapidity with which different receptor organs adapt varies. The proprioceptors, which are concerned with the automatic maintenance of posture and knowledge of the position of the limb segments of the body, adapt quite slowly, as is necessary in order to maintain sustained positional attitudes and reflexes. Touch receptors, on the other hand, adapt very rapidly, which is compatible with the innocuous nature of the stimulus and yet allows for the receptor to remain ready to receive new impressions. Pain receptors adapt very little and continue to generate pain impulses for the duration of the painful stimulus. This is consistent with the protective function of pain.

Under special circumstances the phenomenon of adaptation to pain may come into play and create permanent elevation of pain thresholds. This was the case in a number of Allied prisoners of war subjected to 3 years of imprisonment and torture by the Japanese during World War II. Some of these survivors had varying degrees of persistent anesthesia, and one had complete insensitivity to all sensations except those on the cornea.

Socioeconomic and Cultural Factors

In addition to situational and environmental factors producing alterations in reaction to pain, social, economic and cultural factors may be of significance. An interesting project in this regard was carried out by Richard A. Sternbach and Bernard Tursky, in the Department of Psychiatry, Harvard Medical School. They attempted to determine whether the tolerance for pain was different for various ethnic groups. They obtained their subjects in response to classified advertising in local papers. All the subjects were housewives who had at least one child of school age, so that the process of transmitting attitudes toward pain could be explored in interviews. Ethnic membership was defined as follows: Yankees were Protestants of British descent whose parents and grandparents were born in this country; Irish, Italians, and Jews were those whose parents came to this country as immigrants, were Roman Catholic in the case of the Irish and Italians, and Orthodox or conservative in the case of Jews. Each subject participated in an interview lasting about an hour in which the purpose of the study was explained, family history was gathered, and the specific incidence of reactions to injuries was collected. The pain stimulus was produced by electrical stimulation delivered through an annular disc electrode on the treated dorsal surface of the left forearm. Standard psychophysical procedures were employed, including a notation of the level at which the subject asked that stimulation be stopped in response to the instruction, "We will gradually make it stronger until you tell us you don't want any more." This level was referred to as the "unmotivated upper threshold." Then some subjects who asked to stop before a certain current had been reached were coaxed to try higher levels referred to as the "motivated upper threshold." The mean upper (unmotivated and motivated) thresholds for the 4 ethnic groups were as follows:[3]

Response	Yankee	Irish	Jewish	Italian
Unmotivated upper threshold	9.74	8.68	8.83	6.12
Motivated upper threshold	10.23	9.35	10.16	7.11

Subjects also performed a "magnitude estimation" test as follows: Given a measured stimulation, they were told to call this stimulus "10" and to assign appropriate numbers to other intensities according to their subjective impression of each.

The findings of this study were correlated with and tended to support certain hypotheses regarding the attitudinal dissimilarities among those subcultural groups. It is felt that each group has its own configuration of attitudes toward painful stimuli and toward the expression or response to pain.

The fact that the Italian women showed significantly lower pain thresholds (and that fewer of them would accept the full range of stimuli) is quite consistent with the finding of a present-day orientation in this group with respect to pain, a focusing on the immediacy of the pain itself. This concern may be contrasted with that of the Jewish . . . subjects, who similarly display distress when in pain, but for the future-oriented reason of concern for the implications of the noxious stimulation. In our laboratory situation, where the stimuli carried no implications of future impairment, no activation of this concern would be expected for the Jewish group, and therefore no difference would be expected between them and the Yankees and Irish, who tend to be undemonstrative with respect to pain. But one would expect the Italian group, who are primarily concerned with the avoidance of the unpleasant stimuli, to be reluctant to accept the stronger intensities.[3]

The relatively undemonstrative Yankees had an adapting matter-of-fact orientation toward pain, but the similarly undemonstrative Irish subjects considered a painful stimulus a burden to be endured and suffered in silence.

Thus, the similar demonstrativeness of the Italians and Jews in response to pain arises from dissimilar attitudes, as does the similar undemonstrativeness of the Yankees and Irish.

Athletics

Another attempt to evaluate reaction to pain was carried out by Ryan and Kovacic from the University of California, who attempted to measure pain tolerance and athletic participation.

From observation of everyday experiences in athletics, it would be expected that ability to withstand pain should be related to participation in certain types of athletic events. In many sports, such as football or boxing, the ability to withstand pain appears to be essential to successful performance, while in sports such as tennis or golf, the ability to withstand pain would be less important. Thus, it is not inconceivable that an individual's ability or inability to tolerate pain may well determine the category of participation he selects. An individual with a high pain threshold might be oblivious to bumps and bruises received in a football game, whereas the individual with a low pain threshold might avoid such contact.[2]

For this reason, pain threshold and pain tolerance were studied in 3 groups of subjects: contact athletes, noncontact athletes, and nonathletes. That the study was related to athletic participation was not known by the subjects.

Three methods were used to deliver controlled pain:

1. Radiant heat was focused on the sub-

ject's forehead, and the time of radiation was used to measure the subject's pain threshold.

2. Gross pressure was used to measure pain tolerance by means of a plastic aluminum-tipped football cleat secured to a curved fiber plate and fitted to the leg. The cleat was placed against the anterior border of the tibia, midway between the ankle and the knee, and a sphygmomanometer was used to secure the cleat properly in place. Cleat pressure was obtained by slowly inflating the sphygmomanometer armlet at a slow, constant rate until the subject indicated verbally that he was no longer willing to endure the pain.

3. Muscle ischemia was the third method of evaluating pain tolerance. After the sphygmomanometer cuff was applied to the upper arm and the pressure elevated to 300 mm. of mercury, the subject flexed his fingers and extended his fingers at a rate of one per second until he was unwilling to proceed.

Each test was carried out twice. After the first trial, the examiner remarked to each of the subjects that the score was quite a bit lower than the average of the group tested and the subject was asked to take the test a second time and do better, if possible.

Examination of the results indicated a definite relationship between the subject's willingness or ability to tolerate pain and the type of athletic activity in which he chooses to participate. The contact athlete . . . tolerated more pain than the athlete who participated only in noncontact sports such as tennis or golf, and both groups of athletes are willing to tolerate more pain than the nonathlete. In addition, after being told that his initial effort was poor, the contact athlete showed marked improvement on the second attempt, while the noncontact athlete improved some, but the nonathlete tolerated less pain than on the first attempt.

The question of cause and effect—whether a boy learns to tolerate pain because he engages in contact sports, whether he engages in contact sports because he can more easily tolerate pain (either for physiological or psychological reasons) . . . is unanswered by these data.[2]

Body Area

The body area of the pain is sometimes a factor in determining the patient's reaction. For example, many patients are reluctant to complain about rectal pain or genital pain. Headache is more popularly considered a socially acceptable form of discomfort. In this respect, I recall a patient who had been referred to me by another physician for long-standing headaches. Because of the intractable nature of his headaches, this patient was eventually hospitalized for a complete neurological work-up. In the course of a complete physical examination carried out by the intern, very severely thrombosed hemorrhoids were noted. I noted this on the chart and asked the patient about his hemorrhoids. After some equivocation, he admitted that he had suffered quite severely from rectal pain for more than a year, and despite the fact that he was going to a physician at regular intervals for headaches, he had never mentioned the rectal pain. The reason, of course, was that he was "ashamed of having a painful rectum" but considered the headache socially acceptable.

Psychosis

Most psychotic patients do not differ from sane patients in their reactions to pain. However, many of them complain of severe pain in various portions of their anatomy as a part of their mental illness. On the other hand, some schizophrenic patients have amputated their genitals, fingers, or ears, or have extensively mutilated themselves in other ways without expressing a reaction to pain.

ABSENCE OF PAIN

A number of papers have described persons born without a sense of pain. In spite of the lack of this important modality these rare individuals usually are able to cope with the routine problems of daily living and avoid burns and other injuries, which the adult who develops syringomyelia (which causes loss of pain and temperature sensations) is likely to incur. Because this condition is extremely uncommon and postmortem confirmation is not available, the site of any possible organic lesion is not documented. Some workers believe that this condition represents a form of sensory agnosia or an aphasiclike inability to formulate an appreciation of pain.

PAIN AND SENSORY DEPRIVATION

At one time the ability to withstand pain was considered a possible factor in evaluating men for future space travel. One of the potential problems of prolonged travel in space is a form of sensory deprivation resulting from isolation and confinement. Studies of persons subjected to prolonged sensory deprivation have demonstrated a deterioration in performance capabilities due to the impoverished sensory environment. In addition, a number of personality aberrations have resulted from experimental sensory deprivations such as increased anxiety, feeling of insecurity, and in some cases, hallucinations. In all cases, motor coordination and precision of motor performance are impaired.

Because pain is a sensory phenomenon, one might speculate that those persons who were hypersensitive to pain and had low pain thresholds reacted in this fashion because they were extremely sensitive to all sensory stimuli. Because of this presumed hypersensitivity, such individuals should have a less detrimental reaction to prolonged sensory deprivation. An analogy of this concept is that of a powerful radio receiver (hypersensitive) picking up the faint signals of a distant broadcast (sensory deprivation) while the ordinary low power set (hyposensitive) would not register the signal.

This hypothesis was advanced by Dr. A. Petrie, who postulated that sensitivity to pain is the reverse of sensory deprivation sensitivity. To carry this hypothesis further, since there might be a negative relationship be-

tween sensitivity to pain and performance under reduced sensory input conditions, astronauts who are most sensitive to pain ought to be selected for prolonged space travel because they would be able to endure reduced sensory input conditions for a longer time without degradation in performance. On the other hand, those with higher pain thresholds would not be able to endure reduced sensory input conditions and would manifest an inferior performance.

Studies were carried out by Dr. J. Peters and his associates of the Space Environment and Life Sciences Laboratory of the Republic Aviation Corporation in Farmingdale, Long Island, New York, on a number of volunteers who were first tested for their ability to tolerate pain. After this had been established, the subjects were then placed in an environment of sensory deprivation.

Each volunteer rested on a contour couch in a full scale model of a multiman space capsule. The subjects could communicate with the observer at any time during the experiment, but the observer only responded when a subject requested termination of his stay in the cabin. Each subject donned ear defender headsets with built-in ear phones such as are typically worn by workers at airfields. "White" noise was fed into the headsets at a low decibel load sufficiently above ambient noise to shut out any orientation to the world outside, yet the subject obviously had monotonous and continuous hearing stimulation. The subject wore goggles modified to allow light to come through translucent but not transparent lens surfaces. Thus, the subjects were visually stimulated by incandescent light which always illuminated the cabin, but the illumination was unchanging and unpatterned. The subjects wore heavy leather gloves, similar to those worn by electric arc-welders, and they were instructed to keep the gloves on at all times. Thus, sensations normally received by the fingers and hands were diminished, and the threshold for discernable patterns of sensation was raised. This tended to make the sensory input from the hands monotonous. Similarly, the subjects wore heavy wool socks to diminish sensory input from the feet. Because of the attached sensors and wires, the movement of the subjects was restricted.

They were instructed not to leave their contour chairs and advised that the electronic wiring allowed only limited movement. Thus, the subjects would only turn from side to side, flex and unflex their limbs, and sit up or lie down. The food, Sustagen, was a bland, high caloric liquid, neither markedly pleasant nor unpleasant in taste. The subjects were encouraged to take nourishment whenever they desired, but when they did so, to take at least several ounces of the liquid. Thus, oral stimulation tended to be minimized.[1]

This study seemed to indicate a direct and positive correlation between the ability to endure pain and the ability to endure reduced sensory input conditions. The original thinking—that there is a negative relationship between the ability to endure pain and the ability to endure reduced sensory input conditions—was not supported. The evidence suggested that subjects who were most able to endure pain were better able to tolerate reduced sensory input conditions, suffered less anxiety with attendant headaches and nausea, and remained in good functional condition for longer periods of time than those who were least able to endure pain.

EVALUATION OF PAIN

From time to time most well-adjusted persons will experience occasional aches or pains in various areas of their bodies which will not interfere with activities of daily living. The psychoneurotic person is often prone to seize upon such a nidus of pain and so distort and exaggerate it that the major symptom complex he eventually manifests can hardly be recognized in relationship to the original pain. The various psychologic mechanisms at work in creating this type of distorted clinical picture vary greatly and should always be considered when the symptoms are inconsistent with the findings on examination.

Difficulties in Diagnosis

The evaluation of pain so that it can be treated adequately is made difficult by its being an almost entirely subjective phenom-

enon. It is especially difficult to differentiate organic factors from psychic. The problem is further complicated because in most, if not all, patients both factors contribute to the final expression of pain. Furthermore, the proportion of contribution by the somatic and psychic spheres changes constantly. It is in this area of diagnosis that the "art" of the physician is most severely challenged and is almost impossible to subject to quantitative evaluation and criticism. Estimation of the intensity of pain is likewise difficult for the physician. Nevertheless, he must evaluate the intensity in order to determine what therapy is justified for relief of pain. Such questions as the constancy of pain, its interference with performance of duties and how it affects vital functions, such as sleep, must be answered and clearly evaluated by the examiner.

A careful history is the principal basis for establishing a diagnosis of the pain syndrome and its severity. It often requires considerable time and patience to elicit the findings that permit the diagnosis of a specific organic syndrome or to demonstrate that none exists.

An understanding of a patient's personal conception of the workings of his body or of his medical idiosyncrasies can be instrumental in evaluating the clinical picture. A patient with a spinal cord tumor seen some years ago had been hospitalized on two previous occasions for the same complaint of pain radiating into the epigastrium. Because this patient experienced temporary relief of pain following enemas, he was thought to have gastrointestinal disease. It was not until he developed long-tract signs with weakness of both lower extremities that disease of the spinal cord was considered. Subsequent questioning revealed that the patient held to an "auto-intoxication" theory and believed that most body ills were related to chronic constipation.

The patient with a medical history of multiple surgical procedures, frequent hospitalizations and short tryouts of a parade of physicians should increase the physician's caution before a diagnosis of organic disease is made. In a large number of pain problems the factor of litigation and secondary gain is present and must be evaluated as a possible motivating force. As a general rule, it is necessary to rest an organic diagnosis upon clear objective changes or on the conformity of the complaints to a known syndrome. Again, only a careful, and often time-consuming, history and examination by an unprejudiced observer will permit a true evaluation of the patient's complaints. Often the behavior of the patient is so bizarre that a firm opinion regarding the existence of any underlying pathologic change cannot be offered. In such instances it is generally wise not to initiate therapy that may cause permanent changes and thus avoid an iatrogenic contribution to the clinical picture.

MANAGEMENT OF PAIN

Overtreatment

The most important principle in the management of pain is avoidance of overtreatment. This pitfall is a great source of potential danger and often tests the physician's critical judgment. The aphorism, "Excess always carries its own retribution," is particularly relevant to the management of pain, for violation of this principle may have unfortunate results.

Still vivid in my memory is the picture presented by an unfortunate man who was a living monument to the hazards of overtreatment. This patient had originally complained of severe pain in the low back and lower extremity for which he was subjected to 6 myelograms and 3 lumbar laminectomies. Each successive diagnostic and surgical procedure served only to increase the original pain. The diagnosis of adhesive arachnoiditis of the cauda equina, secondary to the multiple myelograms and surgery, was made and in an attempt to control nerve root pain an alcohol block of several lumbar roots was performed. As a complication of this procedure the patient became paraplegic but continued to complain of his original pain. By

this time, the patient was a confirmed narcotic addict, and in an effort to control the addiction and to alleviate his pain, a prefrontal lobotomy was carried out. A craniotomy wound infection developed, necessitating removal of the entire frontal bone flap before healing could occur. This extensive bony defect involved the upper half of the forehead and resulted in a particularly unfortunate cosmetic result.

The patient then developed severe crossed adductor spasms involving his lower extremities. These were a form of the "mass reflex" involving bladder and bowels so often seen in paraplegia. Because these spasms prevented him from sitting in a wheelchair, and in other ways interfered with his general nursing care, a decision was made to section all the lumbar and sacral nerve roots. It was at this stage, when I was a neurosurgery resident in 1950, that I first saw the patient and, in fact, performed this last operative procedure. After the massive rhizotomy, the mass reflex spasms improved but his original pain persisted.

This patient's history revealed that each of his operative procedures was performed by a different surgeon, with the exception of the first and third lumbar laminectomies. There is no question that these physicians were not only well-intentioned but also of outstanding professional competence. Obviously, each was convinced that the patient's symptoms were nonorganic after he had performed surgery and seen the results. Then another surgeon would be besieged until he was convinced that the patient "deserved another look." The phrase, "We must do something for this suffering patient," has often led to a result much worse than the original ailment.

Target Fixation

In World War II, some of the bravest and most courageous young men this country has ever produced were selected for training as fighter pilots. When these fledglings engaged in their first few "dog fights," they sometimes so riveted their attention on the enemy that even after the object of their pursuit had been destroyed they were unable to collect themselves in time to veer from a midair collision; or they sometimes followed close on the tail of their victim as he crashed into the ground. This phenomenon was called "target fixation." With experience, pilots learned to maintain that important sense of objectivity even while in the heat of deadly combat so that this catastophe could be avoided.

In his desire to relieve suffering, no matter what the source, the physician sometimes develops a form of "target fixation" as he becomes enmeshed and entangled in the dependent demands of the patient for relief of a symptom which is largely nonorganic and involves major psychologic dysfunction. This physician-patient entrapment may progress from drugs of increasing potency through a variety of physiotherapeutic measures and sometimes even to surgery. If the physician is able to stand off and view the problem objectively, he is more apt to be of benefit; whereas such a problem improperly managed may only compound the progressive nature of the symptoms, causing additional suffering.

SECONDARY LOSS AND SECONDARY GAIN

An adequate evaluation of any pain problem requires an understanding of the effect the pain is producing upon the patient's total life style in terms of secondary loss as well as secondary gain. If the low back dysfunction prevents gainful employment, threatens the family's standard of living, or makes the patient dependent upon others, the usual response is depression and anxiety. When dealing with such secondary loss, the physician must be on the alert for denial of existing symptoms in this patient who is so strongly motivated to recover.

Secondary gain factors may exist if the pain gratifies some deep-seated masochistic need to suffer or to be dependent on and cared for by others, if financial gain is a consideration, or if the low back dysfunction removes the patient from a disliked job.

Prolongation of Symptoms and Secondary Gain

Prolongation of symptoms in the face of secondary gain is a fact acknowledged by all physicians. At one time I believed that such prolongation of symptoms was entirely due to malingering but in the past ten years have gradually reversed my opinion. When these suspected patients have been observed surreptitiously, many of them continue to exhibit signs of low back dysfunction. I am convinced that a significant number of these patients have prolongation of their symptoms from the effects of psychological conditioning resulting from the secondary gain situation.

The factors involved are complex and vary from case to case. In work-connected injuries where compensation is involved, all of the underlying resentment of an employee toward the employer (company) may surface and come to light in the course of the illness. Particularly in large organizations, many workers tend to feel that their labors are undervalued and unappreciated. Any overtime or extra duties they have performed in the past may not have been sufficiently acknowledged.

Now that they have incurred a physical injury in the course of their work they may feel that the plant physician turns a deaf ear to their complaints and is unsympathetic to their suffering. The injury may have occurred as the result of someone else's carelessness or somewhat inadequate safety controls on the job site, and this further intensifies their resentment. The injury-producing job may be unpleasant or hazardous and until the time of the accident the patient had no valid mechanism whereby he could react against this job. Prolongation of symptoms now provides the patient with an opportunity for an honorable and socially acceptable retreat or withdrawal from a vexatious task, without suffering scorn or criticism from either fellow workers or his family. He may attempt to utilize his symptoms to work under less hazardous circumstances and more comfortable surroundings.

Although a significant percentage of compensation-related low back patients consciously prolong their symptoms for self-serving purposes, a greater proportion are unaware of the psychological mechanisms associated with and possibly affecting their persisting symptoms. Confronted with such a schema, most patients would react with genuine astonishment and indignation. An explanation of this nature would only tend to increase patient resentment and exasperation over their plight and increase their feeling of abandonment. Rather than pursuing this "elucidative" approach, a generous "lump sum" early settlement may be more effective in terminating the undue prolongation of symptoms. From an industrial compensation point of view an early settlement of this nature might well be less costly.

A similar secondary gain situation, associated with prolongation of symptoms, is seen with low back problems resulting from vehicular accidents. The adversary proceedings of an interminable legal contest often result in the defense hard at work minimizing and deprecating the symptoms as opposed to the plaintiff-patient who must repeatedly document a persisting disability. Such prolonged legal sparring, which often involves an attack on the patient's validity, may serve to create a more firmly fixed symptom complex than would occur in a nonadversary situation. Those states where the so-called "no fault" vehicular insurance plans are in operation, which reduce the number of cases brought to adversary proceedings, have demonstrated a significant reduction in duration of symptoms.

PLACEBOS AND THE PLACEBO EFFECT

I was once called in consultation to see a patient with a pain problem and, upon asking about the efficacy of placebos, was told by the attending physician that this type of "deception" was never practiced on his patients. The physician who made this statement was extremely able and conscientious and because of his obvious sincerity and concern for the health of his patients enjoyed their trust and confidence to an unusually high degree. It is certain that whatever medications he prescribed, the results were frequently augmented by a placebo effect based on his splendid personality.

Viewed realistically, many types of treatment, other than the traditional capsule filled with lactose, can create the placebo effect, since this is based upon trust in the physician and faith in medicine generally. We have all seen patients whose intractable pain from malignant disease was temporarily relieved by an injection of sterile water. This is completely in accordance with our present understanding of psychosomatic medicine and the interrelationships of the mind and somatic illness. It has been shown that placebos can actually cause changes in laboratory data, such as the sedimentation rate, carbon dioxide combining power and the white blood cell count. The faith of the prescribing physician in a drug may have a definite effect on its action.

Double-blind Method

Knowledge of the placebo effect has led to the use of the double-blind method of testing drugs in which the physician as well as the patient is unaware whether the drug being administered is a placebo or the medication being tested. Just as many executives maintain that the best salesmen are not necessarily the brightest men but usually those who are the most enthusiastic about the product, so may the physician who actually believes in the curative properties of the drug he is giving create a greater effect than the doctor who is realistically uncertain about the merits of the medicine prescribed. In addition to drugs, physical measures including diathermy and massage create a positive psychologic effect that is sometimes the basis for the cures achieved by many healing cults, such as chiropractic and naturopathy.

Probably surgery has the most potent placebo effect that can be exercised in medicine. The detailed preliminaries, the rendering unconscious by anesthesia, and the removal or manipulation of vital organs within the body all create an almost mystic and profound emotional effect on the patient. This effect, of course, varies greatly from patient to patient. But in evaluating the results of any large series of surgical procedures, this placebo effect must certainly be considered. A well-known physician, an outstanding pioneer in the field of neurosurgery, when faced with a problem case of low back pain which he believed to be nonorganic in etiology, occasionally resorted to having the patient prepared and anesthetized for laminectomy and merely made the skin incision, which he then promptly sutured. Although several cases were reportedly "cured" by this method, I would guess that the long-term results were not uniformly happy.

Mechanism of Action

How can we explain the action of a placebo? The explanation most commonly accepted is that the patient's faith in the physician and in the medicine he prescribes is responsible for placebo action. Somewhat allied to this explanation is the staunch conviction that many patients entertain regarding the necessity for active treatment of their symptoms with no expectation of spontaneous improvement, making the placebo a sort of required precondition before they can expect to improve.

Also responsible for many placebo effects noted in clinical medicine are the spontaneous remissions characteristic of most illnesses. Any drug given at an opportune time may coincide with symptomatic improvement which would have eventuated regardless of treatment, and this improvement is attributed by both patient and physician to the medication. Such symptom fluctuations, implicit in the natural history of most disease states, emphasize the importance of evaluating a new drug not only with a placebo-receiving group but also with a separate control group receiving no treatment.

Most experienced clinicians are aware of the deliberately falsified response as a factor which must be considered in the evaluation of all drug effects including placebo effects. Reasons for such deliberate falsification vary but most often relate to the patient's desire to please the physician by acknowledging the desired response.

"Placebo-Reactor Type": Fact or Fancy?

Are some patients likely to respond to placebos with consistency while others never do and respond only to the pharmacologic actions of medications, or is reaction to placebos a factor potentially possessed by all depending upon the particular environment and the personal predisposition present at the time the placebo is administered?

Considerable discussion has been directed toward this question and evidence has been cited both for and against the concept of a "placebo-reactor type." The bulk of informed opinion, at this time, considers placebo reactivity a potential tendency that can be exhibited by anyone and is not a specific attribute possessed by some but not by others.

NONORGANIC BACKACHE

APOCRYPHAL DIAGNOSIS

A large percentage of patients complaining of low back pain have symptoms which are recognized as nonorganic or functional, but for a number of reasons the physician is hesitant to label the patient with such a diagnosis. In "off-the-record" conversations, most doctors will readily admit the frequency of this type of symptom in their practice but shy away from imparting their clinical impressions to the patient. It would be well to examine the reasons for the reticence of physicians to be dogmatic on this subject.

1. Often both patient and family will not readily accept a diagnosis of nonorganic disease; and frequently when such a diagnosis is proposed the patient may not return and will seek medical opinion and aid elsewhere.

2. When a diagnosis of nonorganic low back pain is submitted, under the present insurance system the cost of completely evaluating and managing the problem may not be underwritten. When an incident occurring during work was the alleged cause of low back symptoms, the workman's compensation carrier may attempt to avoid payment of the hospital and doctor bills. When industrial compensation is not a factor, many hospitalization insurance plans may object to accepting the cost of hospitalization with a final diagnosis of functional low back pain.

3. In medicolegal problems, mention of nonorganic symptoms is anathema to the patient's attorney, since this will weaken his bargaining position at settlement or in court.

4. Most doctors are concerned about erroneously considering the patient's complaint as nonorganic in the presence of organic disease. An obviously neurotic patient can also be organically ill, and in many instances it is difficult to separate the organic from the nonorganic.

Proper patient management of a suspected nonorganic backache demands a thorough and, in some instances, an exhaustive evaluation. Every experienced physician is able to recall a number of patients initially identified as neurotics who turned out to have hidden organic disease causing their symptoms. Before committing a patient to a diagnosis of functional illness, every effort is made to uncover organic disease. In most cases, hospitalization for some portion of this investigation is necessary.

HYPOCHONDRIAC AND MALINGERER

It is usually possible to identify the hypochondriac or malingerer with a nonorganic low back syndrome. Sometimes the zone of demarcation between these separate entities is indistinct and perplexing, but there are some distinguishing features which may be helpful in attempting to establish a working differential diagnosis.

Hypochondriac

These persons are often intelligent and may be subjected to considerable tension at work and in their home life as well. They may be involved in work that requires unusual abilities with pressures and can be successful in their occupational endeavors.

The history of most hypochondriacs is distinctive. They have usually seen many physicians in the past and have a tendency to be rather critical of each one in turn. They will discuss their previous physician's deficiencies at some length without much urging.

Previous hospitalizations have been necessary for a variety of complaints, often for symptoms involving different anatomical systems; the 3 most common being gastrointestinal, cardiac or chest and musculoskeletal. Objective findings are rare and results of tests and studies performed during previous hospitalizations and on an outpatient basis are nonrevealing or inconclusive.

As symptoms from one system clear, after a short period of time, symptoms from a new system will appear.

Each doctor they have seen, in turn, will prescribe a new medication; and none of these seems to be particularly helpful. They are familiar with the names of the medications and are aware of their action, "Oh yes, I have tried Butazolidin alka." "No, the Valium was not helpful." They are not unhappy to be hospitalized, and gladly undergo all sorts of tests and studies and are eager to try out all varieties of treatment. The latest ultrasonic or fancy new diathermy machine will be eagerly embraced and may have some short-term beneficial effect. Occasionally, the patient may buy his own diathermy machine.

In many cases, the spouse, either husband or wife, enters completely into the spirit of the exercise and is just as conversant with the symptoms as the patient. During the taking of the history, they will sit eagerly by the side of the patient and prompt them, interject with a forgotten symptom, correct them on dates, and, in general, take an active role. One such husband of a hypochondriac wife, who was not particularly wealthy, fitted out his entire basement with a variety of mechanical devices, including a diathermy machine and a traction apparatus, so that it resembled the physiotherapy department of a small hospital.

In addition to backache, the hypochondriac usually manifests symptoms of irritability and nervousness, such as excessive perspiration or tremor of the hands. A telephone ring or an intercom buzzer may produce a striking startle reaction.

Other illustrative symptoms are the tension type of headache with a sensation of "a tight band around my head," "difficulty swallowing," a "constant lump in my throat." There may be voice changes with inability to speak above a whisper. Gastrointestinal symptoms are common and may be categorized as an "irritable colon" or "spastic colitis." Insomnia is a frequent complaint as is shortness of breath and any or all of these may be aggravated by increased intensity of the backache.

Some of these patients have had a number of surgical procedures carried out for indications which were less than classical. They may be willing to submit to surgery, and this may alleviate their symptoms for several months.

Malingerer

This condition is not possible without involvement of secondary gain in some form. Secondary gain does not necessarily have to be financial. It may involve changes in the work status. This commonly includes less physically strenuous work and jobs that involve less traveling in the case of salesmen. This could also include less hazardous work such as in the case of a police officer, an inside job rather than patroling a "beat." Sometimes these changes may be so subtle and may seem so unimportant to the physician that he may not be aware that he is dealing with a secondary gain situation. I recall such a patient who complained of back pain, which was not particularly severe and did not prevent him from working. I was not able to "cure" this patient until the third visit when it was revealed to me that he was acutely concerned with his car parking privileges. He had developed an emotional commitment to parking in a smaller parking lot close to the factory which was reserved for higher ranking personnel, while the larger parking lot for the rest of the employees was a greater distance away. After he was satisfied that he could continue to park his car in the closer lot, his symptoms improved to the point where I did not have to see him again.

There is no specific type of personality or character makeup that relates to this syndrome.

There is no relationship whatsoever between the severity of the injury and the intensity or duration of symptoms. I recall a middle-aged secretary who was struck in the midlumbar region by a gum eraser that had been tossed playfully by a young secretary who meant to hit another young office worker. The intended victim had ducked, causing this small missile to strike my patient. The prolonged duration and intensity of her symptoms prevented her from returning to work for 5 months and were probably nurtured, in part, by the unconscious resentment and hostility she had for her prankish younger fellow workers.

The symptoms, as a rule, are somewhat vague and usually variable, changing from time to time. It is well to document the symptoms carefully and in the patient's own words as much as possible. Several weeks later the symptoms may be quite different; and oftentimes the patient denies having stated what was recorded in the first session.

The characteristics of the low back pain may be unusual in several respects. That improvement came with bed rest or inactivity is denied, a response which is somewhat unusual since most backaches do improve with rest and inactivity. The area of pain is often nonphysiologic, and complaints will be heard of pain that runs "from the bottom of my spine up to the top of my neck," or will radiate forward through the umbilicus or extend into the inguinal areas causing severe genital discomfort. If the pain extends into the lower extremities, the patient is very vague when attempting to point out the exact course or distribution of the pain as it radiates down the leg. Most patients with valid root compression syndromes are quite specific about the course of their pain; and if the physician acts as though he did not understand and points to the lateral aspect of the thigh, when the patient had indicated the pain coursing down the posterior thigh, and states "You mean it hurts here?" the patient with organic pain will almost always correct the physician; the malingerer is more likely to accept the different site suggested by the physician with the thought that perhaps this is the spot that "should be hurting." If you ask "Which leg hurts?" the answer may be vague and all-encompassing with bilateral leg pain not limited to a specific dermatome but rather generalized. Their description of the pain may be unusual, and terms such as "like a shock of electricity" or "sharp, like a knife" are often heard.

A differentiating characteristic between malingering and hypochondria is that the malingerer tends to emphasize symptoms related to the injured area and is not as likely to press what are thought to be irrelevant symptoms.

The malingerer in a work-connected accident is often reticent to resume the job at which the accident occurred; and this may be realistic, particularly if it was a somewhat hazardous occupation. A frequent source of symptom prolongation is a valid concern over being fired if he goes back to work. In the meantime, he has a "sure thing," with his compensation check coming in every week. If "layoffs" are occurring and his job seniority is such that he is afraid of being "laid off," as soon as his symptoms subside and he is pronounced fit to go back to work, he may continue to see the physician who will experience some difficulty in curing this man.

A serious sign, and possibly the onset of a pattern that may be difficult to deal with, occurs when a man's wife takes a job to supplement the loss of income caused by his disability. She may make a fairly good salary, and he may get used to doing a little housework; and when his disability check is combined with her pay, this gives them a fairly adequate income which may leave a lot of time for fishing, "visiting the boys at the volunteer firehouse," and other such activities. After a time his friends may get used to his carrying on various time-consuming nonpaying duties in civic and social organizations and an irrevocable "way of life" has become established.

Oftentimes, the malingerer has been given a low back support, which he claims to need very desperately and which he has supposedly been wearing constantly for the past year; and yet, if this appliance is closely examined, relatively little wear may be noted.

Physical examination of a malingerer claiming low back pain is often helpful and revealing.

Gait changes may be significant. Prior to the formal examination, the patient may walk into the office without noticeable dysfunction, but when asked to walk during the examination, an obvious and striking abnormality may develop.

Inspection of the lumbar spine may reveal a relaxed lumbar lordosis, whereas in the presence of persisting low back pain one would expect some paraspinal muscle spasm with flattening of the normal lumbar curvature. Minimal stimuli, such as light pressure over the lumbar musculature, will cause intense discomfort and trifling, inconsequential touches may cause some patients to jump with pain. When asked to bend forward, the patient is often unable to bend more than 5°, despite the absence of paraspinal muscle spasm to digital palpation. In the absence of muscle spasm, patients with practically complete lumbar fusions can bend forward to the point where they may touch their toes, since considerable rotation at the hips is possible despite almost total lack of mobility of the lumbar spine. Tenderness to pressure may be elicited over the sacrum, rarely a tender site, unless there is an underlying sacral malignancy or cyst. Sacroiliac compression may be very painful. Straight leg raising may be limited while lying supine on the table and, if this is noted, one should attempt the same maneuver with the patient seated. In the seated position, 90° elevation may be painlessly achieved. If straight leg raising is painful, the physician should first flex the knee and then the hip. If 90° hip flexion causes the same degree of pain with the knee flexed, sciatic radiation is eliminated. The pain is explainable either by hip disease or nonorganic symptoms. In performing voluntary straight leg raising, the development of tremors or "spastic jerking" of the elevated leg is usually indicative of functional disease.

Sensory changes are often very helpful in evaluation of functional backache. A frequently encountered form of nonorganic sensory change in the lower extremity is the stocking type of hypesthesia.

Testing of motor strength is often quite revealing. Lower extremity weakness of long-standing duration is invariably associated with some objective evidence of atrophy or loss of muscle tone. When testing some muscle strength, if the patient is resisting against the opposing arm or finger of the physician, a quick unexpected release of opposing pressure will cause even a weakened muscle to rebound immediately. If the patient is not resisting with full strength, the tested member will not rebound.

Complaints of a weak, tender, numb leg in the face of normal reflexes and no atrophy or loss of muscle tone are of questionable organic significance.

Bizarre reactions to drugs may be seen in both malingerers and hypochondriacs. They may be tranquilized by stimulants or vice versa. Both may also have unhappy reactions to injection therapy, "I was pretty good until you stuck those needles in my back, and now I can't even get out of bed."

Both male malingerers and hypochondriacs are likely to complain of sexual dysfunction. Normal sexual functions "have been impossible since that accident, doctor."

MANAGEMENT

It must be recognized that the management of this type of patient often requires more time and thought than of one with average organic low back problem. I believe it is helpful in every regard to get these patients back to work as soon as possible. Return to a work program and resumption of the normal activities of daily living is often associated with improvement, both physically and mentally. Intractable problems of functional low back pain may require psychiatric guidance. In selected instances, this may be helpful but my experience with low back dysfunction patients requiring psychiatric management is generally disappointing.

REFERENCES

1. Peters, J., Benjamin, F. B., Helvey, W. M., and Albright, G. A.: Study of sensory deprivation, pain and personality relationships for space travel. Aerosp. Med., *34:*830, 1963.
2. Ryan, E. D., and Kovacic, C. R.: Pain tolerance and athletic participation. Percep. Mot. Skills, *22:*383, 1966.
3. Sternbach, R. A., and Tursky, B.: Ethnic differences among housewives in psychophysical and skin potential responses to electric shock. Psychophysiology, *1:*243, 1965.

Conservative Treatment

NONSURGICAL MANAGEMENT OF LOW BACK PAIN AND SCIATICA

Rest

    Limitied Activity Program
    Mattress
    Bed Rest

Traction

Physiotherapy

    Heat
    Massage

Trigger Points

Manipulation

    Maneuvers

Medication

    Morphine
    Synthetic Derivatives of Morphine

    Synthetic Addicting Analgesics
    Non-narcotic Analgesics
    Anti-inflammatory Drugs
    Muscle Relaxants
    Miscellaneous Drugs

Occupational Changes

Psychotherapy and Hypnotherapy

**Activities of Daily Living
and Faulty Posture**

    Standing and Walking
    Sitting
    Driving
    Lifting
    Sleeping
    Establishing Proper Habits

LOW BACK EXERCISES

Purpose

**Exercises Adapted to the
Patient's Specific Needs**

When to Start

Preexercise Evaluation

Establishing an Exercise Program

Relaxation Exercises

Pelvic "Uptilt"

Exercises for Hip Flexor Elasticity

Low Back Exercises

    Phase 1
    Phase 2
    Phase 3

LOW BACK SUPPORTS AND BRACES

History

General Principles in the Use of Low Back Supports

Low Back Mechanics
Immobilization—Fact or Fancy
Fitting Supports
Purposes of a Spinal Support
Brace Versus Corset

Braces

"Three-Point Pressure" Principle
Knight Spinal Brace

Williams Brace
Taylor Brace

Corsets

Trochanter Belt
Sacroiliac Corset
Lumbosacral Corset
Dorsolumbar Corset

Less Frequently Used Supports

Conservative Treatment

NONSURGICAL MANAGEMENT OF LOW BACK PAIN AND SCIATICA

Certain basic principles can be applied to the conservative management of most lumbar-sciatic syndromes. An understanding of these principles and the mechanisms of action by means of which they may provide symptomatic relief is essential to proper treatment.

REST

Limited Activity Program

Patients who have low back discomfort from almost any cause will instinctively attempt to avoid activity and will "rest." The method and extent of rest largely depends upon the severity and nature of the symptoms. Patients suffering from mild low back discomfort may be well served by a limited activity program, which does not involve heavy lifting, prolonged forward bending, excessive stooping, or prolonged auto trips. Activities can be further reduced by eliminating prolonged standing or extensive walking and curtailing stair climbing. When stair climbing is unavoidable, the patient is instructed to "baby walk" the stairs by placing both feet on the same step before advancing to the next. If such a limited activity program does not provide adequate relief of symptoms, bed rest must be considered.

Mattress

A firm mattress is most important for rest of the patient with low back symptoms. Some physicians strongly advocate a mat-

tress with no springs, consisting of hair stuffing, firm kapok or foam rubber padding. There seems to be no significant clinical advantage resulting from the use of any of these special mattresses other than reasonable firmness. If the mattress does sag when supporting the weight of a body, boards either in the form of individual slats or 3/4" plywood between the mattress and the box spring is helpful.

Bed Rest

Whether bed rest is to be carried out at home or in the hospital, may be the patient's choice. The flat supine position maintains the lumbar lordosis and is less effective in affording symptomatic relief than is a position of slight lumbar flexion. This can be achieved if the hospital bed is adjusted to a 30° elevation of the head and slight flexion of the knee break. The elevated head allows the patient to read, watch TV and greet visitors, making bed confinement more tolerable. The position can be varied by assuming

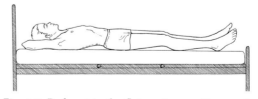

Fig. 4-1. Bed rest in the flat supine position maintains the lumbar lordosis and is less effective in affording symptomatic relief than a position of slight lumbar flexion.

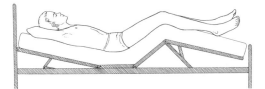

Fig. 4-2. Adjustment of the hospital bed to provide a position of slight lumbar flexion is helpful in affording symptomatic relief.

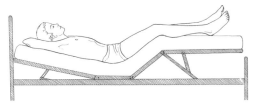

Fig. 4-4. Modified supine position.

the modified supine position with elevation of the legs above the head or a side lying position, keeping the hips and knees flexed. The modern electrical hospital bed has a great advantage in allowing the patient to change the bed configuration without leaving the bed, reducing the need for outside help.

Meals are served to the patient and bed rest is strictly enforced, with the exception of toilet privileges. The use of a bedpan produces at least the same, if not a greater, degree of mechanical stress upon the lumbar spine as allowing the patient to go to the bathroom once or twice daily, and the patient is invariably more satisfied with this ar-

rangement. If a toilet is not reasonably close to the bed, the use of a bedside commode may be helpful.

Many patients prefer to be treated at home, and yet, strict bed rest is less likely to be adhered to in a home situation. Most patients who are not observed tend to get out of bed for a variety of reasons, such as answering the doorbell, taking care of children or general restlessness. The more controlled hospital environment, with meals served at the bed, the use of an electric bed and the usually firmer mattress are all more conducive to symptomatic improvement. If the patient does elect to be treated with bed rest at home, an electric hospital bed should be rented.

In prescribing prolonged bed rest it must be recognized that as a result of lack of activity and muscle disuse a certain degree of muscle atrophy will occur. In addition, there may be loss of calcium from the bones, loss of protein and certain circulatory changes which may give rise to light-headedness and in some cases syncope once the erect position is resumed. An appreciation of these adverse effects of prolonged bed rest will allow the physician to properly estimate the total period of management. After pain relief has been achieved, the patient may require a period of strengthening activities including

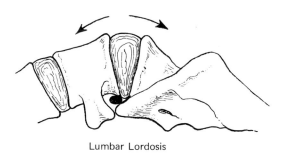

Lumbar Lordosis

Lumbar Flexion

Fig. 4-3. Altered relationship of annulus, nerve root, and intervertebral foramina in lumbar lordosis and lumbar flexion.

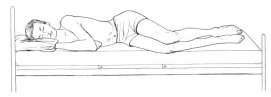

Fig. 4-5. Lateral position, with hips and knees flexed.

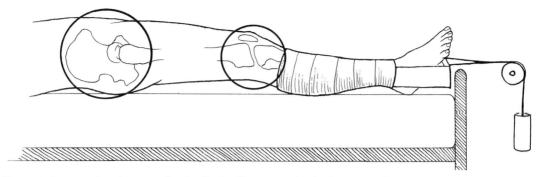

Fig. 4-6. Leg traction is a mechanically inefficient method of traction for low back pain, since the traction force must be transmitted through the knee and hip joints before affecting the low back.

exercises and gradually progressive mobilization procedures before returning to a normal existence. In addition to repairing the adverse effects of prolonged bed rest, some of these measures are important in preventing recurrence of the original symptoms.

It may be necessary to stage the mobilization to the point where total bed rest is reduced to several hours daily in addition to the usual nighttime rest. When the patient is out of bed, a low back support may be necessary. If this program is successful, progressive mobilization can continue until the patient is no longer at bed rest except during hours of sleep.

TRACTION

Traction is a time-honored procedure, having been used in the conservative management of low back dysfunction for the past 50 years. The earlier forms, such as Buck's or Russel's traction, employed the pull directly upon the lower extremities. The most popular form of traction for low back dysfunction at this time is pelvic traction, which employs a snug canvas girdle encircling the pelvis and hips with traction straps leading from this girdle to weights hung at the foot of the bed.

The benefits of traction were originally attributed to a distraction or separation of the vertebrae, permitting a protruding disc to "slip back into place." It is contrary to all reasonable expectation for leg traction, which must transmit a force through the knee and

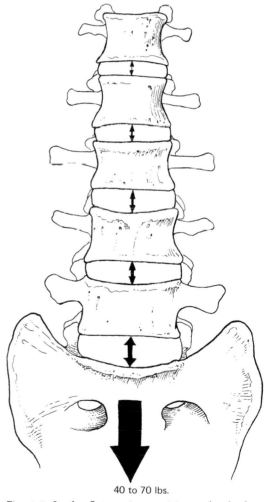

40 to 70 lbs.

Fig. 4-7. In the flat supine position, a load of 40 to 70 pounds is necessary to produce distraction of the lumbar intervertebral joints. Traction effect upon the intervertebral discs progressively diminishes in a cephalad direction.

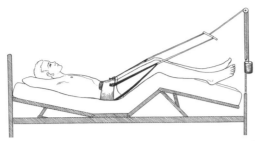

Fig. 4-8. Pelvic traction with the patient in moderate lumbar flexion.

hip joints before involving the lumbar intervertebral joints, to be effective.

Pelvic traction, when utilized on the patient maintained in the flat supine position, requires an intolerable weight of 40 to 70 pounds to exert sufficient force to produce separation of the vertebrae.

When traction is employed on a patient in slight lumbar flexion, it can be adjusted to exert a lever action on the spine to promote further lumbar flexion. The increased mechanical effect of leverage will distract the posterior elements of the vertebral column, reducing compression upon the posterior portion of the annulus fibrosis and increasing the aperture of the intervertebral foramina.

In addition to the mechanical benefits, pel-vic traction, which the patient can control by applying and removing it at will, may alleviate the monotony of enforced bed rest and be of some psychological advantage in imparting to the patient a sense of receiving active therapy. If confined to bed without traction, the complaint, "nothing is being done for me," is frequently voiced. Pelvic traction, using 15 to 30 pounds, allows the patient to move the lower extremities and also turn freely from side to side while in bed so that it does not add to the risk of thrombophlebitis. Any form of traction employing the pull directly upon the lower extremities does increase the risk of thrombophlebitis.

PHYSIOTHERAPY

Heat

Heat applied by a variety of methods is the most commonly used form of physiotherapy. Heat relaxes muscles, is alleged to improve local muscle nutrition by inducing vasodilation and may also be analgesic. It is frequently helpful in alleviating the muscle spasm of low back dysfunction.

Dry heat is often applied in the form of a heat lamp, hot air or heating pad. Dia-

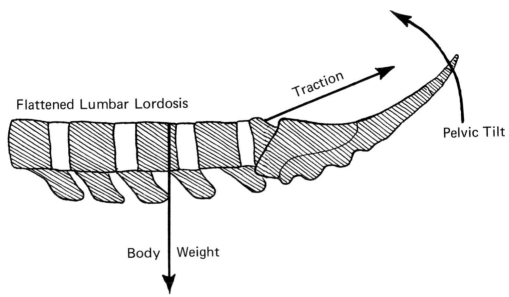

Fig. 4-9. The leverage effect of pelvic traction in a position of moderate lumbar flexion.

thermy and ultrasound are commonly used.

Moist heat can be applied locally by the use of hot compresses or hot paraffin. Warm tub soaks are a form of moist heat.

Massage

The use of massage has its roots in antiquity, and may be helpful in the modern day conservative management of low back dysfunction. Paraspinal muscle spasm can be relaxed by gently performed deep kneading massage. The beneficial effects include increased blood flow, muscle relaxation and improved muscle tone.

Skin rolling, over fibrositic areas, in which a skin fold is raised and rolled along the body surface, may be acutely painful when over the myositic site. Following such a maneuver, the patient may note considerable improvement in symptoms.

When lumbar paraspinal muscle pain is localized to or seems to emanate from a specific and limited site, surface anesthetics such as ethyl chloride spray occasionally are helpful.

Ice massage is another form of temporary surface anesthesia. This is probably best done with an "ice lollipop" which is made by freezing water in a can into which a tongue depressor is inserted during the freezing process. The can is easily removed from the lollipop by running warm water over it.

The patient should not be given physiotherapy at the expense of being moved about too vigorously; and if any of the measures employed are pain producing, they should be stopped.

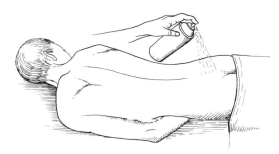

Fig. 4-11. Ethyl chloride spray.

TRIGGER POINTS

Patients with long-standing chronic and recurrent muscle pain develop tender, tense areas in the painful muscles. These tender sites occasionally can be palpated as nodules, the exact nature of which is speculative. Some investigators have reported microscopic changes including increased fibrous tissue, waxy degeneration of muscle fibers, destruction of fibrils and increase in number of nuclei of muscle fibers and fatty infiltration. To refute the claims by some that these nodules are essentially areas of localized muscle spasm, some investigators report that the nodules do not change even when the patient is under general anesthesia and, in fact, remain unchanged after death. Somewhat similar local hardened areas are produced in animal experimentation by tetanic stimulation of the leg of a rabbit and by local freezing of animal muscles.

The existence of areas of tender nodules is generally accepted but most investigators have been unable to confirm the histologic changes in these areas noted above. Whatever the exact nature of these lesions, it

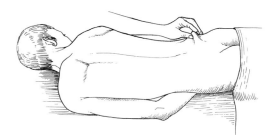

Fig. 4-10. Skin rolling.

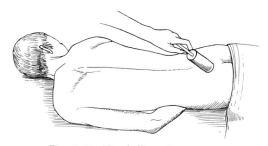

Fig. 4-12. "Ice lollipop" massage.

seems certain that they do constitute a clinical entity characterized by the presence of painful tender areas situated either in the muscle belly or at the ligamentous attachment of the muscle. Exposure to cold and exertion are factors in producing these lesions, and emotional tension seems to augment their formation. In palpating the relaxed muscles of the low back, one can often feel small hard nodules which, when pressed upon, will produce either local or radiating pain. Occasionally, ultrasound current over these areas may produce localized pain and will help identify these trigger points, although the examiner's experienced hand is more reliable. They are found often in the sacrospinal muscles from the lower thoracic region to the sacrum. Ligamentous trigger points are sometimes palpated at the spinous processes of the lumbar spine, the sacroiliac joint, iliac crest and greater trochanter.

Although a number of nodules may be palpated in examining the muscles of the low back, they should not be considered true trigger points if pressure upon them does not produce pain and injection of these sites is not indicated.

To inject these trigger point nodules approximately 10 cc. of Xylocaine are used and one can sometimes feel an increased resistance when the needle enters the nodule. If after injecting one or two trigger points the patient appreciates significant relief of pain, it may be helpful to repeat the injection 2 or 3 times.

MANIPULATION

Manipulation is one of the oldest forms of therapy, having been employed by Hippocrates and a long line of practitioners of the healing arts. During the 18th and 19th centuries, the bone setters in England were well known for this form of treatment and maintained their special methods within families from generation to generation. A certain cloak of secrecy surrounded the practice.

Today, many physicians are antagonistic to manipulation therapy and condemn it on all counts. There are a number of authenticated cases in which a severe exacerbation of signs and symptoms has occurred as a result of manipulation of the lumbar spine. Occasionally, these complications present serious neurological problems, such as a cauda equina syndrome, requiring emergency surgical intervention. It must also be realized that people with low back dysfunction are prone to sudden, acute exacerbations of their condition occasioned by a cough, a sneeze, bending forward to pick up a piece of paper, leaning over a sink to wash the face or sometimes spontaneously for no known cause whatsoever. Undoubtedly manipulative therapy has played a role in exacerbating some patients with preexisting lumbar spine pathology, but the question that must be considered is, would not these patients have worsened without manipulative therapy, purely from the stress of daily living?

In recent years there has been an awakened interest in manipulation among the medical profession, especially among those who are active in the treatment of low back dysfunction.

Manipulative therapy to the low back is effective in certain conditions and may be a helpful adjuvant when used in conjunction with other forms of available therapy. The improvement resulting from manipulation, in addition to stretching of muscles and tendons that have become contracted and shortened as a result of spasm, may be related to some alteration in the lumbar articular facets. The fibrous tissues surrounding these joints may become contracted and even develop adhesions after prolonged immobility of the lower back. Manipulation may be helpful in stretching such adherent tissues. There is no basis to claims that manipulation produces an "adjustment" or realignment of subluxated vertebrae.

Many patients who have chronic intermittent low back pain will routinely seek manipulative therapy when their pain becomes acute. A significant number of these patients derive some symptomatic relief from the treatment and occasionally the improvement will be striking. Occasionally a patient in such acute pain that he has difficulty walking into the office will stride out comfortably, almost immediately after a manipulative session.

Patients who have received manipulative therapy on a somewhat regular basis manifest two differentiating qualities which may be significant. First, the incidence of "clicking or cracking" sounds during manipulation is elicited in almost 90 percent in these cases, while in those patients who had not been previously manipulated the incidence was less than 25 percent. Second, the effects of manipulation are much more successful in the previously manipulated patients than in a "fresh" case. This personal experience has caused me to consider the possibility that, as the person who habitually "cracks" his knuckles can set up a fusillade of "pops" at will, so can a duplication of this effect be established in the frequently manipulated spine. Does repetitive manipulation stretch the facet synovial linings and capsules and make it easier for a facet to slip back and forth, predisposing the patient to more frequent low back symptoms? The exact cause of the clicking sound has never been clearly explained to my satisfaction. It may be produced by a vacuum phenomenon at the facet, similar to the "pop" which occurs when "cracking the knuckles."

One of the disadvantages of manipulative therapy is the practice necessary to acquire some skill in its use. Some doctors with little or no instruction in it attempt to manipulate a patient. After a few unsuccessful attempts they may then condemn manipulation as being of no value. Before attempting a series of manipulative procedures on a patient with low back pain, the manipulator should practice on several normal subjects so that he will be completely familiar with the normal resistance and mobility of each maneuver. No properly performed manipulation should cause discomfort to the normal subject, and the session should not be a particularly painful one to the low back patient. If a specific maneuver causes discomfort, it is preferable to perform it gently, short of pain, and to repeat it at a subsequent session.

Before considering manipulation, a complete evaluation of the patient is necessary, including lumbar spine x-rays. Contraindications to manipulation include spinal tumor suspects, vertebral fractures and dislocations and the stenotic lumbar spinal canal syndrome. Patients with lumbar disc disease may be considered for manipulation if frank radicular symptoms are not present, but this should be done on an individually selective basis in view of the possible complications.

Manipulation can be carried out with the patient awake or under anesthesia. Anesthesia will, of course, provide muscle relaxation in those patients with such severe muscle spasm that without it the treatment would not be tolerated. I am of the opinion that a program of bed rest, medication and patience will allow most patients to become controlled to the point at which manipulation may be tolerated without anesthesia.

Maneuvers

1. Spinal Thrust. The patient lies on an examining table in the prone position. Standing at the patient's right and facing him, the physician places his right palm on the patient's back, perpendicular to the spinal axis with the spinous processes just proximal to the fifth metacarpophalangeal joint. Using the left hand for reenforcement, he makes a short rapid thrust, starting at the lumbosacral joint and progressing along each interspace to the midthoracic spine. The direction of the trust is downward and toward the head.

2. Paraspinal Thrust. With the patient and the therapist in the same position as for Maneuver 1, the physician places his hands on either side of the spinous processes with the fingers pointed toward the patient's head. Starting in the lumbosacral region, the phy-

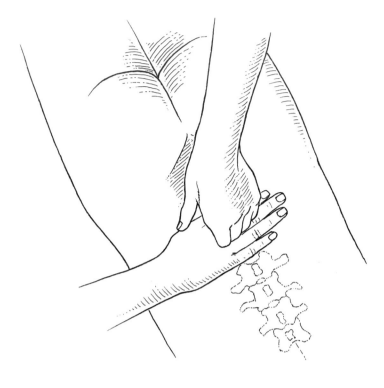

Fig. 4-13. Spinal thrust. The palm of the right hand is placed on the back, perpendicular to the spinal axis with the spinous processes just proximal to the fifth metacarpophalangeal joint. Using the left hand for reinforcement, make a short rapid thrust, starting at the lumbosacral joint and progressing along each interspace to the midthoracic spine. The direction of the thrust is downward and toward the head.

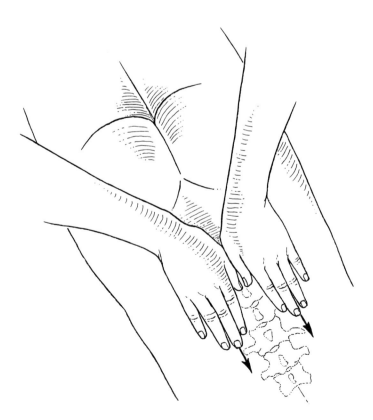

Fig. 4-14. Paraspinal thrust. The hands are placed on either side of the spinous processes with the fingers pointed toward the patient's head. Starting in the lumbosacral region, make a series of short rapid thrusts, using the "heels" of the hands, at each interspace up to the midthoracic spine. The direction of the force is downward and toward the head.

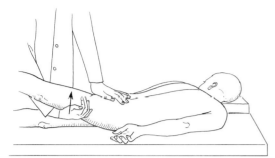

Fig. 4-15. Hyperextension of the thigh. With the left hand exerting a steady, firm, downward pressure upon the right buttock, the left thigh is hyperextended with the knee in extension. This maneuver is repeated on the opposite side.

sician makes a series of short rapid thrusts, using the palms of the hands, at each interval up the midthoracic spine. As in the spinal thrust, the direction of force is downward and toward the head.

3. Hyperextension of the Thigh. With the patient in the prone position, the manipulator places his left hand over the right buttock, exerting a steady, firm, downward pressure. With the patient's knee in extension, the right thigh is hyperextended. This maneuver is repeated on the opposite side.

4. Spinal Hyperextension and Pelvic Rotation. With the patient in the prone position, the manipulator stands at the foot of the table. While the patient maintains the lower extremities in extension, the physician grasps both feet and elevates the extremities in wheelbarrow fashion, causing hyperexten-

sion of the spine. Maintaining one extremity elevated, the physician lowers the other to the table; the same maneuver is repeated with the opposite leg.

5. Backward and Forward Spinal Torsion. The patient is placed on his left side with the left lower extremity extended and the right hip and knee flexed. The patient's right hand is placed over his right breast. Standing behind the patient, the physician places his right hand over the right iliac crest and his left hand upon the right shoulder. A forward torsion movement is then performed by simultaneously drawing the right shoulder backward and exerting a sudden forward and downward thrust on the right ilium. This movement, which is often associated with a clicking sound, produces stretching of the right posterior sacroiliac ligament and the right iliolumbar ligament as well as rotation of the interlaminar joints of the lumbar and lower thoracic vertebrae.

The manipulator then performs a backward torsion movement by thrusting the shoulder forward and drawing the right ilium backward. This manipulation stretches the right anterior sacroiliac ligament and rotates the vertebral interlaminar joints in the opposite direction. The same maneuver is repeated with the patient on his right side.

6. Pelvic Rock. With the patient lying in a supine position, the hips and knees are flexed until the thighs approximate a 90° angle with the trunk. The knees are grasped by the therapist and rocked gently

Fig. 4-16. Spinal hyperextension and pelvic rotation. While the patient maintains the lower extremities in extension, grasp both feet and elevate the extremities in wheelbarrow fashion, causing hyperextension of the spine. Maintaining one extremity elevated, lower the other to the table. Repeat the same maneuver with the opposite leg.

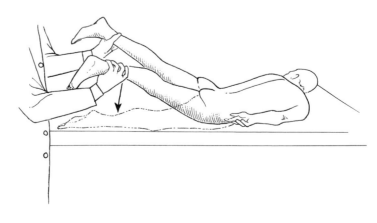

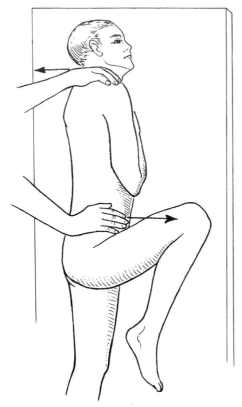

Fig. 4-17. Backward and forward spinal torsion. The patient is placed on his left side with the lower left extremity extended and the right hip and knee flexed. The patient's right hand is placed over his left breast. Standing behind the patient, the physician places his right hand over the right iliac crest and his left hand upon the right shoulder. A forward torsion movement is then performed by simultaneously drawing the right shoulder backward and exerting a sudden forward and downward thrust of the right ilium. A backward torsion movement is then carried out by thrusting the shoulder forward and drawing the ilium backward. The maneuver is repeated with the patient on his right side.

from side to side. If pain is experienced in the low back after several such rocking movements, the manipulation is stopped. If no pain is appreciated, progressive hip hyperflexion is superimposed on the side-to-side movements so that the knees are gradually rocked closer and closer to the axillae. This maneuver is directed toward releasing

locked facet articulations at the L5-S1 and L4-5 levels.

7. Passive Straight Leg Raising. With the patient in a supine position, the lower extremity is slowly elevated with the knee extended. This maneuver is performed short of producing pain or to an angulation of 90°. The maneuver is repeated with the opposite leg.

The patient should experience definite improvement of symptoms following the manipulative session. If no relief occurs after a properly performed manipulation, the underlying disease will not respond to this treatment and there is no need for a repeat session. Prompt ambulation following such manipulation is the rule. Muscle reeducation by means of postural exercises may be helpful when used in conjunction with this treatment.

MEDICATION

The basic principle in prescribing analgesic medication is to give an adequate amount commensurate with the patient's pain. A common error is to dole out sparing doses of drugs, particularly narcotics. Oftentimes, one or two substantial doses of Demerol or morphine will be sufficient to alleviate a severe paraspinal muscle spasm which is exacerbating the pain, after which a less potent, nonaddictive drug will maintain the patient in reasonable comfort. Low back pain associated with muscle spasm may give rise to a pain cycle with the muscle spasm producing pain and pain increasing the severity of muscle spasm. Interruption of such a cycle may require potent analgesic medication.

To maintain the patient as pain free as possible, if the initial pain is severe, have no hesitation about giving the patient a strong analgesic drug such as Demerol or morphine and then gradually reducing this analgesic medication until none is necessary. The quicker one can interrupt the muscle spasm pain cycle, the more efficacious will be the improvement in the overall pain complex.

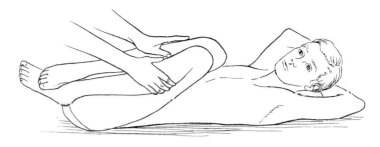

Fig. 4-18. Pelvic rock. The hips and knees are flexed until the thighs approximate a 90° angle with the trunk. The knees are grasped and rocked gently from side to side. After several such rocking movements, if pain is experienced in the low back, this is the full extent of the manipulation. If no pain is appreciated, progressive hip hyperflexion is superimposed on the side-to-side movements so that the knees are gradually rocked closer and closer to the axillae.

Morphine

Morphine, the principal alkaloid of opium, remains the standard to which other analgesics are compared. However, because of its undesirable qualities it has lost the preeminent status which it long enjoyed.

Action. Morphine relieves pain, causes euphoria, and in large doses may induce sleep. In therapeutic doses, it depresses the respiration and constricts the pupils. The action of morphine consists mainly in a descending depression of the central nervous system. Its apparent stimulant effects are attributable to depression of inhibitory mechanisms but its emetic action is caused by stimulation of the chemoreceptor trigger zones of the vomiting center. Morphine exerts its analgesic action not only by increasing the pain threshold (i.e., the magnitude of the stimulus necessary to evoke pain), but also by dulling the sensibility (i.e., the reaction to pain).

Side-effects. Side-effects associated with the use of morphine include nausea and emesis, itching, particularly of the nose and cheeks and constipation. Morphine also slows the heart, increases the tone of smooth muscle, inhibits the secretion of the gastrointestinal tract and, in susceptible individuals, may induce convulsions, excitement and delirium. The most serious drawback to the use of morphine is its tendency to induce tolerance, necessitating the increase of the dose to attain a therapeutic response, and to develop addiction, a liability shared by all morphinelike analgesics.

Therapeutic Use. Morphine is a reliable analgesic when given parenterally, although considerably less effective by mouth. No other established drug equals its analgesic

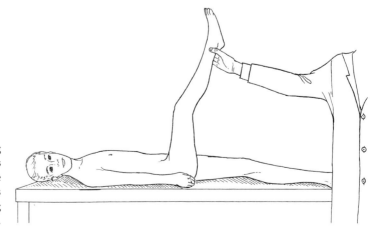

Fig. 4-19. Passive straight leg raising. The lower extremity is elevated slowly with the knee extended. This maneuver is performed short of producing pain or to an angulation of 90°.

capacity and at the same time is free of undesirable qualities. The analgesic dose-response curve for morphine reaches a plateau at about 10 mg. for a 70 Kg. person and this represents the optimal dose. A dose of 15 mg. provides somewhat longer relief of pain but counterbalancing the gains from the higher dose is a significant increase in side-effects. The interval between the subcutaneous injection and the onset of some degree of pain relief is 10 minutes and the duration of analgesia about 4 hours.

Synthetic Derivatives of Morphine

Hydromorphone (Dilaudid). Hydromorphone is 5 to 10 times as potent as morphine but its duration of action is less than that of morphine, and it is also more toxic. It is used in the same manner as morphine but in smaller doses (1 to 2 mg.) for acute pain of short duration. It is administered by injection, orally or as a rectal suppository.

Oxymorphone (Numorphan). A 1 mg. injection of oxymorphone is equal to 10 mg. of morphine as an analgesic. But at this dose oxymorphone is at least as likely as and perhaps more likely than morphine to produce untoward effects.

Levorphanol (Levo-Dromoran) Tartrate. Levorphanol tartrate resembles morphine in action but is somewhat longer acting and is less likely to cause constipation than morphine. It is administered in doses of 2 to 3 mg. (for adults) orally or subcutaneously for the relief of severe pain. As with most morphine substitutes, doses several times larger are required orally than by injection to attain the same analgesic effect.

Codeine

Codeine, one of the most widely used of all analgesics, is an effective analgesic when used in adequate dosage. It is less effective when administered orally than parenterally. When given in the ordinary dose of 32 mg. by mouth, it is no more effective than the usual dose of aspirin (650 mg.) in relieving pain. In fact, for short-term use, it would appear that aspirin is more reliable and effective. When either drug alone is ineffective, the combination of codeine plus aspirin may be effective. There is a summation of effect when 32 mg. of codeine are combined with 600 mg. of aspirin. Codeine by injection in doses of 60 mg. approaches, but is not equal to, 10 mg. of morphine and also possesses most of the disadvantages of morphine. Hence, when used parenterally, 10 mg. of morphine is superior.

Codeine rarely causes addiction. It depresses respiration and causes other undesirable morphinelike symptoms such as constipation, nausea and itching.

Synthetic Addicting Analgesics

A number of synthetic compounds have been prepared as substitutes for morphine and its derivatives in the hope that such compounds might be devoid of the undesirable actions of morphine, particularly its addiction property. As morphine, they are not only potent analgesics but also highly addicting.

Meperidine (Demerol). Meperidine in doses of 60 to 80 mg. parenterally can be substituted for 10 mg. of morphine as an analgesic, but in equianalgesic doses produces many of the side-effects seen with morphine, including respiratory depression.

Meperidine is often prescribed by physicians instead of morphine under the mistaken assumption that it is less addicting. As a matter of fact, experience has shown that this is not the case and addiction to meperidine is far less amenable to cure than addiction to morphine.

Methadone (Dolophine). When used in comparable analgesic doses, methadone is as toxic as morphine, exerting the same depressing effects on the circulation and respiration. Methadone is addicting, but because withdrawal symptoms following prolonged administration of the drug come on more slowly and are of less intensity, it has proved useful in the treatment of morphine and heroin addiction. For this purpose, methadone is substituted for the latter drugs and subsequently withdrawn. In equianalgesic doses, the occurrence of side-effects is similar to morphine.

Methadone is an effective analgesic for most forms of moderate to severe pain. It is administered orally in doses of 2.5 to 10 mg. every 3 to 4 hours. When oral administration is undesirable, the drug may be injected subcutaneously or intramuscularly, but it should not be given intravenously.

Alphaprodine Hydrochloride (Nisentil). Alphaprodine hydrochloride acts promptly and is a potent, short-acting narcotic useful in intense pain of brief duration. It can be used prior to low back manipulative therapy.

Alphaprodine is administered by subcutaneous injection in doses of 40 to 60 mg., depending upon the weight of the patient. Analgesia is induced within 5 minutes and lasts for about 2 hours. Overdosage may be counteracted by nalorphine. Alphaprodine may also be administered intravenously in doses of 20 to 30 mg. (when very rapid and brief analgesia is desired). Analgesia is produced within a few minutes and lasts from half an hour to an hour.

Anileridine (Leritine). Anileridine is intermediate in analgesic potency between meperidine and morphine. As meperidine, it exerts mild antihistaminic and spasmolytic actions but lacks the constipating action of the opiates. Its sedative and hypnotic actions resemble those of meperidine.

From 30 to 60 mg. of anileridine can be substituted for 100 mg. of meperidine and equivalent doses of morphine in most clinical situations. It has one advantage, namely, that it is more efficacious by the oral route in comparison to its parenteral potency than morphine and many of the morphine substitutes, but milligram by milligram is not as potent by mouth as by injection. In doses of 30 to 60 mg. it has significant pain-relieving capacity by either route of administration. In other respects the drug has no superiority over older drugs and side-effects may possibly be greater than those of equianalgesic doses of other agents.

Anileridine hydrochloride is administered orally in the form of 25 mg. tablets every 6 hours, but dosages up to 50 mg. may be used at more frequent intervals in cases of severe pain. Anileridine phosphate is administered by subcutaneous, intramuscular, or intravenous injection in doses of 25 to 50 mg. (1 to 2 ml.) at intervals of 4 to 6 hours.

Phenazocine (Prinadol). Phenazocine in doses of 3 mg. by injection can be substituted for 10 mg. of morphine in the control of pain, but by mouth much larger doses are less effective than this standard dose given by injection. The depression of respiration is possibly greater than with morphine when both are given in equianalgesic dosage. It can also cause addiction, since it is a completely adequate substitute for morphine in addicted persons.

Phenazocine is administered orally in doses of 1 to 3 mg. every 4 to 6 hours. Since its depressant effects are potentiated by such central nervous system depressants as the barbiturates, phenothiazines or anesthetics, smaller doses are indicated when these drugs are being used with phenazocine.

Non-narcotic Analgesics

Analgesics which are nonaddicting and relatively nontoxic have been available for many years, and being procurable without prescription, are used widely for low back pain not requiring the attention of a physician. These drugs exert an antirheumatic action, which renders them particularly valuable as analgesics in many low back dysfunctions.

Aspirin. Aspirin is one of the most widely used of all drugs, as evidenced by the fact that over 60 million pounds are consumed annually throughout the world. It is versatile in its actions, being an effective antipyretic, analgesic, and antirheumatic; it exerts a specific therapeutic effect in rheumatic fever; and, in large doses, it exerts antiallergic, cholesterol-lowering, uricosuric, hypoglycemic, litholytic, anticoagulant and other actions. The mechanism responsible for so wide a spectrum of activity is unknown.

The effectiveness of aspirin in painful states has been repeatedly demonstrated, and it is particularly suited for use as a universal analgesic. It is absorbed from the stomach but for the most part from the small intestine. Peak blood levels are reached within 2 hours, at which time it exerts its maximum analgesic action. It is one of the safest of all drugs but potentially dangerous allergic reactions may attend its use in patients sensitive to the drug. Hematemesis and melena may occur when it is taken in large doses for prolonged periods.

Aspirin, administered in doses of 300 to 600 mg. every 2 to 4 hours, preferably after meals, is effective for mild and moderate degrees of low back pain. Combined with phenacetin, caffeine or codeine, it exerts a synergistic action. Various combinations of these drugs are marketed, as in the APC (aspirin, phenacetin, caffeine) formulation, to which codeine and other analgesic, antihistaminic or tranquilizing drugs are also added.

Anti-inflammatory doses are higher than those needed for analgesia and usually have to be given in a range of 900 to 1200 mg. every 4 hours, depending upon the size of the individual. A good rule of thumb to obtain maximal beneficial anti-inflammatory effects without severe toxicity from side-effects is to give the patient a total daily dosage of $\frac{1}{2}$ to $\frac{3}{4}$ grain per pound of body weight in divided doses administered every 4 hours. One should attempt to obtain a serum salicylate level of 20 to 25 mg. per 100 ml. for full anti-inflammatory activity. In most instances exceeding this therapeutic level will cause unpleasant side-effects such as tinnitus, partial deafness, vertigo, nausea, vomiting, diarrhea, and occasionally both auditory and visual hallucinations. Aspirin may be utilized as the plain aspirin tablet, in an enteric-coated form, or as a timed-release preparation, the latter two causing less local gastric irritation.

Other Salicylic Acid Derivatives. A number of other derivatives of salicylic acid are also available for use as analgesics. Sodium salicylate resembles aspirin in action. Methyl salicylate (oil of wintergreen) is used externally as a rubefacient over surface areas of low back pain.

A timed-release preparation of aspirin (Measurin) is also available, which is claimed to have a prolonged analgesic effect and less adverse gastric effects than aspirin.

Therapeutic use. The use of salicylates is contraindicated in patients with severe renal disease and should be used with caution in patients with a history of allergic reations.

Phenacetin (Acetophenetidin). The use of phenacetin and mixtures containing the drug has come under scrutiny during recent years as possible causes of certain cases of pyelonephritis. The etiologic role of phenacetin in renal disease remains unproven.

Phenacetin is rarely used alone but is usually administered in combination with aspirin and caffeine to which codeine and other drugs are at times also added.

Propoxyphene Hydrochloride (Darvon). The effectiveness of propoxyphene hydrochloride does not approach that of codeine. It is usually used in combination with aspirin, phenacetin and caffeine (Darvon compound), but its superiority to the APC formulation has been questioned. It is administered orally in doses of 65 mg., 4 times daily alone (Darvon), but more often in combination with aspirin, phenacetin and caffeine (Darvon Compound).

The main side-effects of propoxyphene include dizziness, rash, drowsiness and constipation, but these are uncommon. Although not considered a narcotic by the Federal Bureau of Narcotics, the World Health Organization recommends that it be under the same control as codeine. Thus far only in one instance has addiction been reported.

Ethoheptazine Citrate (Zactane). Ethoheptazine citrate is available as a 2-layered tablet (Zactirin Compound-100), which contains 100 mg. of ethoheptazine citrate, 227 mg. of aspirin, 162 mg. of phenacetin, and 32.4 mg. of caffeine. One tablet of the latter drug is administered orally 3 or 4 times daily for low back pain and sciatica. Side-effects include nausea, with or without vomiting, epigastric distress and dizziness, but these symptoms are rarely observed.

Methotrimeprazine (Levoprome). Methotrimeprazine is a potent, nonaddicting analgesic, comparing favorably with morphine and meperidine. In doses of 20 mg. it is equal in analgesic action to 10 mg. of morphine or 75 mg. of meperidine and equals these drugs in speed and duration of action. Tolerance to the analgesic effects of the drug has not been reported.

Addiction has not been noted and the drug is therefore not subject to the restrictions of the Harrison Narcotic Act. In normal subjects it does not depress the respiration as the narcotics do. Excessive sedation, orthostatic hypotension, dizziness and fainting constitute the major side-effects of the drug and restrict its use to nonambulatory patients. Other adverse effects noted with phenothiazine derivatives should be considered when the drug is used for a month or longer.

Methotrimeprazine is available only for intramuscular injection in a solution containing 20 mg. per ml. The initial dose in adults is 10 to 15 mg. and may be increased for greater relief of pain, if tolerated. The drug is indicated especially for severe pain in addiction-prone patients where sedation is desirable and depression of respiration is to be avoided. The drug should not be used concurrently with antihypertensive drugs or depressants of the central nervous system in patients with clinically significant hypotension, or in patients under 14 years of age.

In addition to hypotension, other adverse reactions occasionally encountered include amnesia, disorientation, dizziness, drowsiness, excessive sedation, weakness, slurring of speech, abdominal discomfort, nausea and vomiting, dry mouth, nasal congestion, difficulty in urination, chills, uterine inertia and pain at the site of injection. As with other phenothiazines, the possibility of blood dyscrasias, hepatotoxicity and extrapyramidal effects should be considered possible reactions. Administration for more than 30 days is not advised.

Pentazocine (Talwin). This drug manifests potent analgesia without addicting properties. Pentazocine is not subject to narcotic controls. Unlike morphine, tolerance to the drug does not develop. Side-effects to pentazocine consist of nausea, which occurs in

about 5 percent of patients, and to a lesser degree, vertigo, dizziness, vomiting and euphoria. Respiratory depression is noted in about 1 percent of patients. It is relatively free from the severe respiratory depression, urinary retention, and constipation associated with the use of morphine.

Pentazocine is used in place of morphine and other narcotic analgesics. The recommended dose is 30 mg. by intramuscular, subcutaneous, or intravenous routes, repeated, if necessary, every 3 to 4 hours. The drug should be used with caution in patients with myocardial infarction who have nausea or vomiting, in patients with impaired renal or hepatic function and in patients with respiratory depression.

Mefenamic Acid (Ponstel). Mefenamic acid is a non-narcotic analgesic for oral administration. It is indicated for short-term administration for the relief of back pain. Its use is contraindicated in patients with intestinal ulceration, in women of childbearing potential and in children under 14 years of age. Patients with diarrhea must have the drug promptly discontinued and are usually unable to tolerate the drug thereafter. The drug should also be administered with caution in patients with abnormal renal function or inflammatory disease of the gastrointestinal tract and should be withdrawn promptly if rash or diarrhea occur. It should also be used with caution in asthmatics.

Mefenamic acid is administered orally in capsules of 250 mg. in doses of 500 mg. initially, followed by 250 mg. every 6 hours as needed. It should not be used for periods exceeding one week. Adverse reactions most frequently observed are drowsiness, nausea, dizziness, nervousness, gastrointestinal discomfort and headache.

Anti-inflammatory Drugs

Phenylbutazone. Both phenylbutazone (Butazolidin) and its derivative, oxyphenbutazone (Tandearil), are effective anti-inflammatory agents. Both drugs, however, must be administered with care, since potential toxicity (gastrointestinal tract bleeding, agranulocytosis, decrease in red cell count and aplastic anemia, in addition to nausea, vomiting and skin rash) is great. An advantage is that they are usually more easily tolerated than an equivalent pharmacologic dose of silicylates.

Indomethacin. Indomethacin (Indocin) also has antipyretic and analgesic effects. The drug is given in a dosage range of 75 to 200 mg. per day in 3 to 4 divided doses. Its primary side-effects are gastrointestinal: the drug is capable of causing peptic ulcers and associated gastrointestinal bleeding. In addition, it may cause severe headaches that are unresponsive to aspirin as well as nausea, vomiting, rashes, vertigo and rarely, hematologic and hepatic reactions.

In terms of anti-inflammatory activity, indomethacin lies between salicylates and phenylbutazone when all are used in appropriate pharmacologic doses. Patients using the drug for long-term therapy may develop a tolerance to it and so its initial effectiveness may be lost. As with phenylbutazone, the drug may be used in combination with salicylates to obtain a greater anti-inflammatory effect with decreased toxicity.

Corticosteroids. The corticosteroids are the most potent of the anti-inflammatory drugs and potentially the most dangerous. The synthetic compounds are the most common in use today, having replaced cortisone and cortisol almost completely. The drugs appear to be equally effective in their anti-inflammatory capabilities, although the newer dexamethasone, betamethasone, and paramethasone groups have been found to have less mineralocorticoid activity. Both prednisone and prednisolone, however, have the advantage of producing less muscle wasting and nitrogen loss than the newer derivatives.

The biologically active corticosteroids will suppress inflammation regardless of the cause. The anti-inflammatory effect consists of reversal of the increased permeability associated with inflammation, marked suppression of diapedesis of inflammatory cells, inhibition of fibroblast destruction and preservation of endothelial cells. In this fashion, the signs of the active inflammatory process are obliterated but the causative agent is not affected. Such action may benefit the secondary changes of inflammation and edema of the nerve root but would not affect the primary compression from a protruding disc, which is the underlying cause of these secondary changes.

The undesirable side-effects of corticosteroid therapy may be either of secondary or of more serious importance. Among the secondary type are "facial mooning," obesity, hirsutism, striae and steroid diabetes. The more serious side-effects include osteoporosis, peptic ulcer and increased susceptibility to infection.

In general, oral corticosteroids should be given only when other more conservative measures have failed, and should be given only after a careful search for infections and other contraindications has proved to be negative. They should always be used in the smallest dose possible, and it should always be remembered that corticosteroids do not cure any disease—they only suppress inflammation.

Intrathecal Use of Corticosteroids. For a number of years several clinics have injected corticosteroids intrathecally on a semiroutine basis in an attempt to promote remissions in patients with multiple sclerosis. Between 1956 and 1959, I participated in such a program at the Taylor Hospital in Ridley Park, under the direction of Dr. Arthur Baker. It was apparent that the incidence of postspinal headaches in these patients was reduced, despite the fact that many of these patients remained in the hospital less than 8 hours and were discharged the day of injection. In the hope that it might similarly decrease the number of postspinal headaches, 20 to 40 mg. of methylprednisolone acetate (Depo-Medrol) were injected after myelography. This was introduced, following Pantopaque withdrawal, through the lumbar puncture needle that had been left in place during the procedure. In addition to reducing the frequency of postspinal headaches it also relieved some of the pain that was present prior to myelography. This effect was greatest on the radicular symptoms.

Postmyelography, I routinely inject 40 mg. of Depo-Medrol intrathecally when the myelogram is normal and when surgery is not immediately contemplated.

If the symptoms are primarily related to inflammatory changes involving the nerve root, pain may be alleviated on a long-term basis. If severe nerve root compression is producing symptoms, some temporary relief may be obtained of less than 1 or 2 weeks' duration.

Intrathecal injection of corticosteroids is not recommended for routine use in treatment of low back dysfunction. The disadvantages of lumbar puncture and injection of a foreign substance intrathecally outweigh the possible benefits. However, in patients who have undergone previous surgery with radicular symptoms attributable to postoperative scarring, its use may be considered.

Muscle Relaxants

As a general group, the muscle relaxants are not very potent, but they do play a definite role in the treatment of low back dysfunction. The objective is to use a drug which abolishes spasticity without interfering with normal tone and movement.

Chlormezanone (Trancopal). This drug is probably one of the more widely used for relief of skeletal muscle spasm. The usual dosage is 200 to 600 mg. per day in divided doses. Side-effects—drug rash, nausea, drowsiness—are mild.

Carisoprodol (Rela; Soma carisoprodol). Carisoprodol also has some analgesic properties and appears to modify the central perception of pain. The usual adult dosage is 350 mg. 3 to 4 times per day. The major side-effect is drowsiness, but the drug has also produced dizziness, rash and nausea. **Methocarbamol (Robaxin), orphenadrine (Norflex), and chlorzoxazone (Paraflex)** are other useful muscle relaxants.

Mephenesin. Mephenesin is the oldest and perhaps best known of the skeletal muscle relaxants. As with the previously described drugs, the action is mediated by way of the central nervous system, although the basic mechanism of action is not known. Its pharmacologic action is selective depression of subcortical, brainstem, and spinal polysynaptic transmission. The drug has been largely replaced in modern medicine by the newer synthetic drugs already described.

Miscellaneous Drugs

Although not classified as analgesics, a number of other drugs are often used to relieve pain and hence will be discussed briefly with reference to their analgesic action.

However, in view of the availability of safer and more potent analgesic agents, the usefulness of these drugs as analgesics would appear to be of minor significance.

Alcohol. Alcohol has been used occasionally by intravenous injection as a sedative and analgesic, but other agents are usually to be preferred. Its vasodilatory effects may prove deleterious in the presence of impending shock or cardiac insufficiency.

Procaine Hydrochloride (Novocain). Novocain has been administered in intravenous drip for the relief of severe low back pain associated with muscle spasm, but its potential toxicity renders its use as an analgesic undesirable.

Trichlorethylene (Trilene). Trilene, administered by inhalation, has been used as an analgesic just prior to manipulative therapy of the low back. Its effectiveness is to be attributed to its anesthetic action rather than to any specific analgesic action.

OCCUPATIONAL CHANGES

In the management of low back dysfunction it is most important to carefully delve into the patient's work history. Oftentimes a patient can relate low back symptoms to specific activities performed either at work or in activities of daily living. Occasionally, a modification of such activities may serve to alleviate or improve symptoms to the point where more intensive management is not necessary.

One must keep in mind that it is often the patient's activities that precipitated low back dysfunction to the point where treatment was necessary. Such activities should be modified for the future. If a patient has had long-standing low back dysfunction and is performing heavy activities which involve great stress on the low back, treatment of the presenting symptoms without attempting to modify the stress-producing activities is unrealistic. When the patient is free of pain following treatment, it is a bit shortsighted to allow him to return to the same conditions that originally produced the pain.

PSYCHOTHERAPY AND HYPNOTHERAPY

The daily psychic stresses from family problems and work may generate emotional tension and aggravate low back pain involving muscle spasm. Sometimes emotional guidance may be helpful, but with few exceptions psychotherapy is neither necessary nor helpful. Occasionally in very refractory cases hypnosis has been effective. Hypnotherapy is most effective in those individuals complaining of an anatomically limited specific area of persisting pain. A generalized intermittent low back ache is not as receptive to this form of management.

ACTIVITIES OF DAILY LIVING AND FAULTY POSTURE

The fundamental principle of treating faulty posture and physical activities productive of low back pain is directed toward the goal of reducing the lumbar lordosis. Since increased lordosis primarily depends upon the lumbosacral angle that relates to the pelvic position, our endeavors are directed toward education of the patient in attainment of decreased pelvic angle. This involves alteration of habitual postural patterns which are well-established and not easily altered.

Such a retraining program involves a combination of corrective exercises in association with altered postural attitudes, but it has many pitfalls and is not easily achieved. The corrective exercises are time-consuming and require diligence on the part of the patient, who may not possess the psychological resources for this task. If the patient is capable and willing to devote an adequate period of time to these exercises, the manner in which they are performed may require interval rechecking by the physician. Patients occasionally modify or embellish the exercise program, in some cases producing an adverse effect. When the patient is faithful in the performance of the corrective exercises, but in the remainder of the day continues to maintain a position of increased lumbar lordosis during activities of daily living, no decrease in low back dysfunction will be realized. (For description of low back exercises, see pages 117–124.)

All activities involving daily living must be carefully reviewed in an effort to avoid ex-

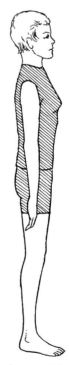

Fig. 4-20. A satisfactory "flattened low back" erect posture.

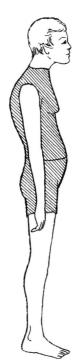

Fig. 4-21. A posture of increased lumbar lordosis.

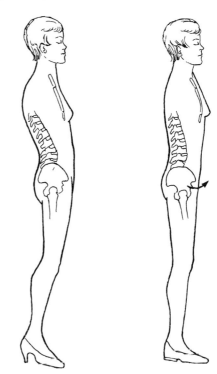

Fig. 4-22. Wearing high heels results in a compensatory increase in lumbar lordosis.

cessive stress on the low back with an appreciation of the body mechanics involved.

Standing and Walking

Standing and walking should be done in an erect position with the chest uplifted so that it, rather than the abdomen, becomes the most anterior portion of the trunk. In an effort to decrease lumbar hyperlordosis, women should be dissuaded from wearing high heels, particularly for prolonged periods of standing or walking, since this results in a compensatory increase in the lumbar lordosis.

The patient can practice proper erect posture by standing against a wall and pressing the belt line against the wall but not the head and shoulders so that the lumbar spine is as close to the vertical plane as is comfortably possible.

When initially performing this exercise, the patient is instructed to place the feet a foot from the wall, facilitating flattening of the lumbar spine against the wall. With time, lumbar flattening can be accomplished with

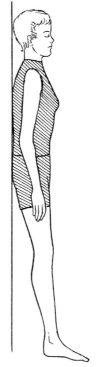

Fig. 4-23. Proper erect posture can be practiced by "flattening" the low back against a wall.

less effort and the feet can be positioned closer to the wall.

The patient should occasionally check his posture in front of a full-length mirror, viewing the body position from the side as a reminder to avoid the protruding abdomen and substitute the uplifted chest.

Individuals with occupations involving prolonged standing may achieve comfortable flattening of the lumbar lordosis by placing one foot on a low stool 6 to 8 inches high. Such a posture, which flexes one hip, reducing iliopsoas and hip flexor pull upon the lumbar spine, results in a relaxed reduction of lumbar lordosis. The flexed hip should be alternated from time to time. Tavern keepers, whose livelihood is directly related to the length of time their clientele remain standing at a bar, have intuitively appreciated this postural truth for the past century. The well-known "brass rail" permits their patrons to comfortably stand at the bar for many hours.

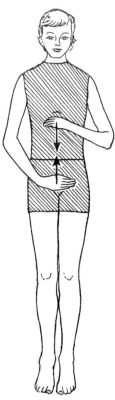

Fig. 4-25. Instruct the patient to place one hand on the symphysis pubis, the other on the xiphoid, and attempt to bring both hands closer together to flatten the lumbar lordosis.

It is sometimes difficult to convey to patients the concept of maintaining a flattened lumbar spine in the erect position. They may "flatten" their lumbar spine against a wall and immediately upon withdrawing from this firm surface will resume the lumbar lordotic position. Such terms as "tuck in the pelvis" may be meaningless to patients, and they are unable to grasp what is desired. Occasionally, it is helpful to have the patient place one hand on the symphysis pubis and the other on the xyphoid and attempt to bring both hands closer together, which will result in an "upward tilt" of the pelvis.

Another teaching aid is to have the patient imagine that he must hold a coin between the buttocks by "squeezing them together." Such a maneuver will also result in an "upward" pelvic tilt and a reduction of the lumbar lordosis.

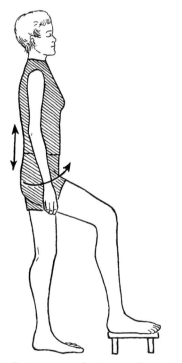

Fig. 4-24. Resting one foot on a low stool will flex the hip, reducing iliopsoas the hip flexor pull upon the lumbar spine, resulting in reduction of lumbar lordosis.

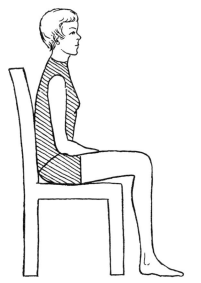

Fig. 4-26. Good "flat backed" sitting position in chair of satisfactory height with a firm seat and back.

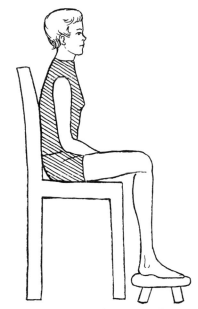

Fig. 4-28. Correction of excessively high chair with a short stool beneath the feet.

Sitting

Sitting is done by first flexing the lumbar spine and then performing a flexion in both the hips and knees. When sitting, the lumbar spine should be slightly flexed; if the chair is too high to sit in this fashion, a short stool may be necessary beneath the feet. Because of the shorter height of most women, chairs are often a bit too high to sit in this position and a compensatory correction may be achieved by crossing the knees.

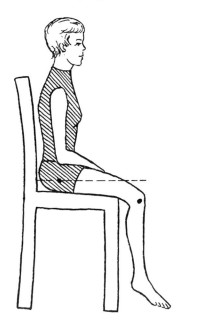

Fig. 4-27. An excessively high chair allows the feet to dangle, causing the knees to be lower than the hip joints. This will result in increased lumbar lordosis.

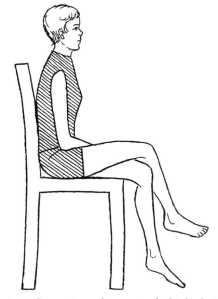

Fig. 4-29. Correction of excessively high chair by crossing the knees to flatten lumbar lordosis.

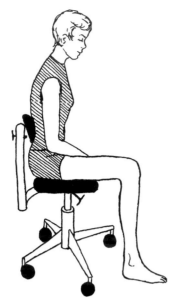

Fig. 4-30. Poorly constructed typist's chair with a narrow back rest producing increased lumbar lordosis.

Driving

When driving, the seat should be advanced forward so that the knees are at a slightly higher level than the hips, which tends to reduce lumbar lordosis. The car seat should not be pushed so far back that the knees are lowered with extension of the lower extremities, resulting in a compensatory increased lumbar lordosis.

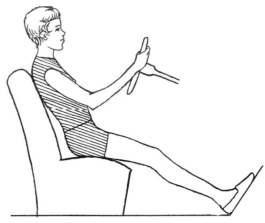

Fig. 4-32. Incorrect driving posture.

Lifting

Lifting any significant load is done with a slight flexion of the hips and knees and a flexion of the lumbosacral spine. The load should not be lifted with the knees and lumbosacral spine in extension.

Sleeping

The patient with low back dysfunction should sleep on the side with hips and knees in flexion. If sleeping on the back is habitual, a sizable blanket roll beneath the mattress at the level of the knees is advisable since a pillow placed in that position will become displaced from normal movements occurring during sleep. Sleeping on the abdomen tends

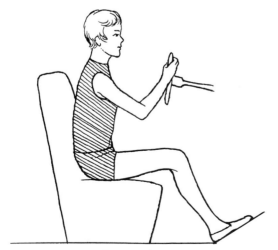

Fig. 4-31. Correct driving posture.

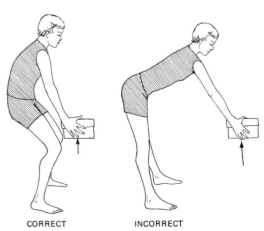

Fig. 4-33. Correct and incorrect lifting postures.

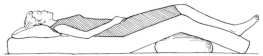

Fig. 4-34. If sleeping in a supine position is habitual, a blanket roll beneath the mattress at the level of the knees will decrease the lumbar lordosis.

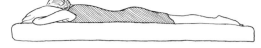

Fig. 4-35. Sleeping on the abdomen increases lumbar lordosis and is best avoided by patients with low back dysfunction.

to increase the lumbosacral angle and often causes increased discomfort. It is best avoided.

With long-standing low back dysfunction, it may be necessary for a patient to obtain a hospital bed with the various adjustments available for proper sleeping position.

Establishing Proper Habits

Every task the patient does from household chores, such as using a broom or carpet sweeper, or getting in and out of a car, must be analyzed in terms of body mechanics. The patient must practice these defensive and protective movements until they become second nature.

A frequent deficiency in the management of a conservative treatment program is that the physician will prescribe a low back support shortly after pain has subsided. The patient will wear this support for an indefinite period of time without any specific instruction or corrective exercises.

The greatest barrier to a satisfactory end result is the formidable task of convincing a patient who is no longer suffering from severe pain to carry out an ongoing exercise and a daily living program which will permit resumption of activities with reasonable expectation that the future will not be marred by recurrent attacks of low back dysfunction.

In many cases the patient has a protuberant abdomen with inadequate abdominal and lumbar musculature. The program will be directed toward reducing obesity with a combination of diet and exercise, in addition to improving lumbar mobility by progressive stretching and elongation of the hamstring muscles and hip flexors so that a well-distributed but not excessively lordotic curvature of the lumbar spine may be eventually achieved. Most physicians must take time to stress the advantages of this program to the patient, recounting the potential evils of what may occur in the future if such a regimen is not followed.

LOW BACK EXERCISES

PURPOSE

Many physicians, including those who devote considerable time and interest to patients with low back dysfunction, may not clearly appreciate the intended purpose of a low back corrective exercise program. The word exercise, in this regard, may be misleading, giving rise to imagery of gymnastics or strenuous athletics. Although there is certainly no objection to the improvement of general body muscle tone and rehabilitation of an overweight person to a more suitable habitus, this is not our specific object. The

fact is that many patients suffering from low back dysfunction are quite trim and may be splendid tennis players or golfers with no need to be "built up" physically. It must be constantly borne in mind that the express intention of the exercises is to help achieve an improvement of the faulty posture which is productive of low back dysfunction.

The vast majority of patients manifesting a faulty posture usually exhibit an increased lumbar lordosis so that much of our exercise program is designed to obtaining a flattened or reduced lumbar lordosis.

EXERCISES ADAPTED TO THE PATIENT'S SPECIFIC NEEDS

Often a standard set of "back exercises" may be handed to the patient with little instruction, and he is left to devise his own regimen. Sometimes, the entire exercise program is turned over to a therapist who may have been trained to give the same set of exercises to all "low back problems." As in any low back therapy, whether it be rest, the wearing of a low back support or medication, exercises must be in keeping with the patient's individual needs.

In planning a low back exercise program an understanding of the role played by the principle muscle groupings upon the lumbar spine is mandatory. To meet the individual needs of the patient, 4 factors must be considered:

1. The specific postural impairment manifested by the patient

2. Preexercise evaluation of the strength and flexibility of the principal muscle groupings

3. The special action each of the various exercises exerts upon the principal muscle groupings

4. The degree of muscle strength and flexibility demanded by each exercise in accordance with the limitations imposed by the patient's present clinical status.

WHEN TO START LOW BACK EXERCISES

The program is instituted as soon as pain relief has been achieved with bed rest, and this may be initiated with several sessions of massage and diathermy, both to the abdominal and low back musculature, in preparation for exercises which can be initially carried out on a flattened bed. When compatible with the patient's condition, a firmer surface, such as a mat- or rug-covered floor, is preferable because it provides easier maneuverability and permits greater awareness of points of body contact.

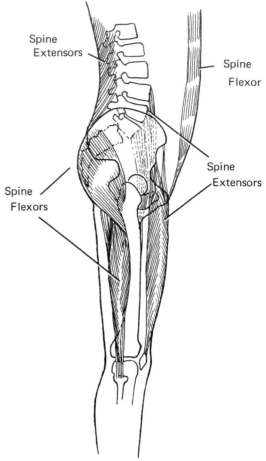

Fig. 4-36. Diagrammatic illustration of the principle muscle groupings involved in flexion (lordosis) and extension (flattening) of the lumbar spine. The spine extensors (erector spinae, etc.) and the iliopsoas muscles extend the spine by direct action. The gluteal and hamstring muscles flex the spine and the quadriceps extends the spine by tilting the pelvis. The abdominal muscles flex the spine by approximating the distance between the thoracic cage and the pelvis, thereby tilting the pelvis also.

PREEXERCISE EVALUATION

The first step in prescribing low back exercises is evaluating the strength and flexibility of the muscles related to the low back using the following tests.

1. Abdominal Strength. Lying supine, hands clasped behind his neck, the patient

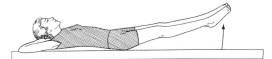

Fig. 4-37. Testing "lower abdominal" muscle strength.

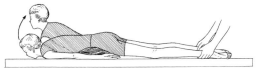

Fig. 4-39. Testing "upper back" muscle strength.

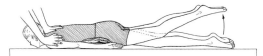

Fig. 4-40. Testing "lower back" muscle strength.

is instructed to keep his knees straight and lift his feet 12 inches off the table. The ability to maintain this position for 10 seconds is indicative of normal *lower abdominal* muscle strength. Mark from 0 to 10. Zero is indicative of inability to lift the feet off the table, and 10 is normal.

Lying supine, hands clasped behind his neck, with his feet held down against the table by the examiner, the patient is instructed to perform a "sit-up" by raising the trunk from the supine position to a 90° sitting position without assistance. The ability to perform this is indicative of normal *upper abdominal* muscle strength. Mark from 0 to 10.

2. Lumbar Strength. Lying prone, with a pillow beneath his abdomen, his legs held down on the table by the examiner, the patient is instructed to raise his chest from the table. The ability to maintain this position for 10 seconds is indicative of normal *upper back* muscle strength. Mark from 0 to 10.

Lying prone, with a pillow beneath his abdomen, his chest held down against the table by the examiner, the patient is instructed to lift his legs off the table. The ability to maintain this position for 10 seconds indicates normal *lower back* musculature. Mark from 0 to 10.

The nonanatomical terms *upper* and *lower*

abdominal and *back musculature* employed in the preceding section are admittedly generic and indeterminate but are used for want of a more designate description. However, they serve as an approximate scale for prescribing corrective low back exercises.

3. Lumbar and Hamstring Elasticity. The patient is asked to stand erect in stocking or bare feet, put his feet together, keep his knees straight and bend forward and attempt to touch the floor with his fingertips. The ability to touch the fingertips to the floor indicates normal lumbar and hamstring muscle elasticity. Deficiency in elasticity is determined by an approximate percentage. For example, when the distance from the floor to the fingertips is 24 inches, then if the patient is 12 inches short of touching the floor, he would have a 50 percent deficiency. Mark from 0 to 10; a 50 percent deficiency is a 5.

Long-standing muscle tension will result in a lack of mechanical elasticity or a relative muscle contracture, making the muscle less

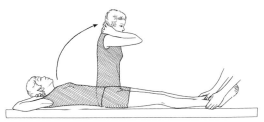

Fig. 4-38. Testing "upper abdominal" muscle strength.

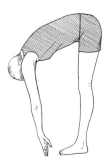

Fig. 4-41. Testing lumbar and hamstring elasticity.

flexible. Some believe that such tension and spasticity affecting the low back musculature causes this region to be more vulnerable to mechanical trauma, leading to the so-called recurrent lumbosacral strain syndrome.

ESTABLISHING AN
EXERCISE PROGRAM

Neither the muscle strength tests nor the exercises should be performed during a period of acute pain. When pain has subsided, however, the patient must establish a habitual regularity in performing the low back exercises twice daily. It should be emphasized that even in days that involve considerable emotional stress or increased work activity, time should be set aside for these exercises. It is probably in such times of increased stress that the exercises are most helpful. An erratic exercise program is ineffectual.

RELAXATION EXERCISES

Low back exercise programs should include relaxation and limbering exercises.

The following exercises are described in the form of instructions to the patient:

1. While lying on the floor, raise your arms slowly over your head as you inhale deeply; then exhale as you allow your arms to return slowly to the floor. Repeat 10 times and with each exhalation allow your arms and legs, head and shoulders to rest limply on the floor, making your entire body as flaccid as possible.

2. Breathe deeply again and with each slow inhalation, bring your legs and feet tightly together, arms tightly at your sides, make tight fists, tighten the muscles of your body, tighten your buttocks; with each exhalation relax as completely as possible allowing your arms and legs to "drift away" from your body. Close your eyes and allow your jaw to sag. Repeat 10 times.

Alternating muscle contractions with relaxation is a helpful device to emphasize and accentuate relaxation by directing the patient's attention to the difference between muscle tension and muscle relaxation. If done properly, each succeeding period of relaxation is a bit more profound and produces total physical and mental relaxation prior to starting the low back exercises.

PELVIC "UPTILT"

The most essential of all the corrective low back exercises is some variation of the pelvic "tuck or uptilt." It is this maneuver that will train and habituate the muscles to maintain reduction or flattening of the lumbar lordosis. If the patient is confined to bed for the treatment of an acute attack of low back pain, the exercise may be initially performed in bed after the low back pain and muscle spasm has eased. As soon as the clinical status permits, the maneuver should be carried out on a firmer surface. After the "pelvic tuck" has been mastered in a supine position, it is practiced in the erect position keeping in mind that the eventual object of the exercise is to flatten the lumbar lordosis.

The exercise is performed in a supine position with a pillow beneath the patient's head. When first practiced the hip and knees are well flexed, both feet flat on the floor, with the heels fairly close to the buttocks. The patient then presses his lumbar spine firmly against the floor by contracting the gluteal and abdominal muscles. After the lumbar spine is pressed against the floor, the pelvis is "tucked" or "uptilted" by raising the buttocks off the floor but maintaining the pressure of the lumbar spine against the floor.

The most common patient error in this exercise is to elevate the lumbar spine from the floor along with the buttocks, thus effecting an adverse position of lumbar extension (lordosis) rather than the desired flexion (flattening). This maneuver should be performed 10 times twice daily and in time the number of "tucks" should be gradually increased until a fatigue plateau is reached. Patients over 50 years of age should have no difficulty doing 20 tucks 2 times daily. Younger patients may be able to do 40 tucks twice daily.

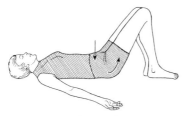

Fig. 4-42. "Pelvic uptilt." 1. Supine position with hips and knees flexed. 2. Press lumbar spine firmly to the floor. 3. Maintaining pressure of the lumbar spine upon the floor, elevate the buttocks, "uptilting" the pelvis.

Gradually, over a variable period of time, the hip and knee flexion is reduced until complete extension of both legs is achieved. Extension of the lower extremities increases the lumbar extension action of the iliopsoas. As a result of the necessity to overcome this muscle antagonist, not only is greater exertion required to perform the exercise but also a lesser degree of lumbar flexion is achieved than is possible in the flexed leg position. Only after the exercise has been performed with extended lower extremities for at least 2 weeks should it be practiced in the upright position.

Decreased elasticity of the iliopsoas group of hip flexors maintains the lumbar lordosis and works against flattening of the lumbar spine. The following exercises designed to promote hip flexor elasticity are companion exercises to the pelvic "uptilt."

EXERCISES FOR HIP FLEXOR ELASTICITY

Two exercises designed for stretching the hip flexors are given to patients.

1. In the supine position, extend one leg and flex the hip and knee of the opposite leg in the knee-chest position 10 times. With each flexion, press the lumbar spine firmly against the floor. Repeat, alternating legs. The stretched hip flexors are those on the side of the extended leg.

2. Kneel on one knee, place the opposite leg forward in a position of hip and knee flexion and position both hands on the floor

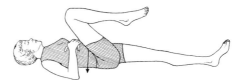

Fig. 4-43. Iliopsoas muscle stretching in supine position.

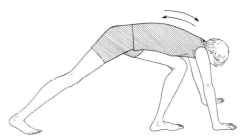

Fig. 4-44. Iliopsoas muscle stretching in crouching position.

in front of the flexed leg. Using the hands for balance, completely extend the posterior leg and rock back and forth 10 times. Repeat, alternating legs. The stretched hip flexors are those on the side of the extended leg.

The extent to which the "pelvic uptilt" and the iliopsoas stretching exercises are performed should be modified in accordance with the patient's clinical status.

LOW BACK EXERCISES

The following exercises are graded into 3 phases on the basis of mechanical stress.

Phase 1

These exercises are prescribed to patients who have recently recovered from a bout of low back pain.

Exercise 1. Lie flat on your back, flex your knees and slowly allow them to fall to the floor in an extended position, limp and re-

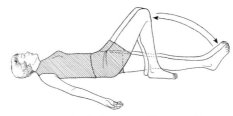

Fig. 4-45. Low Back Exercise. Phase 1, Exercise 1.

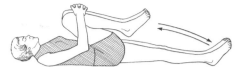

Fig. 4-46. Phase 1, Exercise 2.

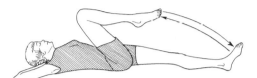

Fig. 4-47. Phase 1, Exercise 3.

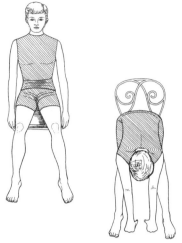

Fig. 4-49. Phase 1, Exercise 5.

laxed. Repeat 5 times. Purpose: To promote lumbar and hamstring elasticity.

Exercise 2. Lie on your back, flex your knees. Then bring both knees up to your chest, and with your hands clasped pull your knees toward your chest. Hold this position for a count of 10 and then return your legs to the starting position of lower extremity extension. Repeat this exercise 3 times. Purpose: To promote lumbar and hamstring elasticity.

Exercise 3. Lying on your back with legs flat on the floor, hands clasped behind your neck, raise one knee up as far as you can toward your chest. Maintain this position to the count of 10. Return the flexed leg to the neutral position and repeat the movement with the opposite leg until each leg has been flexed 5 times. Purpose: To promote lumbar, hamstring and iliopsoas elasticity; increase "lower" abdominal muscle strength.

Exercise 4. Lie on your back with your arms above your head and your knees bent. Flatten your back against the mat; at the same time contract the abdominal muscles. Maintain this position for a count of 10 and

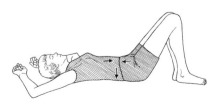

Fig. 4-48. Phase 1, Exercise 4.

repeat 5 times. Purpose: To increase *upper* and *lower* abdominal muscle strength.

Exercise 5. Sit in a chair with your hands at your sides, drop your head down between your knees and allow your hands to rest on the floor. Maintain this position for a count of 3. Bring your body back up into a sitting position. Relax. Repeat the exercise 5 times. Purpose: To promote lumbar and hamstring elasticity; increase *lower back* muscle strength.

Phase 1 exercises should be done twice daily for a period of 4 weeks. If, at the end of that period of time, no difficulty is encountered in carrying out the exercises, the patient may go on to the next set of exercises in Phase 2. However, the Phase 1 exercises should be done as preliminary exercises so that a longer period of exercises will be necessary thereafter.

Phase 2

Exercise 1. Lying on the back, bring both knees up to a bent position with feet resting on the floor. Rotate the pelvis and legs to the right and then to the left side of the body. Repeat 5 times. Purpose: To promote lumbar and hamstring elasticity.

Exercise 2. Lying on the back, raise feet 12 inches from the floor. Maintain this for a count of 10. Then slowly lower feet to the

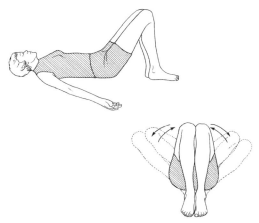

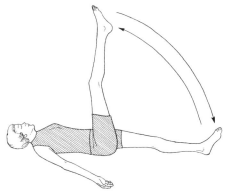

Fig. 4-53. Phase 2, Exercise 4.

Fig. 4-50. Phase 2, Exercise 1.

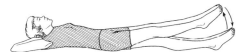

Fig. 4-51. Phase 2, Exercise 2.

floor. Repeat 5 times. Purpose: To increase "lower" abdominal muscle strength.

Exercise 3. Stand erect while holding onto a table or chair. Squat down, straighten up again. Repeat 5 times. The table or chair should be used merely to maintain balance not to help pull the body up into the erect position. Purpose: To increase quadriceps and hamstring muscle strength.

Exercise 4. Lying on the back with legs outstretched, straight leg raise one leg as far as possible without producing discomfort. Lower it slowly to the floor and straight leg raise the opposite leg. Repeat 5 times with each leg. Purpose: To promote lumbar, hamstring, and iliopsoas elasticity.

Exercise 5. Lying on the back with both legs extended, bring right foot up to left knee, resting the heel and sole of the foot on the knee, and slowly rotate the flexed knee laterally as far as comfortable and then rotate the knee medially as far as is comfortable. Repeat the exercise with the opposite leg, alternating sides until the exercise has been done 5 times with each leg. Purpose: To promote hip rotator elasticity.

Exercise 6. Stand erect, relax your body by inhaling and exhaling deeply. Slowly flex the head and neck and allow the trunk to slowly bend forward from the hips with the knees

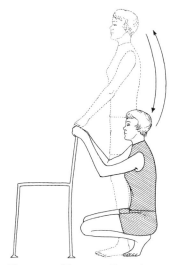

Fig. 4-52. Phase 2, Exercise 3.

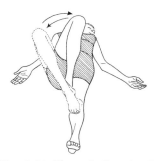

Fig. 4-54. Phase 2, Exercise 5.

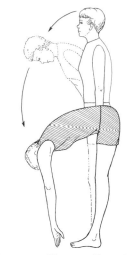

Fig. 4-55. Phase 2, Exercise 6.

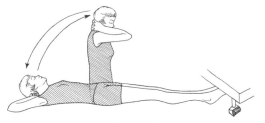

Fig. 4-56. Phase 3, Exercise 1.

time, if these exercises can be done comfortably, the patient may go on to Phase 3.

Phase 3

The Phase 3 exercise is fairly strenuous and is done to maintain the low back and abdominal musculature.

Exercise 1. Lie on the back with hands clasped behind the head, tucking the feet under a heavy object. Perform a "sit-up" until the trunk is at 90° to the outstretched legs and then slowly lower the trunk to a lying position. Repeat 10 times.

straight. Try to touch the floor with your fingertips. Repeat 5 times. Purpose: To promote lumbar and hamstring elasticity.

The exercises in Phase 2 should be done twice daily for 4 months. At the end of that

LOW BACK SUPPORTS AND BRACES

HISTORY

The use of low back supports in the form of braces or corsets must certainly extend beyond the limits of recorded history. It is almost instinctive for those who carry out heavy activities to wear heavy leather belts or to use other supporting measures. The Colorado State Historical Museum in Denver contains a tree bark corset dating to about A.D. 900, originating from the pre-Columbian Indian cliff dwellings.

The earliest spinal braces were cumbersome, but in the twelfth century, surgeons of the Bolognese School of Italy had constructed fairly effective spinal supports of simple design made of wood and metal.

During the past 150 years a voluminous literature has detailed a great number of braces and corsets made of a variety of materials.[1]

In the nineteenth century, braces were

designed in this country for the two most widely prevalent diseases of the spine, Pott's disease and scoliosis. The best-known spinal brace of American origin was designed by Charles Fayette Taylor in 1863, and was popularly referred to in that time as the "spinal assistant." The basic design and function of this brace is still utilized in various modifications in a number of braces today. He utilized the now familiar "3-point principle" of support to produce hyperextension of the spine by exerting force backward at the hip and shoulders and forward in the middle of the back. Another commonly used brace of American origin is that designed by James Knight in 1884. This brace was originally designed as a supporting brace for tuberculosis; a later modification of this brace was used by Knight for treatment of scoliosis. The Taylor brace was one which produced hyperextension of the spine while the Knight brace provided lateral support, preventing lateral and rotary movements and, therefore, is widely used for support of the lower lumbar spine. There are many modern modifications of this brace, and it is designated by various names. It is often referred to as the "chair back brace."

GENERAL PRINCIPLES IN THE USE OF LOW BACK SUPPORTS

Low Back Mechanics

The spine stripped of its musculature may be considered a modified elastic rod. It has an intrinsic stability resulting from the pressure of the nucleus pulposus pushing the vertebral bodies apart and opposed by the annulus which holds the bodies together. When the isolated spine is maintained in the erect position, the heaviest load it can sustain without buckling is 4 or 5 pounds. This is illustrated by the anesthetized patient who cannot maintain a sitting position unless ex-

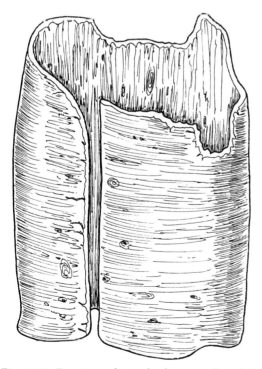

Fig. 4-57. Drawing of tree bark corset found in pre-Columbian Indians' cliff dwellings (The Colorado State Historical Museum, Denver).

ternally supported. The spine, thus, cannot function without the extrinsic stability provided by the back and abdominal musculature.

Compression tests have been carried out on isolated spinal segments. In a young adult, the intervertebral disc will yield and be deformed at pressures exceeding 1400 pounds and in older individuals will yield at about 350 pounds. The vertebral body of a young adult will yield at a compressive force of between 1000 and 1300 pounds, whereas in the elderly, failure can occur at only 300 pounds. Vertebral body fracture will take place before failure of the intervertebral disc.

These tests clearly demonstrate that single severe stresses subjecting the spine to a compressive force of 300 to 1000 pounds are likely to produce vertebral body fracture. Yet with strenuous activity, forces theoretically far exceeding 1400 pounds may be applied to the lower lumbar vertebral bodies and intervertebral discs. An understanding of the mechanism whereby the spine can withstand these forces derives from study of the trunk musculature. By increasing the pressures within the thoracic and abdominal cavities during strenuous activities, trunk muscle contraction can convert the trunk into a fairly rigid cylinder. With the accompanying increase in intercavitary pressure, the load on the lower lumbar intervertebral discs is diminished by at least 30 percent. Based on the same principle, the load on the low lumbar spine can be reduced drastically by wearing a tight abdominal corset.

Electrical activity of trunk musculature was studied during lifting. Muscle contraction and intercavitary pressure were found to increase proportionately with the load being lifted. However, when wearing a corset results in abdominal compression, the electrical activity of the abdominal muscles markedly decreases. This would indicate diminished contraction of the abdominal muscles in the presence of external support. It may also be true that prolonged wearing of such a support will result in muscle atrophy. This suggests that a proper program for a patient with low back dysfunction should include abdominal and postural exercises with the corset being considered a temporary expedient to be ultimately supplanted by the strengthened abdominal and trunk muscles.

Immobilization—Fact or Fancy

A spinal support exerts some immobilizing effects upon the spinal segment which it contains. However, Norton and Brown have shown that motion tends to be increased in the segments adjacent to the ends of the appliance. They further demonstrated increased lumbosacral motion in some subjects when a long spinal brace was worn.[3] It follows that the use of a brace following lumbosacral fusion may actually increase motion at a site where immobilization is being sought. In an effort to hold down this compensatory increase in motion, supports have been designed to extend well down onto the pelvis and grip it firmly. This is an important consideration in prescribing an appliance for lumbosacral pathology.

Fitting Supports

In fitting supports consideration should be given to comfort, convenience and patient acceptance. Pressure is necessary in order to achieve the effects desired. The discomfort of pressure can be lessened by reducing its force or by increasing the surface area on which it acts. Bony prominences and superficial structures should be avoided or carefully padded. An appliance should be contour-fitted so that no sharp edge concentrates compression. The effects of pressure should be evaluated during motion as well as rest. Sliding movements of spinal supports which apply sheer forces and may produce tension on underlying tissues or produce skin abrasion can be minimized by proper contour and fit. The use of low friction materials or the wearing of the support over some clothing is helpful. Moisture adds to the undesirable effects of friction and can be minimized by the use of a brace rather than a corset and by the use of perforated or absorbent material. An appliance should be designed to permit easy application and removal. Buckles and straps used today are of improved design. The increasing use of Velcro to fasten the apron of the brace permits easy removal for laundering. Materials should be lightweight and durable as well as easy to keep clean and odor-free. The patient should be carefully instructed in the application and removal of the appliance, as well as how to clean it.

Cosmetic considerations deserve attention in the design so that the appliance will be as inconspicuous as possible. Female patients in particular may either refuse to wear a brace or wear it only sporadically unless it is cosmetically acceptable.

Purposes of a Spinal Support

A spinal support is designed to:

1. Limit spinal motion
2. Correct posture
3. Diminish mechanical stress on lower lumbar spine.

A corset or brace is indicated when it is desired to achieve one or more of these effects.

Brace Versus Corset

A brace differs from a corset only in having horizontal rigid elements. In all other respects they are similar. Corsets may be made fairly rigid by the addition of paraspinal steels. A brace and a corset may be combined to obtain the advantages of both.

Advantages of a brace:

1. Limits motion to a greater degree.
2. Better lumbar positional control.
3. Limits lateral and rotary motion.

Advantages of a corset:

1. More acceptable cosmetically, especially under a dress.
2. Better control over obesity; improved support when patient is obese.
3. Usually lighter than a brace.
4. Long-term use thought, by some, to be less likely to weaken muscles.
5. Often more acceptable to elderly patients.

6. More likely to provide abdominal compression.

A consideration of the characteristics of specific braces and corsets in relation to the particular low back dysfunction and the type of patient will permit selection of the proper appliance.

BRACES

"Three-Point Pressure" Principle

Braces designed to support the lumbar spine are constructed in accordance with the "three-point pressure" principle described

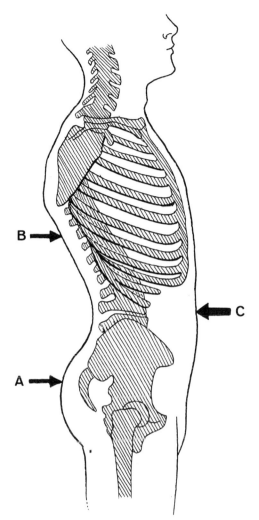

Fig. 4-59. Diagrammatic illustration of the "three-point pressure" principle in design of the Williams lordosis brace.

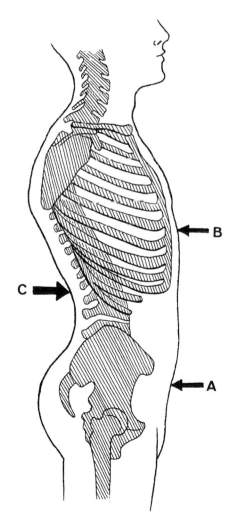

Fig. 4-58. Diagrammatic illustration of the "three point pressure" principle in design of spinal braces.

by Henry H. Jordan in his text, "Orthopedic Appliances."[2] He proposed that the supporting forces of an effective brace must be applied from 3 directions. For example, the 3 forces may consist of (*a*) a backward thrust against the pelvis anteriorly, (*b*) a backward thrust against the thoracic cage anteriorly, (*c*) a forward thrust over the lumbar spine posteriorly.

The particular location of the 3 forces may vary. In the Williams Lordosis Brace, for example, the components are reversed with 2 forces posteriorly at the (*a*) low thoracic level, and the (*b*) sacral region, opposing the

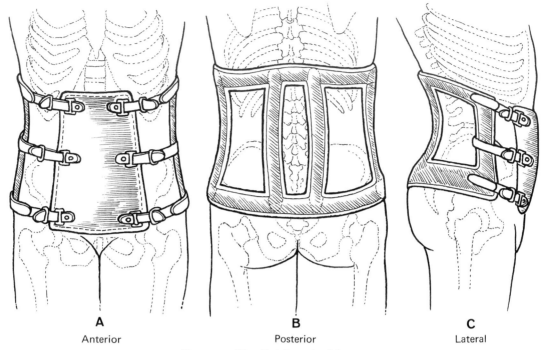

A
Anterior

B
Posterior

C
Lateral

Fig. 4-60. The Knight spinal brace.

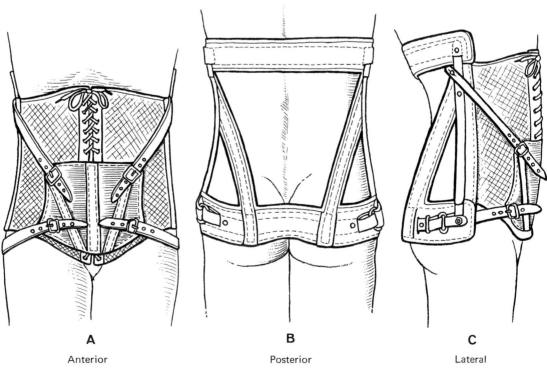

A
Anterior

B
Posterior

C
Lateral

Fig. 4-61. The Williams lordosis brace.

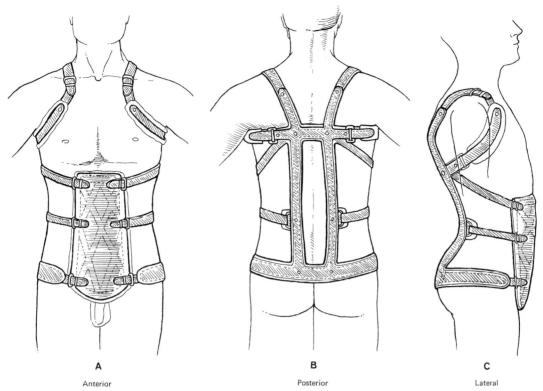

A

Anterior

B

Posterior

C

Lateral

Fig. 4-62. The Taylor spinal brace.

single force anteriorly at the (c) lower abdomen.

In all instances, however, the sum of the 2 forces should be equal to the single force which should be located approximately midway between the 2 opposing forces.

Knight Spinal Brace

The Knight spinal brace, currently the most widely used brace, is a metal frame made up of 2 lumbar posterior and 2 lateral uprights attached to a pelvic band below and a thoracic band above. It has an abdominal apron fastened with 3 pairs of straps. The Knight spinal brace limits flexion, extension and lateral trunk motion, as well as providing abdominal compression.

Williams Brace

The Williams brace, also called the Williams Lordosis Brace, consists of a pelvic band, a thoracic band, a pair of lateral up-

rights pivoting on the thoracic band and a pair of oblique lateral uprights pivoting on the vertical lateral uprights and rigidly attached to the pelvic band. There is an abdominal or corset front and a pelvic strap. This rather unusual support limits lumbar lordosis or extension and lateral tilt. The adjustable "three-point pressure" system restrictively diminishes the lumbar lordosis, and the corset front increases the intra-abdominal pressure. Unlike most spinal braces which are primarily supportive in nature, the Williams Brace is specifically designed to "exert a constant corrective force on the lumbar spine" by restrictively reducing the lumbar lordosis.

Taylor Brace

The Taylor brace is made up of 2 thoracolumbar posterior uprights attached to a pelvic band. The uprights are secured by an intrascapular bar to which axillary straps are attached. There is a corset or abdominal front. This is a hyperextension brace and limits trunk flexion in the thoracolumbar area and slightly in the lumbar area.

CORSETS

Corsets are constructed of fabric reinforced with flexible or rigid stays. They are adjusted by side or back lacing. Side lacing provides firmer back support and permits the addition of heavy steels posteriorly for contouring and reinforcement. The lacing should be capable of being securely tightened with some reserve remaining. A properly fitted corset does not require perineal straps to hold it in place.

Trochanter Belt

The trochanter belt ranges from 1 to 3 inches in width and is worn within the iliac crest and the greater trochanter. It acts to support the sacroiliac joints by strengthening the pelvic ring and preventing excessive stress. Some believe it tilts the pelvis forward. The wearing of such an appliance, or a similarly fitting snug leather belt, has long been a practice of laborers.

Sacroiliac Corset

The sacroiliac corset is somewhat wider but serves much the same purpose as a trochanter belt.

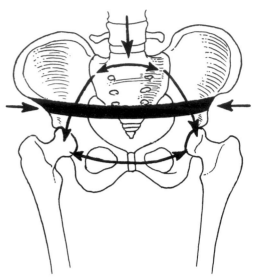

Fig. 4-64. Pelvic arch support furnished by the "hoop action" of an encircling belt about the pelvis.

Lumbosacral Corset

The lumbosacral corset is the most commonly used of all appliances. It should extend well above the dorsal lumbar junction in the back, be contoured to the upper but-

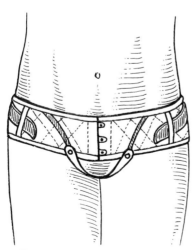

Fig. 4-63. The trochanter belt.

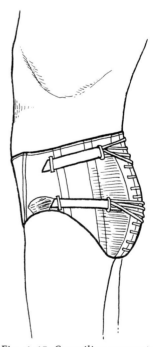

Fig. 4-65. Sacroiliac support.

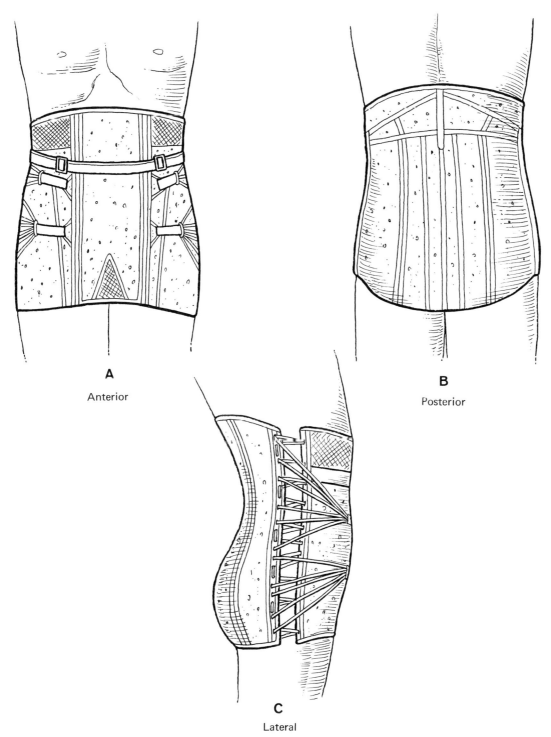

A

Anterior

B

Posterior

C

Lateral

Fig. 4-66. Lumbosacral support.

tocks below and extend down to the upper thighs in women. Side lacing is preferred together with paravertebral steels to diminish the lumbar lordosis.

Dorsolumbar Corset

The dorsolumbar corset is similar in construction to the sacroiliac corset. It extends up the back over the scapulae and is additionally secured by shoulder straps.

LESS FREQUENTLY USED SUPPORTS

Less frequently used supports are those molded of leather, plaster of paris, or plastic materials. These have the advantages of precise fit, the widest possible distribution of pressure, being light in weight and, in the case of plastics, being easy to clean.

The molded leather jacket has the disadvantage, however, of absorbing perspiration with attendant odor and being difficult to clean.

The advantages of a plastic jacket are offset by its high cost. It is chiefly used when a support will be needed permanently.

Plaster of paris jackets are often used for short periods of time. Advantages are: accurately molded fit, rigid support and low cost.

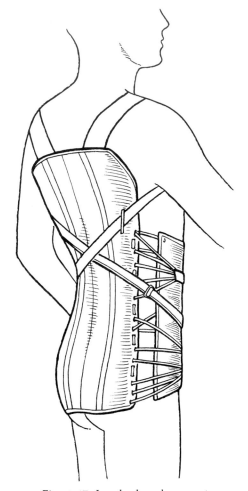

Fig. 4-67. Lumbodorsal support.

REFERENCES

1. Edwards, J. W.: Orthopaedic Appliances Atlas. vol. I. Ann Arbor, American Academy of Orthopaedic Surgeons, 1952.

2. Jordan, H. H.: Orthopedic Appliances. New York, Oxford University Press, 1939.
3. Norton, P. L., and Brown, T.: The immobilizing efficiency of back braces. J. Bone Joint Surg., vol. 39-A, no. 1, Jan., 1957.

5

Lumbosacral Strain

Epidemiology

X-ray Abnormalities

Wastebasket Diagnosis?

Chronic Lumbosacral Strain

Signs and Symptoms
Pathophysiology

Management
Exercise for Shortening Achilles Tendon

Acute Lumbosacral Strain

Signs and Symptoms
Management

5
Lumbosacral Strain

The diagnosis of lumbosacral strain is probably employed more frequently than any other diagnosis relating to low back dysfunction. Despite its common usage, our knowledge of it is considerably less than of many of the less frequently encountered conditions that give rise to back pain. When dealing with such an ambiguous clinical entity, which often is not authenticated by x-ray or laboratory changes, the physician tends to feel unsettled because of his background and training. In many instances, a patient with indeterminate low back dysfunction will be found to have an anatomical or x-ray abnormality, and the physician will seize upon this finding as the cause of the pain, despite the common existence of such abnormalities in many who are symptom free.

EPIDEMIOLOGY

Lumbosacral strain can occur at any age but is most common between the ages of 25 and 50 years, men being affected approximately twice as frequently as women. Statistically, persons who work at heavy labor are no more prone to this condition than are sedentary workers; they are affected about equally. No particular somatotype is specifically prone to this disease, with the exception of the grossly obese whose problem is associated with an increased incidence of lumbosacral strain. However, when obese patients reduce their excess weight, often low back pain persists. Though inequality of leg length often is found in persons who have never experienced low back dysfunction, when seen in a patient with lumbosacral strain, heel lifts are often helpful in compensating for this difference.

X-RAY ABNORMALITIES

(For discussion of lumbosacral strain and x-ray abnormalities see pp. 57–58.)

WASTEBASKET DIAGNOSIS?

Although many patients are labeled with a diagnosis of lumbosacral strain the diagnosis eventually is found to be a completely different entity. They may have early lumbar disc disease prior to the onset of obvious nerve root signs or symptoms; occult malignancies have occasionally been so misdiagnosed before the true nature of the disease process became evident; and a host of medical, genitourinary, and gynecological conditions can give rise to low back dysfunction as the presenting symptom. Because of frequent indistinguishable symptoms in the early stages of these other entities, lumbosacral strain is considered by some as a sort of wastebasket diagnosis into which any low back dysfunction which is not readily identified may be placed. Though our factual knowledge of this disease is wanting, and we are not even sure what causes the pain in strain, this condition does exist as a specific entity with special characteristics and findings. It is classified as acute lumbosacral strain and chronic lumbosacral strain.[1]

CHRONIC LUMBOSACRAL STRAIN

Chronic lumbosacral strain is the most common low back problem encountered in practice. It is a disease of mechanical stress upon the lower spine owing to a variable combination of unknown factors but generally including faulty posture and inadequate musculature. The symptoms are apt to occur after the age of 35 when the spinal ligaments begin to lose their normal elasticity and resiliency and becoming progressively more fibrous. Prior to that age, the more elastic ligaments of the spine tend to compensate and adjust to the undue demands of poor posture associated with lack of proper muscular support.

If this condition is allowed to persist, degenerative changes involving the intervertebral joints will eventually occur, resulting in hypertrophic osteoarthritic degeneration of the vertebrae. These irreversible changes will augment preexisting low back dysfunction and create a more serious problem in management.

Signs and Symptoms

The primary complaint is an aching discomfort in the lumbosacral region. The pain often covers a wide area and is not usually of great severity; it is commonly described as "fairly annoying" or even "mild." This discomfort has often been present for a prolonged and somewhat indefinite duration; although a history of a fall or injury may be elicited, careful questioning usually reveals that some low back discomfort antedated the trauma. Aside from pain, the single most common complaint is fatigue, which is constantly present, despite adequate hours of sleep. Frequently, patients may complain of a "tired feeling" in the back instead of pain. Almost any activity can aggravate the pain and bed rest may or may not relieve it. The posture and general carriage are usually poor, the patient is often overweight and the musculature often generally atonic and flabby.

Examination may reveal some mild paraspinal muscle spasm in the lumbar area. The lumbar spine is rarely "fixed" or splinted as a result of spastic paraspinal muscles and mobility may be fairly good. However, any activity involving repetitive hyperflexion or hyperextension tends to produce moderate aching discomfort, and pressure on the lumbar paraspinal muscles following such activities may be associated with moderate tenderness. A significant increase in the lumbar lordosis is usually noted. Reflexes, sensation and straight leg raising tests are usually normal. X-rays of the spine may reveal an increase of the normal lumbar curvature.

Pathophysiology

This condition results from deterioration of muscles and ligaments and may occur when, because of ignorance or indolence, the patient does not properly care for his body. Constipation, poor diet, inadequate rest and a host of other poor health habits are frequently elicited in the history. A somewhat flat effect is sometimes considered characteristic. One is less likely to encounter this syndrome in the person who has established a good health regimen. Erect carriage involves a mental as well as a physical state of health.

Women seem to be more frequently affected by these symptoms, particularly housewives, since the wearing of high heels and girdles may play some role in this syndrome. The routine wearing of high heels requires a compensatory adjustment of the spine in order to maintain erect posture, thus increasing the lumbar curvature which, in the presence of flabby musculature, creates a disproportionate strain upon the lower back. The wearing of a properly fitted corset or girdle could conceivably be of some benefit in lending support to inadequate trunk musculature.

Management

In dealing with a persistent low back problem a thorough work-up is essential. Rectal or pelvic disease must be ruled out. Routine laboratory studies, in addition to x-rays of the lumbar and thoracic spine, are

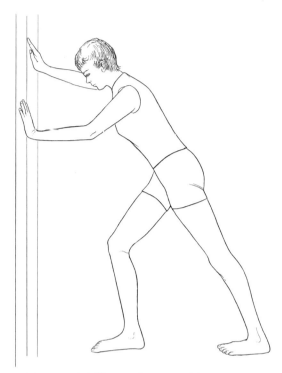

Fig. 5-1. Achilles tendon stretching exercise.

heeled shoes. Any abrupt reduction of heel length may aggravate symptoms by placing the shortened Achilles tendon on stretch.

Exercise for Shortened Achilles Tendon

When shortening of the Achilles tendons adversely affects proper body position, a corrective exercise is available. This is described in the form of directions to the patient:

Stand facing the wall, with the palms resting against it. Position one foot 12 inches from the wall, the second foot 12 inches behind the first. Maintain the heel of the rear foot flat against the floor to stretch the Achilles tendon. Maintain the lumbar spine in slight flexion. To achieve a rhythmic back and forth movement of the body, flex the arm and the anterior hip, knee and ankle. After 20 rhythmic stretching movements, alternate legs. Perform this exercise twice daily.

Adequate rest should include 8 hours of sleep at night supplemented by a 1-hour period of bed rest in the afternoon. The mattress should be firm. A plywood board inserted between the spring and the mattress usually corrects a moderate sag. Many patients sleep on bed boards or even buy a special orthopaedic mattress only to sit in overstuffed furniture during their waking hours. Firm, straight chairs support the back best; and if a great deal of driving is done, the car seat should be moved forward to reduce the lumbar lordosis.

All of the activities of daily living must be carefully reviewed with the patient in an effort to determine how he may avoid excessive stress on the low back. An explanation is helpful describing the body mechanics involved, including standing, walking, sitting, lifting, and sleeping. (See pages 112–117.) Because it is difficult to alter postural habits that have become established over many years, it usually requires at least 6 months to become effective to eliminate symptoms. It is usually necessary to utilize a lumbosacral support designed to sustain the low back and abdominal muscles but as

in order. A careful, painstaking evaluation is the first important step in the management of this syndrome, since it gives a certain degree of confidence to the patient and gives the physician the opportunity to rule out a variety of occult conditions. The patient's trust in the physician and a willingness to follow instructions are of prime importance, since the treatment involves many changes in the patient's mode of living. A detailed explanation of basic lumbar spine mechanisms is of great value in securing the patient's confidence and cooperation.

A properly prescribed series of low back exercises designed to increase the strength of the trunk musculature must be regularly performed. (See pages 117–124.) If the patient is overweight, a gradual weight reduction program is initiated. A moderate decrease in heel length, rather than a sudden shift to a low heel, is advisable in women accustomed to wearing extremely high-muscle tone and strength improve, this support can be discarded.

ACUTE LUMBOSACRAL STRAIN

This condition can result from injury to the low back, such as from lifting excessive loads, lifting in a mechanically disadvantaged position or direct trauma to the back or falls in which the low back musculature is strained.

Signs and Symptoms

The precipitating trauma to the low back region invariably causes immediate discomfort. Often, the initial pain is not unduly severe and is appreciated mainly as a stiffness of the low back region due largely to muscle spasm. The patient may continue to work and remain active in the hope that the activity will serve to "work away" the muscle spasm. Severe acute muscle spasm resulting from trauma frequently worsens with activity, so that the patient may eventually become completely incapacitated. It is not unusual to find the patient lying in bed, or even on the floor, suffering so severely that not only is he unable to move himself, but also the gentlest movement of the stretcher used to transport him to the hospital may cause excruciating discomfort.

The more commonly encountered acute lumbosacral strain syndrome is less severe and is manifested as low back discomfort, usually worse on one side, with the most severe pain often being localized in a rather discrete area.

Examination of the low back reveals severe bilateral or unilateral spasm of the lumbar paraspinal muscles. Forward bending causes increased discomfort with limited mobility of the lumbar spine. If the paraspinal muscle spasm is unilateral, lateral bending of the body away from the side of the spasm is painful, while the same movement toward the muscle spasm is less uncomfortable and may actually relieve the pain. Occasionally, with unilateral muscle spasm, lumbar scoliosis is seen with the con-

cavity toward the side of the spasm. When the spasm is severe and widespread, any body movement, including movement of the lower extremities, may be painful. Reflex and sensory examinations are normal. The x-rays of the lumbosacral spine are often normal but may reveal some straightening of the normal lumbar curvature; and when the muscle spasm is unilateral, lumbar scoliosis may be noted.

Management

A patient who is so incapacitated with an acute lumbosacral strain that he is unable to work should be placed on bed rest. As in all low back problems, a bed board or a firm mattress is necessary. Muscle relaxants are occasionally helpful in reducing the muscle spasm, but it may be necessary to use narcotics in fairly substantial dosages if the pain persists despite enforced bed rest. A natural reluctance to use narcotics for a condition which may eventuate into a long, drawn-out, chronic problem may impel the physician to prescribe small doses, which will often be ineffective. Once the physician decides what narcotics are required, 1 or 2 large doses are more effective in relaxing muscle spasm than several smaller doses.

Physiotherapy in the form of heat and gentle massage is often helpful. If muscle spasm persists, in spite of bed rest and medication, infiltration of the paraspinal muscle with a local anesthetic may offer prompt relief in those patients with discrete localization of pain; and this relief frequently lasts beyond the pharmacologic duration of the drug.

Unless an underlying condition is present, such as a herniated disc or a fracture, the muscle spasm will invariably improve with bed rest, medication and physiotherapy. With the subsidence of muscle spasm, the patient will be comfortable as long as he remains in bed. Before ambulation is permitted, which may aggravate a prompt exacerbation of the muscle spasm, several nonstrenuous low back exercises should be performed while lying in bed. The first 3 exercises described in the section on low back exercises are suitable (pages 121–122). Exercises 1 and 2 are performed several times daily; and if no discomfort is appreciated, exercise 3 is added. After several days of such mobilizing exercises, the patient is ambulated wearing a lumbosacral support or Knight spinal brace to sustain the low back and abdominal muscles. This support is worn for 6 weeks whenever the patient is out of bed for any activity, including resting in a chair. Activities are increased progressively until the patient is able to resume normal endeavors without discomfort. During the period of convalescence, the patient should be carefully supervised. Excessive exercise may cause exacerbation of the muscle spasm while excessive rest may not only prolong the recovery period but may also create a so-called "low back neurosis" in which the patient considers himself an invalid. Such a potentially serious situation, if not properly managed, may eventually progress to permanent disability.

Manipulative therapy to the lower back is occasionally effective in the treatment of the residuals of an acute low back strain. The improvement resulting from manipulation is due chiefly to stretching of muscles and tendons that have become contracted and shortened as a result of spasm. In addition, manipulation may be helpful in stretching the fibrous tissues surrounding the joints of the back which may have become contracted and even have developed adhesions after prolonged immobility of the lower back.

For a more detailed discussion regarding treatment, review Nonsurgical Management of Low Back Pain and Sciatica (pp. 95–117); Low Back Exercises (pp. 117–124); Low Back Supports and Braces (pp. 124–132).

REFERENCES

1. Ford, L., and Goodman, F. G.: X-ray studies of the lumbosacral spine. South. Med. J., *10*:1123, 1966.
2. Horal, J.: The clinical appearance of low back disorders in the city of Gothenberg, Sweden. Acta. Orthop. Scand., Supp. 118, 1969.
3. Hult, L.: The Munk Fords investigation. Acta. Orthop. Scand., Supp. 16, 1954.
4. Splitoff, C. A.: Roentgenographic comparison of patients with and without backache. JAMA, *152*:1610, 1953.

Lumbar Disc Disease

STATISTICAL ANALYSIS

SYMPTOMS

Preexisting Backache

Secondary Gain
History of Trauma
No Secondary Gain

Primary Symptoms

Absence of Sciatica
Sciatica

Sciatic Distribution
Activities and Posture
Radiculitis
Motor Symptoms
Sensory Symptoms
Scoliosis and Posture
Gait

SIGNS

Mobility of the Spine
Reflex Examination
Sensory Changes

Motor Dysfunction
Straight Leg Raising

CONSIDERATION OF OTHER LESIONS

ELECTROMYOGRAPHY

X-RAY FINDINGS

Vacuum Phenomenon
Intervertebral Disc Space Narrowing

Vertebral Body Alignment
Degenerative Changes

FORAMINAL ROOT COMPRESSION SYNDROME

TRANSITIONAL LUMBOSACRAL VERTEBRAL AND ROOT FUNCTION

CLINICAL DIFFERENTIATION OF AFFECTED LEVEL

CLINICAL PATTERNS OF DISC PROTRUSIONS

TREATMENT OF LUMBAR DISC DISEASE

Conservative Management

Rest
Traction
Physiotherapy
Trigger Points
Manipulation of the Low Back
Medication
Occupational Changes
Activities of Daily Living
Low Back Supports and Shoe Lifts

Inadequate Response to Conservative Management

Intractable Symptoms
Persisting Motor Signs
Intermittent Symptoms
Subjective Response

Lumbar Disc Surgery

Indications for Surgery

Contraindications for Surgery
Normal Myelogram

Surgery

Historical Development
Double-check Side of Lesion
Anesthesia
Position
Surface Landmarks
Preparing the Skin and Draping
Skin Incision
Subperiosteal Dissection
Developing the Interspace
Interlaminar Surgery

Vascular and Visceral Injuries During Disc Surgery
Operative Report
Postoperative Management
Cause of Operative Failure

Common Causes of Postoperative Pain

Results of Initial Surgery

EXCEPTIONAL LUMBAR DISC PROBLEMS

Cauda Equina Syndrome
Transdural Excision of Midline Disc Extrusion

THE REPEAT OPERATIVE PROCEDURE

Indications for Repeat Surgery
Technical Considerations in Repeat
  Spinal Surgery

Reexploration Following Complete
  Laminectomy
Results of Repeat Procedures

6
Lumbar Disc Disease

In properly appraising lumbar disc disease, a searching and deliberative history and examination are required. This information is indispensable for establishing an accurate diagnosis as well as for the medical insight furnished by such an evaluation. Without a complete understanding and knowledge of the patient, a proper and suitable course of management is impossible. Conceivably, a number of medical and surgical conditions exist which can be treated quite adequately with a truncated history and physical examination limited to the condition under treatment. Lumbar disc disease is not included in this category.

STATISTICAL ANALYSIS

For purposes of statistical analysis of lumbar disc lesions, I have analyzed 1,000 consecutive cases that I have personally operated upon between 1961 and 1970. The advantage of analyzing an even number of cases is that it may offer an explicit statistical frame of mental comparison, so that when we refer to 643 cases out of 1,000 a more precise image is imparted that can easily be translated into percentages. All of the patients included in this series were brought to surgery. Using exclusively surgical material will load the statistics toward the more severe disorders, but it does have the advantage of establishing both myelographic and visual verification of each lesion. The selection of my most recent group of 1,000 cases must be considered with regard to evaluating the results of surgery. It is said that "experience teaches slowly and at the cost of mistakes." As I look backward, I recognize significant shifts in my judgment and surgical technique.

The patients included in this study ranged in age from 14 to 79 years with a mean age of 42; 769 males, 231 females.

Thirty-one patients had midline lesions with no lateralizing preponderance of symptoms. Of those who had lateralizing symptoms, 540 were left, and 360 were right.

The levels affected were as follows:

L5–S1 = 516
L4–5 = 218
L5–S1 and L4–5 = 243
L3–4 = 16
L2–3 = 3
L1–2 = 2
T12–L1 = 2

SYMPTOMS

PREEXISTING BACKACHE

Prior to the development of signs and symptoms compatible to a diagnosis of lumbar disc disease, most patients have experienced preexisting low back pain and other symptoms that in retrospect can be related to the ensuing lumbar disc syndrome.

For want of a better label these are referred to as "preexisting symptoms." Of 1,000 patients subjected to analysis, 643 gave a history of preexisting backache, and 357 denied this symptom. Exactly what produces these preexisting low back symptoms is uncertain. They may represent early changes in the nucleus pulposus, causing forces to be transmitted to the annulus fibrosis in an asymmetrical fashion and may result in increased tensile stress on the outer layers of the annulus, which contain pain fibers.

One of the most characteristic signs of disc disease is intermittency of the pain. Unrelenting and constantly progressive pain must make one alert to neoplasm. Preexisting backaches were classified into 3 groupings:

1. Severe = 192
2. Moderate = 320
3. Mild = 131

1. Severe. The 192 patients included in the severe grouping complained of almost constant varying degrees of low back pain. The pain would fluctuate in severity from "hardly noticeable" to "extremely severe." It often interfered with the activities of daily living and was a source of considerable disruption in their lives. In all instances, they required treatment for this problem, and most of them (164) had been hospitalized for low back pain on one or more occasions. Almost all of these patients had missed periods of time from their occupations. In the case of housewives, at times the severity of their symptoms confined them to bed so that help was needed to carry out their home commitments. The duration of these preexisting symptoms varied from 18 months to 46 years.

2. Moderate. Three hundred and twenty patients were classified as having moderate preexisting symptoms. They had intermittent back pain which was usually associated with strenuous activities but occasionally was spontaneous in onset. Exertion, such as an unusual weekend of sports, gardening, prolonged stooping, spring housecleaning or heavy lifting are the types of activities likely to precipitate an exacerbation of backache. As a rule, these episodes of pain improved with rest, and often the patient required no active medical treatment; self-treatment, consisting of a few aspirins and avoidance of strenuous activities, was successful. In many instances, the patient saw a physician for other ailments either on a regular or intermittent basis but rarely saw fit to discuss his low back symptoms because the pain was not severe. The general attitude could be summarized by such a statement as "I got used to the idea of living with my backache." Most of the patients classified as moderate had experienced several attacks of low back pain that they considered severe. They were incapacitated for the duration of these attacks, and 102 of them required previous hospitalizations for treatment of severe backache. The duration of these preexisting backaches was from 6 weeks to 12 years.

3. Mild. Of the 131 patients classified as having mild preexisting backache, most of these had to reflect a bit before stating that they, indeed, did have a history of backache. Terms such as "mild ache," "tired feeling in my back," "a weak back" were used. A number of these patients actually denied having backaches; but when leading questions were asked regarding how they fared when carrying out strenuous tasks such as moving furniture, gardening and so forth, a history of some low back dysfunction was elicited. A typical comment might be "I feel a bit stiff on arising the morning; but in a half an hour or so, I've limbered up." Mild discomfort on prolonged car trips, necessitating disembarking from the vehicle and strolling about to "ease the stiffness," is also heard.

The duration of these preexisting symptoms was from 8 weeks to 5 years. Four patients had been hospitalized for low back pain, and in 3 of these patients this hospitalization represented the only severe episode of previous backache.

Secondary Gain

Of the 643 patients with a history of preexisting low back symptoms, 57 claimed in-

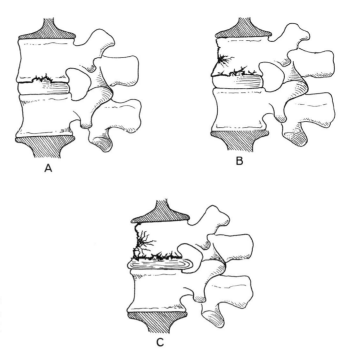

Fig. 6-1. Directly applied stress to the spine will fracture the bony elements before rupturing the intervertebral disc.

jury either while working or as the result of an accident with medicolegal involvement.

This factor introduces consideration of possible secondary gain, either in the form of direct financial reward or time off from work, with financial remuneration. The circumstances of this type of arrangement involve some genuine or implied advantages in having all of the symptoms date from the alleged injury, with some motivation on the part of the patient to negate any previous symptoms that could be related to the present condition.

Secondary gain was a potential consideration in 286 of the 357 patients who denied preexisting backache. Approximately 80 percent of these patients were involved in a secondary gain situation, while less than 9 percent of patients who gave a history of preexisting back pain were in a position to derive possible secondary gain from their symptoms. To ignore the human element in these statistics is to close our eyes to reality.

History of Trauma

A history of trauma in the etiology of lumbar disc disease is elicited in the majority of patients (764 out of 1,000), but the actual clinical significance of this type of information is open to question.

When Harvey Cushing collected statistics on his personal series of meningiomas, he reported a greater than 60 percent incidence of cerebral trauma in association with this tumor. As a result of these statistics, for years, credence was given to trauma as a possible etiology for meningiomas. Of course, trauma to the cranium is a common occurrence; and when questioned carefully, many of his patients could recall instances of varying degrees of cerebral trauma. Since some form of direct or indirect trauma to the low back occurs frequently in the course of daily living, considerable discretion and imagination are needed to properly evaluate such information.

On the basis of our present understanding of the pathophysiology of lumbar disc disease, a single episode of trauma may be a precipitating, but rarely a causative, factor. Augmenting this line of reasoning, if sufficient stress is applied to the spine, a fracture of the bony elements will occur before any damage is done to the disc. Furthermore, it is often minor episodes of trauma, such as picking a light object off the floor or bending forward over a sink to wash one's face, that often precipitates a severe attack.

Out of 1,000 patients, 764 alleged that trauma was the direct cause or played a significant role in the development of their lumbar disc symptoms; 343 were involved in a possible secondary gain situation, in which they were hoping to derive compensation to reap restitution for their injuries. Since trauma is implicit in this situation, 100 percent of these patients gave a history of trauma. The trauma was classified into 3 categories:

1. Severe = 24
2. Moderate = 71
3. Mild = 248

1. Severe. All of the 24 patients classified as having suffered severe trauma were hospitalized as a result of these injuries. In many instances the initial hospitalization was for treatment of symptoms other than the lumbar spine (i.e., long bone fractures, severe head injuries, soft tissue injuries). The trauma included falls from ladders or heights over 10 feet, severe vehicular injuries, or direct trauma to the body from falling or propelled objects.

2. Moderate. The 71 patients classified as having suffered moderate trauma experienced fewer associated injuries than the severe group. In addition to falls, direct trauma and vehicular injuries, a variety of lifting experiences were included. A number of patients reported lifting a heavy object with a partner's help, and either through loss of footing or inadequate hand purchase, the partner released his portion of the load, placing the increased weight unexpectedly on the patient. Of these patients 18 were hospitalized for treatment of their initial injuries.

3. Mild. The 248 patients in the mild trauma classification displayed the greatest degree of variation. In addition to the usual falls, many patients reported losing their footing on a slippery floor; and in preventing themselves from actually falling, they "twisted" the back. Lifting relatively light objects was cited, as was prolonged stooping or working in a cramped position.

No Secondary Gain

Of the 657 patients not involved in a secondary gain situation, 236 (36%) gave a history of trauma.

1. Severe = 12
2. Moderate = 83
3. Mild = 141

There is little in the way of differentiation between the severe and moderate categories of the secondary gain patients and those who are not. In the mild classification, the only significant difference is the considerable uncertainty in the mind of the patient who has no secondary gain regarding this mild trauma as a precipitating factor of their symptoms; in the secondary gain group, most of the patients were quite certain that the episode of mild trauma was the causative factor.

PRIMARY SYMPTOMS

Of the 756 patients who had backache as an initial symptom, 643 had preexisting intermittent low back pain, anatomically diffuse and varied in severity from rather mild backache to occasional severe pain; 113 denied a preexisting history of intermittent low back pain prior to the onset of backache, which persisted and eventually led into clearly definable lumbar disc symptoms.

Of the 643 patients with preexisting back pain, 448 could relate the onset of backache leading to disc symptoms with trauma; 57 claimed secondary gain, and 391 had no secondary gain claim. Of the 113 patients without history of preexisting backache, 104 could relate the onset of their symptoms to trauma; 86 were in a secondary gain situation, and 18 had no secondary gain claims.

Absence of Sciatica

Of 46 patients who had no significant sciatic symptoms, backache, either bilateral or unilateral, was the chief complaint. Included in this grouping are those who com-

plained of numbness or tingling in one or
both feet and mild aching or crampy discomfort in one or both calves or in the buttocks.
I reserve the term sciatica for those who had
symptoms that conformed, at least in part,
to the distribution of a lumbar root. Of the
46 patients without sciatica 31 had midline
disc protrusions. Of the remaining 15 cases,
the disc protrusions were at the following
levels: 2 at the L1–2 interspace, 1 at L2–3
interspace, 7 at the L3–4 interspace, 3 at the
L4–5 interspace, and 2 at the L5–S1 interspace.

Sciatica

Manifesting sciatica, either with or without
backache, were 964 patients; 386 noted a
marked diminution in the low back pain with
onset of sciatica, often appreciated as an
extension of the low back pain into the hip.
The hip pain would then begin to assume
a different character from the low back pain,
described in such terms as "toothache-like"
rather than like the muscle spasm type of
pain noted in the low back. With extension
of the discomfort down the posterior thigh
and eventually involving the entire course of
the involved nerve root, the low back pain
gradually subsided.

Developing sciatica after a bout of backache, were 324 patients and both symptoms
remained acute with no significant subsidence of the backache during the entire
course of illness; but 208 patients developed
sciatica as the primary symptom.

Sciatic Distribution

It is always an unexpected rarity to encounter a sciatic neuralgia that extends every
inch of the way down a specific nerve root
dermatome without a hiatus or gap. In fact,
such a "perfect pattern" may cause one to
worry about the possibility of malingering.
The two most commonly encountered sites
of lumbar disc disease are the L5–S1 and the
L4–5 levels. If the sciatic pain and paresthesia
reaching the foot follows a dermatomal pattern, the specific level affected may be identified. The L5–S1 (S1 root) syndrome extends

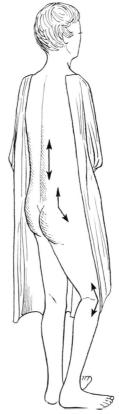

Fig. 6-2. Flattening of the normal lumbar lordosis
in association with severe paraspinal muscle
spasm.

along the lateral aspect of the foot and usually involves the fourth and fifth toes. The
L4–5 (L5 root) syndrome extends over the
dorsum of the foot toward the great toe.
Unfortunately, the pain and paresthesia of
many sciatic syndromes stop at the ankle,
preventing identification of specific root involvement on the basis of symptoms.

Of the 964 patients with sciatica, 585 had
pain and paresthesia within an identifiable
nerve root pattern, enabling a correct diagnosis to be established; 171 had a seemingly
identifiable distribution of pain, but this
clinical localization was incorrect when correlated with the myelogram and operative
findings; 208 did not have sufficient identifiable distribution of pain or paresthesia to
enable a reasonable clinical opinion regarding the involved interspace.

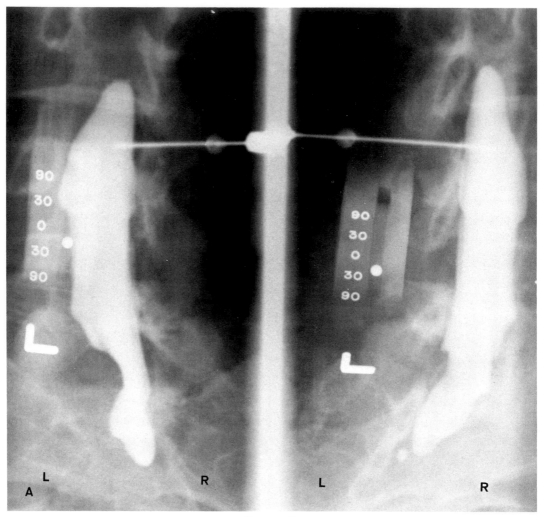

Fig. 6-3A.

Activities and Posture

Most patients with lumbar disc disease appreciate some relief of their discomfort with rest, and increased pain with such activities as prolonged standing or walking, forward bending, stooping and sitting. Climbing in and out of a car, prolonged vehicular driving or even riding are often painful. Occasionally, a patient will be seen who states that bed rest aggravates the pain, and the position of least discomfort is standing. This is often related to muscle spasm which may be appreciated after a period of immobility, so that when the patient first arises from a bed he feels extremely stiff and uncomfortable. Many patients who deny any significant improvement in their symptoms with bed rest at home, when maintained at absolute bed rest in the hospital will after 2 or 3 days appreciate some definite easing of their pain.

Reaction to coughing and sneezing have often been cited as ways of differentiating disc lesions from lumbosacral strains. The presumption in this case is that the sudden increase in intraspinal pressure resulting from these activities will produce a reflected shock or impulse to be transmitted through the root sleeve to the already irritated nerve

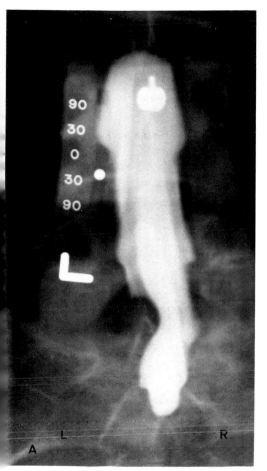

Fig. 6-3A. (*Cont'd*)

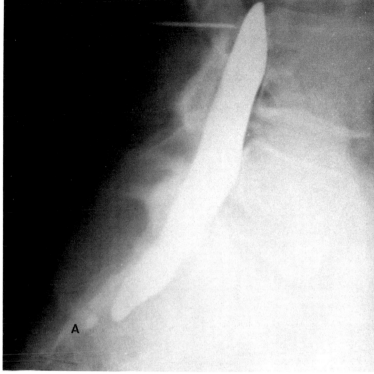

Fig. 6-3A. (*Cont'd*)

Fig. 6-3. A, This 36-year-old female complained of long-standing low back and left sciatic pain. Signs and symptoms were compatible with S1 root compression including an absent left Achilles reflex plus pain and numbness along the lateral border of the foot within the S1 dermatome. She manifested an alternating sciatic scoliosis with the concavity to the left when seen in out-patient clinic and the concavity to the right two weeks later upon hospital admission. On the basis of the alternating sciatic scoliosis, it was presumed that the disc protrusion was within a position beneath the root that would allow the root to slip to either side of the protrusion. The myelogram revealed a large filling defect seen only on the A-P and oblique views with no defect visualized on the lateral "cross-table" view. This is compatible with a lesion directly beneath the root but not producing significant medial elevation of the dural sac.

B, Disc protrusion L5–S1 immediately below the S1 nerve root.

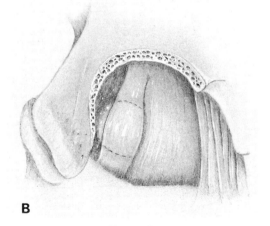

Fig. 6-3B.

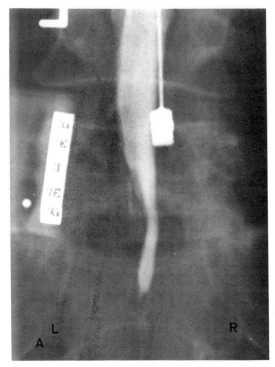

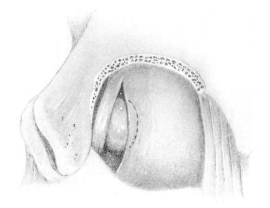

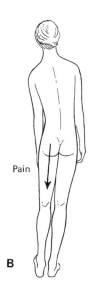

Fig. 6-4. A, This 35-year-old man had long-standing left sciatica compatible with S1 root compression. He had severe sciatic scoliosis with concavity to the left clinically indicative of "axillary" protrusion. Myelogram reveals nerve root cleavage compatible with free disc fragment between nerve root and dural sac.

B, Large free fragment of intervetebral disc within axilla of nerve root.

root. However, any musculoskeletal pain may be aggravated by the sudden movement of the body caused by coughing or sneezing, so that this cannot be considered a pathognomonic symptom of nerve root pressure. Straining at stool, a type of Valsalva maneuver, seems a more valid test of this principle. No associated sudden movement of the body occurs with this maneuver to becloud the issue.

Radiculitis

Exactly what it is that causes the nerve root pain is not clearly understood. It involves more than a simple pressure phenomenon. One can occasionally see a patient with

metastatic carcinoma invading the lumbar spine, with a multiple nerve root pressure syndrome producing numbness and weakness of an entire lower extremity, yet suffering surprisingly little pain. Why is this type of pressure so often not as painful as the radiculitis produced by a protruding disc? Possibly the combination of root compression and associated inflammatory changes involving the root is productive of the typical nerve root pain associated with lumbar disc disease.

Why is the onset of sciatica so often associated with subsidence of low back pain? Possibly the low back pain is caused by the tensile stress on the outer layers of the annulus, which are known to contain pain fibers. Once the annulus has ruptured these fibers are no longer under the same tension reducing the stimulus for low back pain.

It is, of course, the material extruding from this site of rupture that does cause compression and irritation of the nerve root creating acute sciatic pain.

Motor Symptoms

Occasionally, a patient's chief complaint will be a foot drop with very little, if any, pain. Less frequently, weakness of the quadriceps muscle is produced by a disc protrusion at the L3–4 or L2–3 interspaces, resulting in instability of the knee; this will occasionally cause the leg to buckle without warning. One patient complained of falling and was unable to completely understand the true reason for these "attacks." Root compression from disc protrusion rarely causes painless motor dysfunction; usually weakness and pain are associated.

Sensory Symptoms

There is often a discrepancy between the radicular symptoms relating to pain and those involving sensory impairment. As a rule, the pain is appreciated proximally and gradually diminishes as it progresses more distally, so that the average patient with sciatica will note increased pain in the hip and posterior thigh with pain of a lesser intensity in the leg and foot. When numbness is noted, it seems to be more distinct distally, and less so, proximally. Most patients who complain of numbness seem to be more aware of this symptom in the foot or leg, and it is unusual for them to appreciate this sensation in the hip or thigh. The same is true of sensory testing, with the examiner more likely to elicit a zone of numbness distally.

Scoliosis and Posture

The position of the nerve root in relationship to the disc protrusion will determine the posture manifested by the patient. As a rule, the normal lumbar lordosis is flattened, because of paraspinal muscle spasm; in some

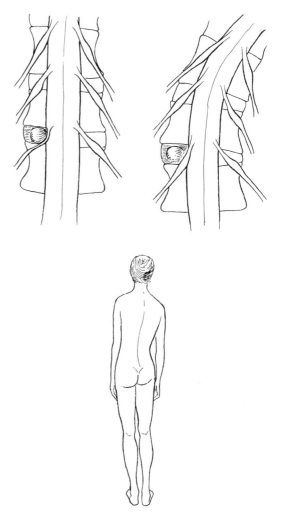

Fig. 6-5. The mechanism of "sciatic scoliosis." Decreased root tension may result in decreased sciatic pain.

cases, with very severe muscle spasm, there is reversal of the lumbar lordosis into a position of slight lumbar flexion. Less frequently, in association with flattening of the lumbar lordosis, a scoliosis occurs to one or the other side. It is not that type of long-standing scoliosis that first occurs in childhood and progressively worsens; it is a "sciatic scoliosis" associated with pronounced spasm of the paravertebral muscles and is a protective measure, allowing the patient to maintain that posture which will allow him some degree of pain relief. It is, of course, involun-

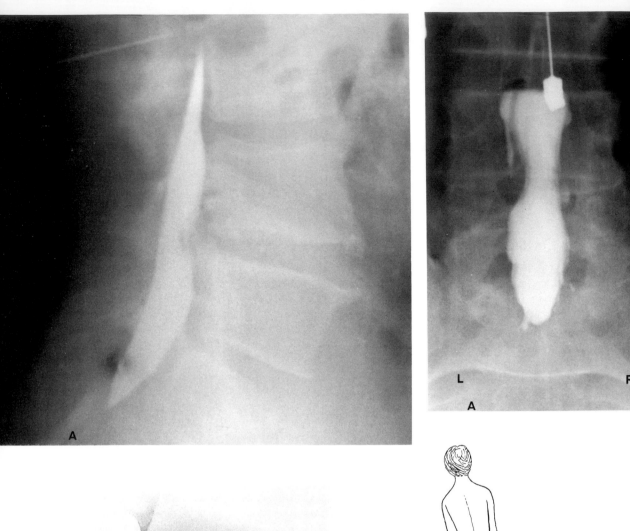

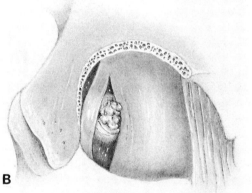

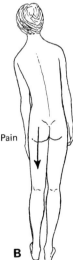

Fig. 6-6. A, This 55-year-old man complained of long-standing low back and left sciatic pain. In addition to typical signs and symptoms compatible with L5 nerve root compression including weakness of great toe extensor power and hypesthesia over the dorsum of the left foot within the L5 sensory dermatome, he demonstrated marked and persistent "sciatic scoliosis" with the concavity to the left. A diagnosis was made of disc protrusion at the L4–5 level on the left. In addition, we presumed on the basis of the scoliosis that the protrusion was within the "axilla" of the root displacing the nerve root laterally. Myelography demonstrated a disc protrusion at the L4–5 level on the left with root cleavage indicative of protrusion discernible between the dural sac and root. Surgery confirmed the protrusion medial to the root within the "axilla".

B, Partially extruded disc within axilla. (See Fig. 6-6C, D, p. 152.)

tary on the part of the patient but does permit reduction of nerve root irritation by decreasing root pressure related to root stretch or tension. If the disc protrusion is on the medial side of the nerve root displacing it laterally, the spine is scoliosed with the concavity toward the side of the lesion, in order to afford relief of radicular symptoms. Conversely, if the protrusion is lateral to the nerve root, displacing the root medially, scoliosis with the concavity away from the side of the lesion will provide relief of radicular pain. When the protruded portion of the disc is directly under the root, the scoliosis may shift from one side to the other. Because the splitting of the lumbar spine by protective muscle spasm and spinal distortion are mechanisms to decrease irritation and motion at the involved interspace, it is not uncommon to observe patients who have a striking lumbar scoliosis with severe muscle spasm experiencing relatively little discomfort. When this is the case, any effort to "straighten out" the low back either by traction, manipulation, exercise or brace may disrupt the patient's protective mechanisms and worsen the pain.

Gait

The gait of a person suffering with a lumbar disc syndrome has considerable variability. In almost all cases, as a result of the paraspinal muscle spasm in the lumbar region, the gait is stiff and a bit deliberate to avoid increasing pain. When root pain is severe, the patient appreciates increased discomfort, with complete straightening or extension of the affected lower extremity. To walk in comfort, the patient may maintain a position of slight flexion at the hip and knee in association with an attempt to maintain the trunk as rigid as possible, producing a characteristic limp with a slight tilting of the entire body toward the side of the pain. In some cases the root pressure is so severe that the foot is maintained in a position of plantar flexion, and the patient is unable to lower his heel to the floor, which is a protective antalgic movement designed to avoid tension on the sciatic nerve. With extremely severe pain the patient is unable to ambulate at all and must remain in a flat position. Any movement, including breathing, will increase the discomfort.

SIGNS

Mobility of the Spine

Lumbar spine mobility in the presence of lumbar disc protrusion depends on two factors: the degree of paraspinal muscle spasm and subsequent splinting of the lumbar spine plus the severity of nerve root pressure. Flexion is, as a rule, more restricted than extension. If the patient has a splinted lumbar spine as a result of severe muscle spasm, on attempting forward flexion, movement will occur at the hip joints and in the thoracic and cervical spines; but the lumbar spine will be maintained in a fixed position. This is noted visually and also can be checked manually by placing the thumb and forefinger on the lumbar spine and determining if a separation of these fingers occurs with movement. Occasionally, when the spine is com-

pletely fixed by muscle spasm, remarkably little pain is produced with forward bending, in view of the splinting action of these muscles. Although flexion is more impaired, extension too will be limited. When extension is attempted at a time when paraspinal muscle spasm is severe, rather than any true extension of the lumbar spine, the entire trunk will be tilted backward; and a slight extension of the thoracic spine and a hyperextension of the cervical spine occurs.

Lateral flexion is tested by having the patient bend laterally to either side and note the distance the extended fingers reach on the thigh and knee. Normally, the extended fingers are able to reach the knee or a few inches below the knee. Even with relatively severe muscle spasm, the spine has fairly

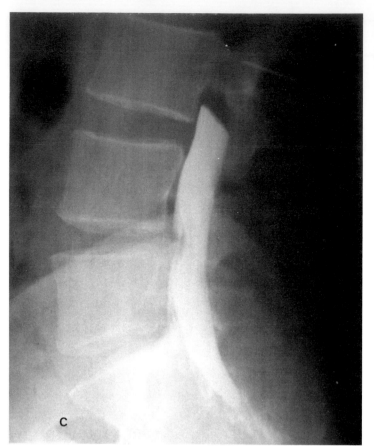

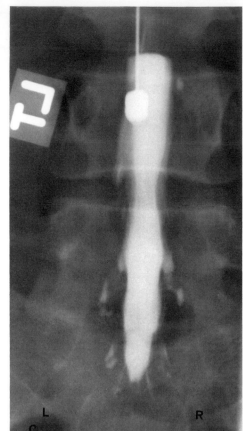

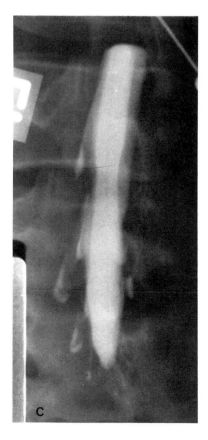

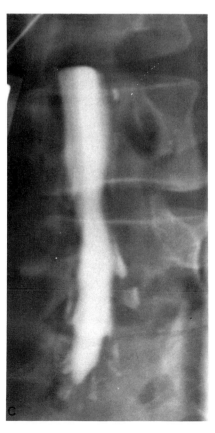

Fig. 6-6. C and D, This 28-year-old man complained of long-standing low back and right sciatic pain. His signs and symptoms were compatible with L5 nerve root compression including marked weakness of great toe extensors and hypesthesia over the dorsum of the right foot within the L5 sensory dermatome. He manifested a persisting sciatic scoliosis with the concavity to the left. A diagnosis was made of disc protrusion at the L4–5 level on the right. In addition, on the basis of the scoliosis, the protrusion was thought to be lateral to the nerve root. Myelography demonstrated a lateral disc protrusion at the L4–5 level. Surgery confirmed the lateral position of the protrusion.

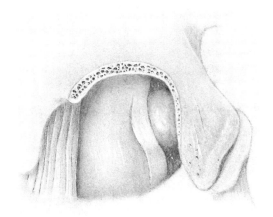

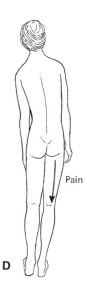

D

good lateral flexion. In some instances, when the disc protrusion is lateral to the root, lateral flexion increases the radicular pain and so will be limited on the side of the lesion. When the lesion is medial to the nerve root, displacing it laterally, root tension is relieved by bending toward the side of the lesion and worsened by lateral flexion away from the lesion. It must be noted, however, that it is the relationship of the protrusion to the root that may hamper lateral flexion and not the paraspinal muscle spasm itself.

Rotation of the spine is determined by having the patient stand erect, with the examiner maintaining the hands on each of the iliac crests, and have the patient turn his head and shoulders as far as possible in one direction and then in the other. Normally, the arc of shoulder rotation is a bit less than 90° to either side and may be diminished slightly with severe paraspinal muscle spasm.

The proper way to palpate muscle spasm is to start at the midline, over the spinous processes, and move laterally to determine the degree of muscle resistance and firmness. This is done gently. It is a common mistake to palpate directly over the muscle mass, which is a less revealing method of evaluating paraspinal muscle spasm and will only determine the grosser degrees of difference.

Reflex Examination

Reflex examination is likely to reveal a diminished or absent Achilles reflex, if the S1 root is compressed from an L5–S1 disc. Reflexes will probably be normal, if the herniation is at the L4–5 level; and herniation at the 3–4 or 2–3 level may reveal a diminished patellar or suprapatellar reflex.

In eliciting reflexes, it must be realized that many patients have reflex changes unrelated to nerve root compression. Many persons have hypoactive or completely absent deep tendon reflexes. Bilaterally absent reflexes are often seen in elderly patients with peripheral neuropathy. Long-standing diabet-

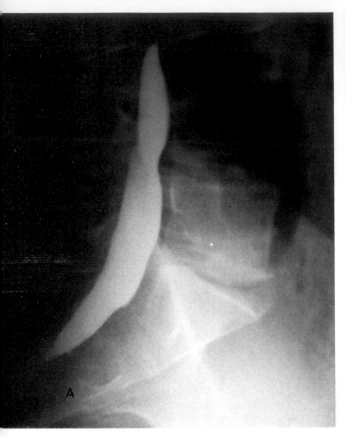

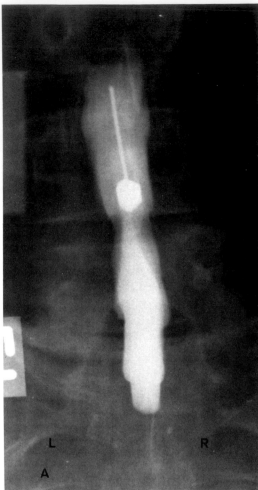

Fig. 6-7. A and B, This 53-year-old woman presented with a long-standing history of low back pain, which in the past 2 years was associated with left sciatica. Six months prior to admission, she developed right sciatica. Clinically, she manifested evidence of bilateral L5 nerve root compression. Myelography revealed changes compatible with bilateral disc protrusions at the L4–5 level. Surgery confirmed the presence of laterally positioned protrusions of the L4–5 intervertebral disc, and these lesions were excised via bilateral interlaminar exposures.

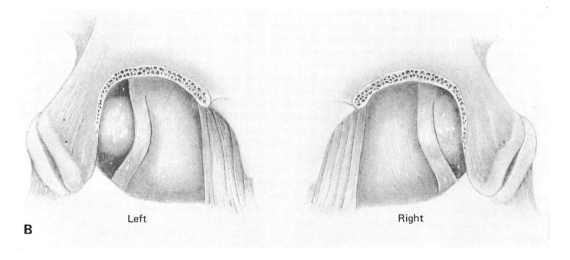

B   Left   Right

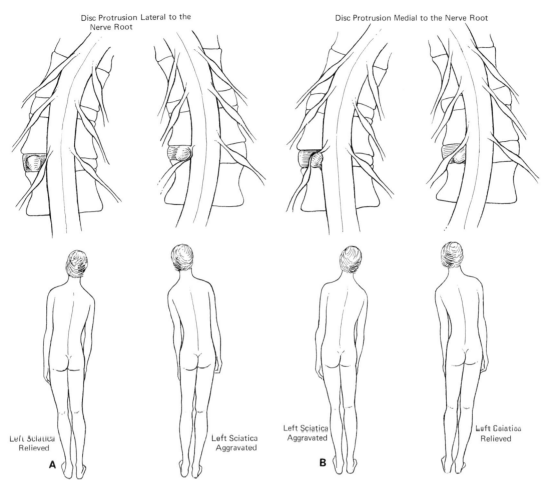

Fig. 6-8. A and B, Relief or aggravation of pain with lateral flexion may indicate if the disc protrusion is lateral or medial to the nerve root.

ics, with peripheral neuropathy, commonly have absent Achilles reflexes. If the radicular symptoms are unilateral, one must look for an asymmetrical reflex diminution or absence on the side of the pain before it is considered significant.

Sensory Changes

Various instruments and gadgets are available to test sensation, such as pinwheels, along the circumference of which are multiple points which can be rolled over the surface of the body. After practicing with one of these instruments, I always seem to return to the humble safety pin. In testing sensation with a pin it is best to test a specific area and compare it with the same region in the opposite extremity. Certain sites tend to be more sensitive than others. For example, the fleshy portion of the calf which indents under the pinpoint is less sensitive to pinprick than the unyielding skin over the anterior tibial region, despite identical pressure. Because of this difference in anatomical sensitivity, it would be a mistake to compare two different sites. Examination may occasionally elicit sensory changes, which do not correlate with the other clinical findings or do not follow a dermatomal pattern. Because of the subjective aspect of sensory testing, an abnormal sensory pattern is considered of clinical significance only if it can be correlated

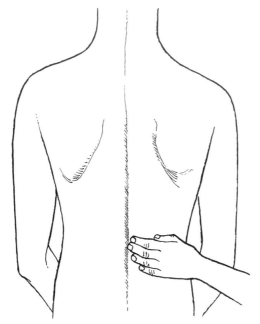

Fig. 6-9. Appreciation of paraspinal muscle spasm is best done by placing the fingers at the midline and palpating laterally.

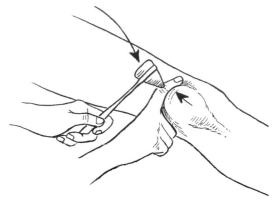

Fig. 6-10. The suprapatellar reflex.

Straight Leg Raising

Pain occurs with straight leg raising on the affected side and usually the opposite leg can be raised without any great discomfort. Occasionally, straight leg raising on the unaffected side is productive of pain in the affected side.

CONSIDERATION OF OTHER LESIONS

Any patient with back and leg pain must have evaluation of peripheral vascular status. The posterior tibial and dorsalis pedis arteries are examined, in addition to comparing skin temperatures in both feet.

One must always be alert to the fact that back and leg pain can occur with metastatic, intra-abdominal and retroperitoneal lesions.

ELECTROMYOGRAPHY

Electromyography is a test which will reveal evidence of motor changes secondary to nerve root involvement. It requires the presence of nerve demyelinization before it will reveal muscle dysfunction, so that it is of no value in the first three weeks after onset of root compression. The muscle fibrillation effect of demyelinization will be noted with this test for a variable period of time after

with the other radicular signs and symptoms.

In carrying out a sensory examination it is important to use the same number of pinpricks in comparing opposite limbs, since the physiological principle of recruitment of stimuli is in effect; and not only each individual pinprick, but the total number of pricks creates an overall sensory impression.

Motor Dysfunction

The most revealing test of motor weakness is the action of muscles under weight bearing. When a patient walks on his toes, if there is some slight calf muscle weakness, there may be a tendency to drop the heel a little closer to the ground on the weaker side with each step. With weakness of the dorsiflexors of the foot, a slight weakness can be demonstrated by having the patient walk on his heels; and the examiner will note a slight tendency for the toes to drop closer to the floor each time weight bearing occurs.

actual root compression has subsided, so that often clinical evidence of improvement is seen long before this can be elicited on an EMG. Electromyography may be helpful in order to differentiate nonorganic weakness from muscle dysfunction secondary to root pressure. Aside from confirmation of a clinical impression, this test is not particularly helpful in evaluating lumbar disc lesions.

X-RAY FINDINGS

X-rays of the lumbosacral spine are necessary in the evaluation of all patients who are considered to have lumbar disc disease. The physician should look for intervertebral space narrowing with or without hypertrophic osteoarthritis of the adjacent vertebral bodies. Occasionally, condensation or sclerosis of the subchondral bone of the vertebral bodies above and below the involved disc may be seen. Calcification either in the nucleus pulposus or the annulus fibrosis may be significant.

Vacuum Phenomenon

The vacuum or pneumatization phenomenon should also be looked for, although the actual significance of this finding is uncertain, and it may occur without any significant symptomatology. The vacuum phenomenon is noted on extension and may last for only a short time, so that the x-ray has to be taken quite promptly. Some authorities imply that this phenomenon indicates gross fissuring of the annulus.

Intervertebral Disc Space Narrowing

Narrowing of the intervertebral disc space is probably the single most valuable plain radiographic finding in lumbar disc disease, although it is often difficult to interpret. In some cases, it may be more apparent than real when the angulation of the x-ray tube is such that a false impression is created, with one interspace appearing wider than the other as a result of improper radiographic technique. Often, these narrowings may be

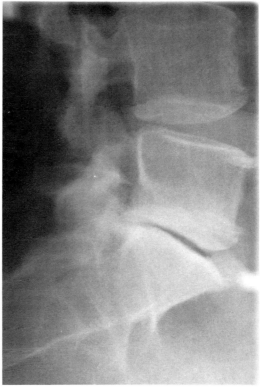

Fig. 6-11. Vacuum phenomenon L5–S1 intervertebral disc.

quite subtle, and it should further be remembered that the L5–S1 interspace is often narrowed after the age of 35, which may be indicative of the usual degenerative process occurring with advanced years and not represent symptom-producing lumbar disc disease. Narrowing will also occur with acute infection, such as pyogenic, or chronic infections, such as TB. Often, such narrowing is related to an old, previously existing infection, which at this time has long since resolved and is not directly related to the presenting symptoms. In addition to narrowing, arthrosis of the intervertebral joints of the lumbar spine with osteophyte formation, sclerosis and condensation of the subchondral bone may be indicative of lumbar disc pathology. These findings are of greater significance when they are limited to one intervertebral space. In elderly patients such

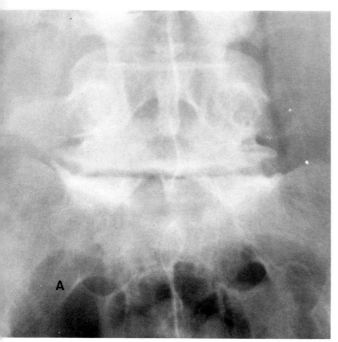

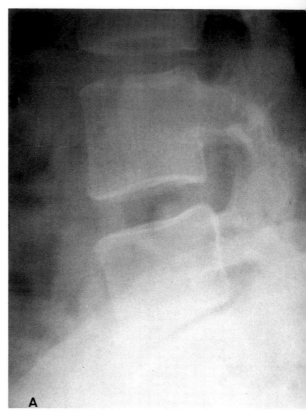

Fig. 6-12. A, This 47-year-old woman complained of long-standing low back and right sciatic pain compatible with L5 nerve root compression. Plain x-ray films demonstrated extensive degenerative changes at the L5–S1 level with considerable intervertebral disc narrowing, sclerosis, and hypertrophic osteoarthritis. The myelogram demonstrated a filling defect at the L4–5 level compatible with a protruding intervertebral disc. Excision of this lesion produced good relief of pain. This case is a good demonstration of the discrepancy between x-ray changes and symptom producing lesions.

B, Disc protrusion beneath L5 nerve root.

alterations are widespread, involving much of the lumbar spine and may not be associated with a specific symptom-producing condition.

Vertebral Body Alignment

Changes in alignment of the vertebral bodies may occur when the posterior facets are in an oblique downward and forward plane, allowing the upper vertebrae to settle in a slightly posterior position in relationship to the lower vertebrae. Often backward displacement of the fifth lumbar vertebra occurs at the L5–S1 level; it can also be encountered at the 4–5 and 3–4 levels, but less frequently.

Degenerative Changes

It is rare to see calcification of the nucleus pulposus, but calcification of the anterior portion of the annulus is common, particularly in elderly patients or those who have considerable intervertebral lumbar arthrosis.

On reviewing lumbar spine x-rays, one can see disc lesions that involve the superior and inferior cartilaginous plates and sometimes protrude anteriorly. Except as an indication of lumbar disc degeneration, in most cases these lesions are not symptom producing. Symptoms usually occur in association with posterior protrusions of the annulus fibrosus and disc.

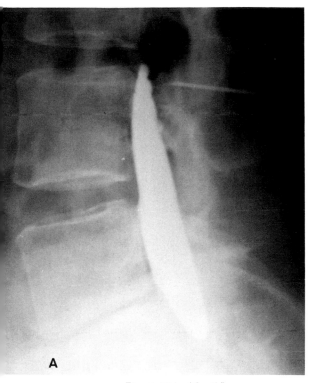

A

Fig. 6-12A. (*Cont'd*)

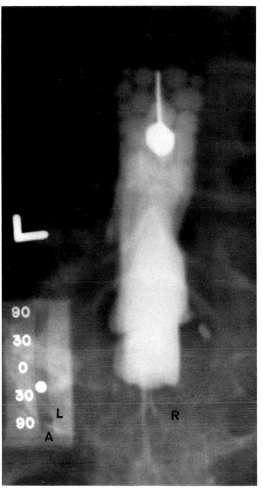

Fig. 6-12A. (*Cont'd*)

Anterior displacement of nuclear material is more common than generally appreciated, because this lesion is not symptom producing. When extruded nuclear tissue penetrates the anterior fibers of the annulus, coming to lie immediately beneath the anterior longitudinal ligament, an erosion of the centrum at the site of the protrusion may occur. Eventually, this type of lesion will form an anterior osteophyte.

Schmorl described extrusions of nuclear material into the spongiosa of the vertebral bodies. This penetration of nuclear tissue usually occurs just behind the center of the cartilaginous plate where it is quite thin and sometimes defective. Reactive formation of a thin layer of dense bone around the displaced material occurs within the spongiosa of the vertebra, allowing diagnosis of this lesion on plain x-rays. Because of his original description of this condition, these are usually referred to as Schmorl's nodes.

Narrowing and stenosis of the inter-

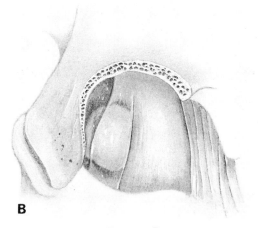

B

Fig. 6-12B.

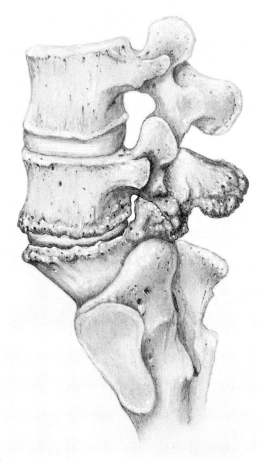

Fig. 6-13. Stenosis of the L5–S1 intervertebral foramen secondary to degenerative changes.

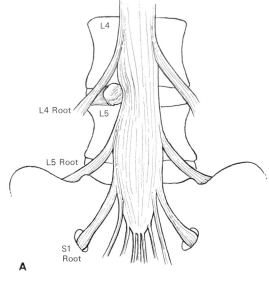

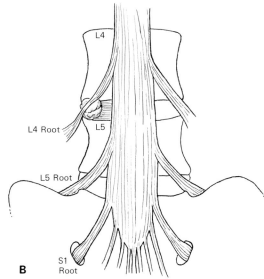

vertebral foramina is best seen on lateral and oblique views of the lumbar spine. Often, this will be seen at many levels and may not be associated with symptoms. However, if a root is irritated and becomes swollen at a level where there is intervertebral foraminal encroachment, radicular symptoms will likely occur.

Prior to myelography about 55 percent of the plain x-rays of patients with suspected lumbar disc disease were interpreted as revealing significant lumbar interspace narrowing, and the next most common abnormality was degenerative changes involving the lumbar vertebrae.

Postoperative review of some of the plain

Fig. 6-14. Foraminal root compression syndrome.

A, The usually situated L4–5 disc protrusion will impinge upon the L5 nerve root.

B, A laterally situated L4–5 disc protrusion will extend into the intervertebral foramen impinging upon the L4 root.

x-rays using hindsight, revealed only 10 percent that were perfectly normal with no congenital defect, no sacralized or lumbarized vertebrae or other evidence of abnormality.

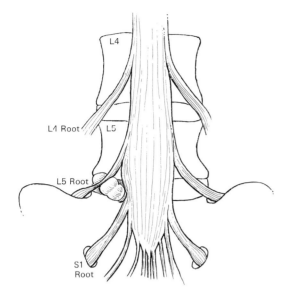

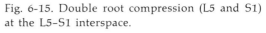

Fig. 6-15. Double root compression (L5 and S1) at the L5–S1 interspace.

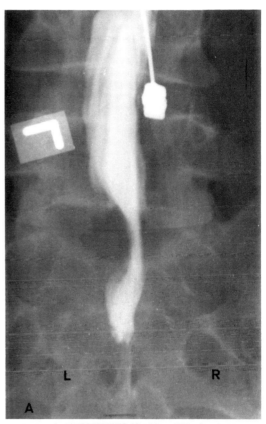

FORAMINAL ROOT COMPRESSION SYNDROME

In the lower lumbar region, the nerve root departs from the dural sac approximately 2 cm. above the point of exit, through the intervertebral foramen. The L5 nerve root exits from the L5–S1 intervertebral foramen, at which point it passes over the lateral aspect of the L5–S1 intervertebral disc. An appreciation of this anatomical relationship productive of the foraminal root compression syndrome will be most helpful in identification of this entity. It usually presents clinically with typical signs and symptoms of L5 root compression, presumably due to lumbar disc protrusion at the L4–5 interspace. Myelography may reveal a defect at the L5–S1

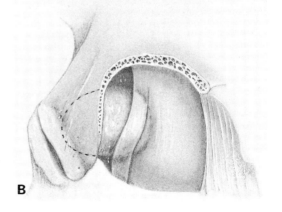

Fig. 6-16. A and B, This 54-year-old man presented with severe long-standing left sciatica. Examination revealed a partial foot drop on the left in addition to an absent left Achilles reflex. Sensory impairment was noted over dorsum of foot within the L5 dermatome as well as the lateral aspect of the left foot. The myelogram revealed a large filling defect at the L5–S1 level and was normal at the L4–5 level. At surgery, a large completely extruded fragment of disc was found compressing both the S1 root within the spinal canal and the L5 root as it passed through the intervertebral foramen.

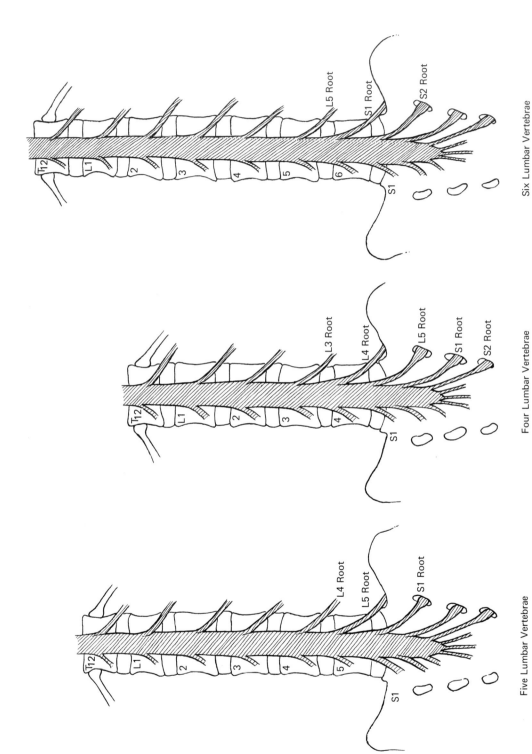

Fig. 6-17. Transitional lumbosacral vertebral and root function.

Five Lumbar Vertebrae

Four Lumbar Vertebrae

Six Lumbar Vertebrae

interspace or may be unrevealing. When the myelogram is positive one interspace below the clinically suspected site, this unanticipated finding may be construed by the physician as documentation of a "prefixed" lumbar plexus, with the S1 root subserving the functions and dermatomal pattern normally fulfilled by the L5 root. Such a root function variance in the absence of transitional vertebrae is extremely rare, and the apparent anomaly is more likely due to lateral root compression at the intervertebral foramen.

A normal myelogram may occur when a completely extruded disc fragment has migrated laterally toward the foramen beyond the edge of the dural sac or when the sac itself is unusually narrow. This set of circumstances can lead to a serious error when, because of persisting pain and despite a normal myelogram, a decision is made to perform surgery; and the surgeon concentrates his exploratory efforts on the L4–5 interspace based on the clinical picture. If the surgeon is not satisfied that the findings of the L4–5 exploration are compatible with the pain

syndrome, he may turn to the L5–S1 interspace. A cursory exploration of that level which omits a facet resection and foraminotomy may overlook the laterally extruded symptom-producing fragment of disc.

A variation of the foraminal root compression syndrome is compression of two roots by an extensively protruding disc. The S1 root is compressed by the medial portion of the protrusion and the L5 root by the laterally extruded fragment.

Three distinctive characteristics may help identify foraminal compression of the L5 nerve root:

1. Straight leg raising is often not particularly painful.
2. Lateral flexion to either side is not painful.
3. The radicular pain may remain quiescent for prolonged periods, but motor dysfunction in the form of great toe extensor weakness persists.

Because of these characteristics, the condition can be confused with peroneal neuritis.

TRANSITIONAL LUMBOSACRAL VERTEBRAE AND ROOT FUNCTION

Transitional lumbosacral vertebrae occur in approximately 6 percent of the population as a whole. This implies that the last (fifth) lumbar vertebra assumes the anatomical appearance of the first sacral segment, resulting in only 4 lumbar vertebrae, or the first sacral vertebra anatomically resembles the last lumbar vertebra resulting in 6 lumbar vertebrae. A sacralized lumbar vertebra is described as sacralization and a lumbarized sacral vertebra, lumbarization.[9]

In considering identification of root func-

tion in the presence of lumbosacral transitional vertebrae, "counting down" from the last rib is usually a more reliable guide than "counting up" from the nonsegmented solid sacrum. In other words, a disc protrusion at the L5–6 interspace will likely be associated with a symptom complex characteristic of an L5–S1 protrusion. However, this is far from an infallible rule and, in the face of transitional vertebra, root localization will remain uncertain.

TREATMENT OF LUMBAR DISC DISEASE

Selection of proper treatment is related to a number of factors, duration of symptoms being of foremost importance. The patient who has had recurrent symptoms of lumbar disc disease for a number of years may be

a suitable candidate for surgery, while the individual, with recently developed back pain and sciatica, requires a suitable course of conservative management. The presence of motor dysfunction, in addition to severity

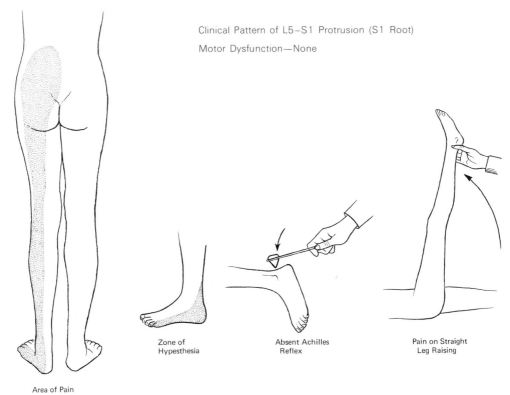

Clinical Pattern of L5–S1 Protrusion (S1 Root)

Motor Dysfunction—None

Zone of
Hypesthesia

Absent Achilles
Reflex

Pain on Straight
Leg Raising

Area of Pain

Fig. 6-18. Clinical pattern of L5–S1 disc protrusion.

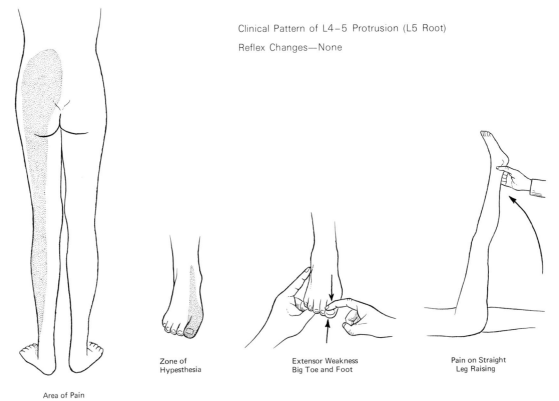

Clinical Pattern of L4–5 Protrusion (L5 Root)

Reflex Changes—None

Zone of
Hypesthesia

Extensor Weakness
Big Toe and Foot

Pain on Straight
Leg Raising

Area of Pain

Fig. 6-19. Clinical pattern of L4–5 disc protrusion.

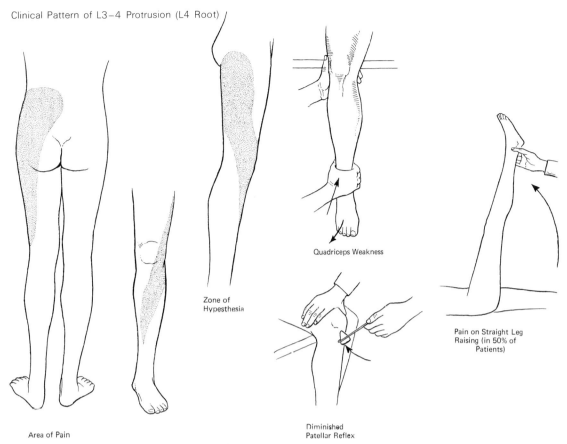

Fig. 6-20. Clinical pattern of L3-4 disc protrusion.

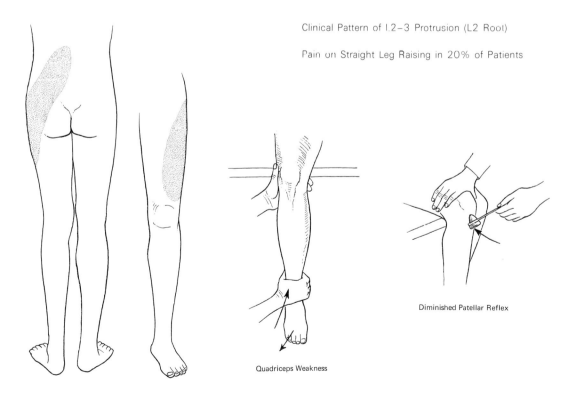

Fig. 6-21. Clinical pattern of L2-3 disc protrusion.

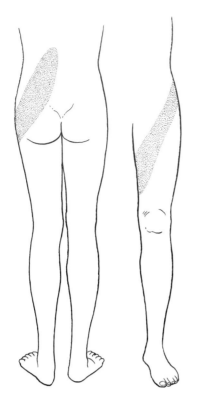

Clinical Pattern of L1–2 Protrusion (L1 Root)

Slightly Weak Quadriceps

No Pain on Straight Leg
Raising

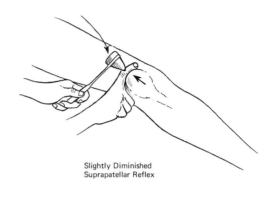

Slightly Diminished
Suprapatellar Reflex

Area of Pain and
Zone of Hypesthesia

Fig. 6-22. Clinical pattern of L1–2 disc protrusion.

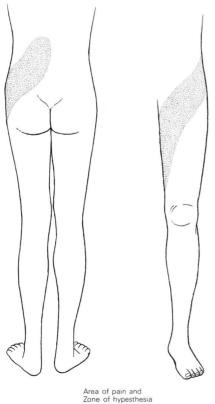

Clinical Pattern of T12

L1 Protrusion (T12 Root)

No Motor Dysfunction

No Reflex Changes

No Motor Dysfunction

No Pain on Straight Leg
Raising

The Clinical Pattern

Area of pain and
Zone of hypesthesia

Fig. 6-23. Clinical pattern of T12–L1 disc protrusion. No motor dysfunction. No reflex change. No pain on straight leg raising.

Table 6-1. CLINICAL DIFFERENTIATION OF AFFECTED LEVEL

Most patients with lumbar disc disease affecting any level, have back pain which is sensitive to mechanical and postural changes. Clinical differentiation of the specific level is principally determined by the area of pain, site of sensory dysfunction, specific motor dysfunction, reflex changes, and response to straight leg raising. The following table is a summary of the principal differentiating characteristics.

	Area of Pain	Sensory Dysfunction (Subjective and Objective)	Motor Dysfunction	Reflex Changes	Straight Leg Raising Test
L5–S1	Low back Buttock Sciatic distribution extending to lateral aspect of foot	Lateral aspect foot	None	Diminished or absent Achilles reflex	Positive
L4–5	Low back Buttock Sciatic distribution extending over dorsum of foot toward big toe	Dorsum foot	Extensor weakness big toe and foot	None	Positive
L3–4	Low back Lateral buttock and hip Posterolateral aspect thigh and anterior tibial area Midlumbar area Lateral hip	Posterolateral thigh and anterior tibial area, rarely below upper third of leg	Quadriceps weakness	Diminished patellar reflex	Patients positive 50%
L2–3	Anterolateral thigh (never below knee) Midlumbar Flank	Anterolateral thigh	Quadriceps weakness	Diminished patellar or suprapatellar reflex	Patients negative 80%
L1–2	Anterior and medial aspect upper thigh Midlumbar Flank	Anterior and medial aspect upper thigh	Slightly weak quadriceps	Slightly diminished suprapatellar reflex	Negative
T12–L1	Inguinal region and medial thigh	Inguinal region and medial thigh	None	None	Negative

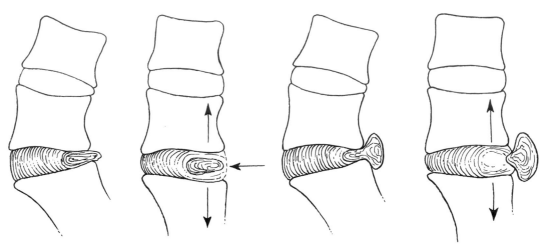

Fig. 6-24. Positive effect of traction upon pro-truding fragment of disc.

Fig. 6-25. Adverse effect of traction upon pro-truding fragment of disc.

of pain, are essential considerations in deter-mining method of management. The pa-tient's ability to tolerate pain, the medication required for pain relief and the existence of secondary gain all deserve attention in mak-ing a decision. The socioeconomic status and the physical requirements of work are also factors. Are we dealing with a patient who is content to rest in bed for an indefinite period of time, hoping that surgery can be avoided? Or, is this a patient with limited resources, who must return to work in a stated period of time; and when returning, must he be able to perform physically stren-uous work for an indefinite period?

If we do elect to treat conservatively with rest and medication, how long should we wait before considering surgery? How long should we wait if there is a partial foot drop? How long before irreversible motor weak-ness will occur so that, despite eventual de-compressive surgery, persisting dysfunction persists? Many patients manifest a symptom complex presenting clear indications for ap-propriate management. Others will have a more provisional clinical picture, and only the physician's judgment, based on his expe-rience and careful evaluation of the individ-ual factors, can be relied upon to determine a proper course of treatment.

CONSERVATIVE MANAGEMENT

Since all of the following methods of treat-ment which comprise the basic essentials of the conservative management of lumbar disc disease are presented in more detail in Chapter 4, it is advisable to review pages 95–117.

Rest

Almost every patient with lumbar disc disease is helped by rest and worsened by activity. Such a direct cause and effect rela-tionship may not be so readily apparent to the patient, who may appreciate some in-crease in the stiffness and discomfort of the paraspinal muscles after a period of inac-tivity, while after walking and performing some light activity will feel more "limber." The muscle spasm and pain are not primary symptoms but are secondary effects of the protruding lumbar disc. Goaded, by this seemingly paradoxical effect, the patient may intentionally increase the level of physical activities, with the thought of "working out the stiffness in my back," which may, all too frequently, result in such an acute flare-up of symptoms as to be completely incapac-itating.

Traction

Pelvic traction is employed routinely in conjunction with bed rest. The traction apparatus is positioned to promote increased lumbar flexion. This spinal position will promote distraction of the posterior elements of the lumbar spine, reducing tensile stress on the annulus fibrosus and widening the intervertebral foraminal apertures at the lower two interspaces. Nerve root compression at these levels may be relieved by so altering the position of the lumbar spine.

Physiotherapy

The use of heat and gentle massage is often helpful in relieving muscle pain and

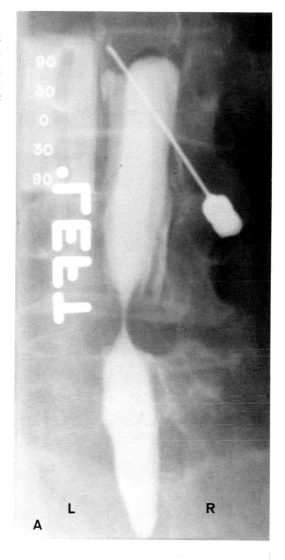

Fig. 6-26. A and B, This 18-year old man was hospitalized with long-standing low back and right sciatic pain. He had typical signs of L5 nerve root compression with weakness of the right great toe extensor and hypesthesia over the dorsum of the right foot within the L5 dermatome. Conservative treatment consisting of bed rest and pelvic traction was instituted; and after two days of traction, he noted left sciatic pain in addition to the original right sciatica. Myelography demonstrated a large bilateral filling defect at the L4–5 interspace. At surgery the disc was completely extruded on the right side and markedly protruded on the left. Traction was probably a factor in aggravating the protrusion on the left side.

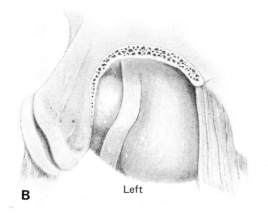

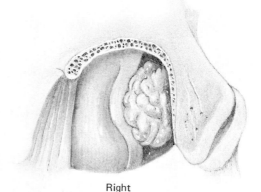

B   Left   Right

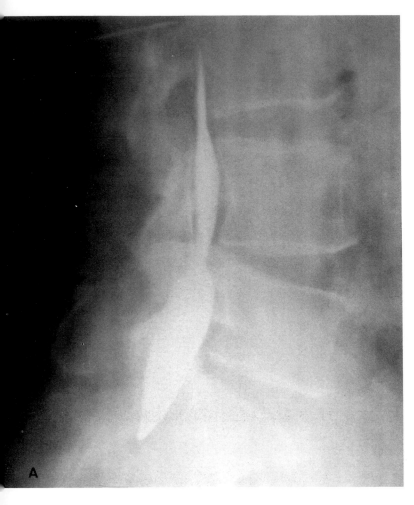

Fig. 6-27. A and B, This 53-year-old man was treated by lumbar manipulation therapy for long-standing low back and left sciatic pain. Following a spinal torsion maneuver the patient suddenly developed a severe right sciatic pain associated with a right partial foot drop. Myelography demonstrated a bilateral filling defect at the L4–5 interspace larger on the right side. Surgery revealed a disc protrusion on the left with an extensive disruption of the annular fibers and a large free fragment of completely extruded disc material on the right side. The annulus on the right side appeared intact and after removing the free fragment on the right, the disc did not appear to protrude. It appeared that the free extruded fragment on the right had originated from the annular lesion clearly visualized on the left.

spasm. However, it must be recognized that the muscle symptoms are secondary to protrusion of an intervertebral disc producing annular distension and root pressure. Moving the patient, especially during a period of acute symptoms, may aggravate this primary condition. If transporting the patient to a department of physiotherapy, or any of the physiotherapeutic measures employed, are pain producing, they should be stopped.

Trigger Points

If a specific localized area of the lumbar region is persistently painful, Xylocaine infiltration of the site is in order. This may be helpful in providing relief of localized muscle discomfort, but it will probably not affect the overall outcome of conservative management.

Manipulation of the Low Back

A clear lumbar disc syndrome with back pain and radicular symptoms should not, in my opinion, receive manipulation. If radicular symptoms are absent, in which case the diagnosis is open to question, manipulation can be considered.

Medication

The dosage and potency of medication should be commensurate with the intensity of symptoms. The patient should be maintained in reasonable comfort. Avoid doling out inadequate amounts of analgesic drugs.

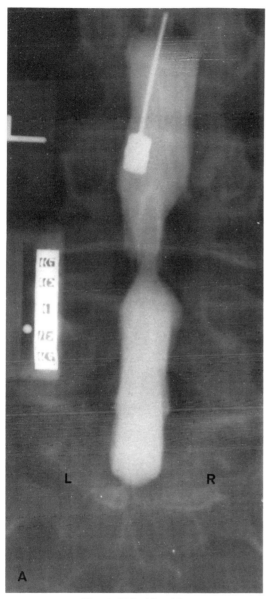

Fig. 6-27A. *(Cont'd)*

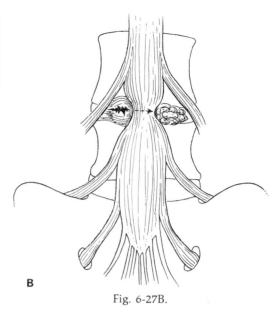

B

Fig. 6-27B.

Anti-inflammatory agents should be used in the presence of radicular symptoms.

Occupational Changes

A number of patients with lumbar disc disease, who are employed in jobs involving heavy labor, manifest a direct and apparent cause and effect relationship involving their work and recurrence of symptoms. Every effort must be made to direct and help the patient to obtain working conditions compatible with his disease. To perform lumbar disc surgery on such a patient and then allow him to return to the same work environment, may eventuate into a disservice to the patient and may reflect poorly upon the surgeon.

Activities of Daily Living

Every routine daily activity that places stress upon the lumbar spine should be thoroughly reviewed with the patient, in order to provide an appreciation of the body mechanics involved, including standing, walking, sitting, driving, lifting and sleeping.

Low Back Supports and Shoe Lifts

Following a 10-day-period of bed rest, if there is significant relief of symptoms, it is usually necessary to fit the patient with a low back support, which should be considered a temporary aid to allow progressive mobilization. This should not be worn more than 90 days, and during this time a corrective exercise and rehabilitation program is instituted to allow this appliance to eventually be discarded. (See pp. 117–123.)

If one leg is significantly shorter than the other, a shoe lift in the short leg may be helpful.

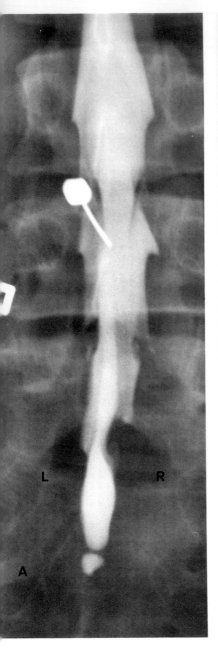

L   R

A

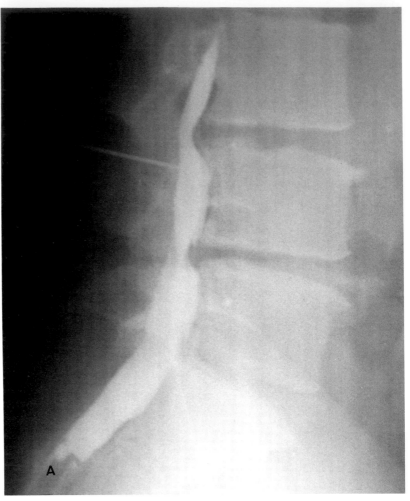

A

Fig. 6-28. A, This 35-year-old man had no significant low back dysfunction until a fall six months prior to admission was followed by severe intractable low back and right sciatic pain. His signs and symptoms were typical of S1 root compression with an absent right Achilles reflex and numbness along the lateral aspect of the right foot. Myelography demonstrated intervertebral disc protrusions at the L3–4, L4–5, and L5–S1 interspaces. The protruding disc at the L5–S1 level was excised via a right interlaminar approach with no attempt to visualize or decompress the presumably non-symptom producing lesions visualized myelographically. The patient has done well since surgery.

It must be recognized that this patient will probably be predisposed to low back dysfunction in the future and with this in mind has changed his work at my request to a job which is not physically demanding. I do not believe that "prophylactic" disc excision is an acceptable concept and think this patient is best served by confining his surgery to the symptom producing lesion.

B, Large disc protrusion L5–S1, right.

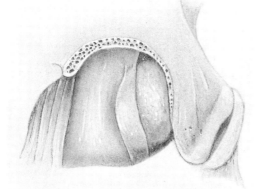

B

INADEQUATE RESPONSE TO CONSERVATIVE MANAGEMENT

Intractable Symptoms

Despite the intensive employment of all conservative means of treatment, some patients' pain will perversely remain unyieldingly fixed. This lack of response is not common and is a clinical indication of severity and irreversibility of the disc protrusion. If after a week to ten days, such a refractory situation prevails, myelography and possible surgery should be considered.

Persisting Motor Signs

When a course of conservative treatment is given to patients who exhibit motor weakness as a component of their radicular symptoms, they will often note, after several days, improvement in their pain but little or no change in motor dysfunction. This inequality, in rapidity of response to treatment, between pain and motor symptoms is usually seen.

The diminution of pain may be considered an indication to persist with conservative management, in the expectation of deriving an eventual motor improvement. If after ten days or two weeks the motor weakness has not changed, myelography should be carried out.

Delay of such duration, in the face of motor weakness, may be considered ill-advised and dilatory by some, but review of my records bears me out in demonstrating a significant number of such patients with motor weakness who responded favorably to conservative management.

Intermittent Symptoms

Many patients will note symptomatic improvement from bed rest and traction and while remaining in bed are quite comfortable, requiring no analgesic medication. However, with assumption of a weight-bearing position, recurrence of pain immediately follows. Under these circumstances, bed rest and traction are continued for several additional days, after which very gradual

and progressive mobilization is attempted. Before further mobilization is ordered, it may be helpful to have the patient fitted with a low back support, which should be worn prior to weight-bearing efforts. If despite these measures, weight bearing is not tolerated, after two weeks, myelography is in order.

Subjective Response

Variations that exist from patient to patient, in response to conservative treatment of lumbar disc disease, is conspicuous to all physicians. One patient may not be happy with an end result that another will gladly accept. These differences relate to individual temperament, mode of living and the underlying disposition to accept and live with some degree of discomfort.

A patient who leads a more sedentary existence may more readily accept some residual dysfunction than one who by inclination or necessity is physically active. The patient who is forced to earn a living by means of physical labor may not be able to tolerate lumbar disc symptoms of moderate intensity, nor will the sports-minded office worker, who is a devoted golfer or tennis player, be happy with the limitations imposed by such disease.

A decision regarding proper management of these controvertible problems must be based on the experience and judgment of the physician.

LUMBAR DISC SURGERY

Indications for Surgery

The results of disc surgery relate to a number of factors, unquestionably the most important being patient selectivity. There are certain specific guidelines that can be established for selecting patients for surgery:

1. Long-standing symptoms, with an inadequate response to conservative management.

2. Intractable pain from a clearly defined single root syndrome confirmed by myelography.

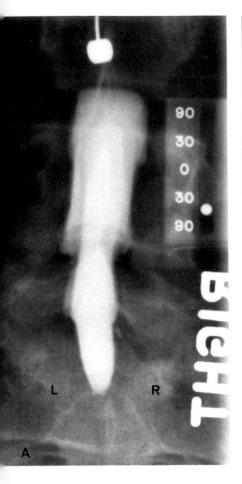

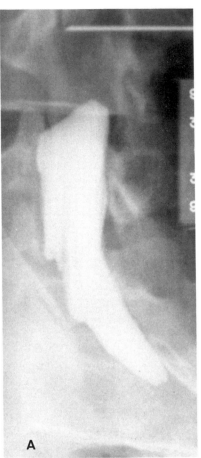

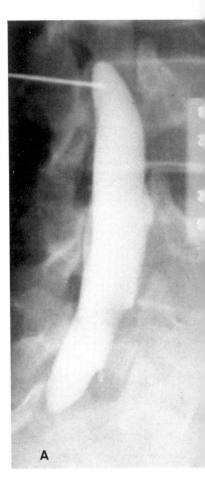

3. Persisting motor weakness, with confirmation of the lesion at myelography.

Contraindications for Surgery

1. A first episode of low back and sciatic pain, without an adequate trial of conservative management.

2. Intermittent low back pain associated with occasional pains of equivocal nature, extending into one or the other lower extremity and an equivocal myelogram.

3. A prolonged history of intermittent low back pain and an equivocal myelogram.

4. Low back and intermittent sciatic pain with a myelogram demonstrating a lesion on the "wrong" or pain-free side. I have seen several patients in whom disc surgery was performed with these criteria, and the two surgeons who elected to proceed on the basis of this information were divided in choosing the side of surgery. The one who operated upon the painful side, used as his justification, myelographic evidence of disc dysfunction at a specific interspace; and since the pain was on the opposite side, decided it would be best to decompress the root on the side of the pain rather than on the side of the myelographic defect. The surgeon who elected to operate on the side of the myelographic defect, rather than on the side of the pain, felt that the disc protrusion might cause a shift of the cauda equina enclosed within its dural sac, pressing the opposite root against the lamina and producing radicular symptoms.

5. Surgery is probably contraindicated in the face of improvement. In the presence of significant motor weakness, if some slight

Fig. 6-29. A and B, This 38-year-old lady presented with long-standing low back and right sciatic pain compatible with L5 root compression from an intervertebral disc protrusion at the L4–5 level. The myelogram was originally interpreted by the X-Ray Department as nonrevealing. Careful review and correlation of the films with the clinical picture indicated a significant elevation and "curling in" of the root sleeve at the L4–5 level on the right in association with a small defect at that level on the oblique views. Surgery revealed a large laterally placed disc protrusion at the L4–5 level.

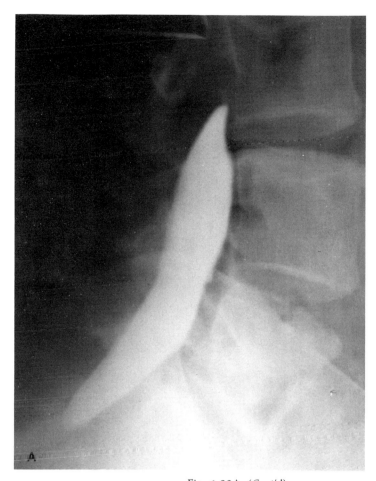

Fig. 6-29A. (*Cont'd*)

improvement occurs after surgery is scheduled, it may be justifiable to proceed. If pain is the primary symptom, improvement is an indication to cancel surgery. I adhere to this principle and have cancelled many scheduled cases on the day of surgery upon being told that the patient no longer had pain or that the pain was markedly improved. Pain surgery performed during an interval of improvement may result in patient dissatisfaction, despite an adequate postoperative result. The patient may be less willing to accept residual symptoms, even of a relatively minor nature, and is more apt to question in retrospect how pressing and indispensable the need was for surgery. If, in the face of improvement, the patient is discharged and subsequently readmitted for surgery with an exacerbation of pain, occasional residual symptoms may present less

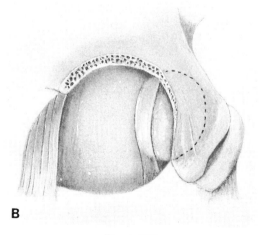

B

Fig. 6-29B.

of a problem and be tolerated more kindly. When contemplating lumbar disc surgery, the indications must be clear to the patient as well as to the surgeon.

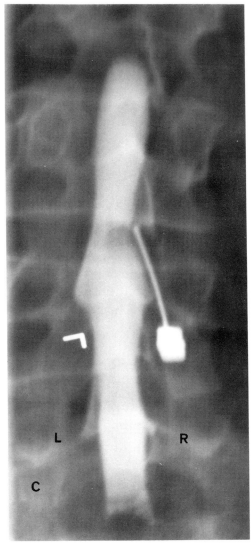

June 25, 1970

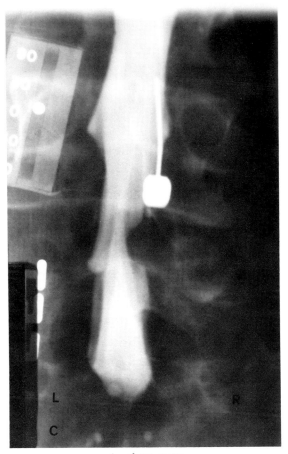

April 10, 1972

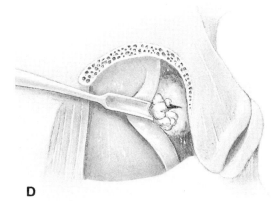

D

Fig. 6-29. C and D, This 34-year-old man presented with a 6-months' history of low back and right sciatic pain typical of an L4–5 intervertebral disc protrusion. A myelogram performed June 25, 1970, was interpreted as non-revealing. He was discharged from the hospital and treated conservatively with inadequate improvement. Because of persisting pain, he was rehospitalized and repeat myelography performed on April 10, 1972. A large filling defect was seen at the L4–5 level. Surgery revealed a protruding intervertebral disc at the L4–5 level with partial extrusion of disc fragments. In retrospect, review of the original films reveal significant root asymmetry which was probably due to a protruding disc. The large defect seen on the second myelogram was likely caused by the extruded free fragment. It must be noted that despite the striking change on myelography, the patient's symptoms remained the same from time of onset.

Normal Myelogram

A number of patients with lumbar disc disease, manifesting clear clinical evidence of single root compression symptoms, who have not responded to conservative management, will have normal myelograms. In such patients, more than the usual efforts are made to persist with conservative management. If postmyelography injection of intrathecal Depo-Medrol results in some improvement in the symptom complex, possibly one or two more injections of this medication should be given. In addition, a more prolonged period of bed rest, the wearing of a low back support, and all other nonsurgical means that can be brought to bear are utilized. If, despite these measures, severe back and sciatic pain persists, exploratory lumbar disc surgery may be indicated. It must be stressed that such cases are not frequently encountered, and many patients with a normal myelogram will eventually improve with conservative management.

SURGERY

Historical Development

Fifty years ago, an occasional laminectomy was performed for lumbar disc disease and the extruded disc fragments were identified as "chondromata," with some question regarding the exact nature of these lesions, although some surgeons did recognize them as consisting of displaced intervertebral disc material. The surgical technique utilized in the removal of such lesions invariably involved an extensive bilateral laminectomy, which was usually followed by opening the dura in the midline, separating the nerve roots to either side and by means of a narrow probe, palpating the anterior spinal canal, until the underlying protrusion was identified. The anterior dura was then incised over the most eminent portion of the hump, and through this anterior dural opening, the protruding portion of the disc was exposed and removed. The entire concept of ruptured intervertebral discs changed after the classic paper of Mixter and Barr.* They conclusively and unequivocally demonstrated the origin of these lesions, laid to rest any lingering doubts that they were neoplasms and documented their etiology as protrusions of the nucleus of an intervertebral disc. They emphasized the indications for surgical treatment of this condition. Shortly after the appearance of this paper, surgical technique for protruding lumbar intervertebral discs underwent an important change, with the dura left intact and the protruding disc removed extradurally, although the widespread bilateral laminectomy was continued. Further surgical refinements followed, including the hemilaminectomy, leaving the spinous process and lamina intact on the pain-free side. Twenty-five or thirty years ago it became common practice to carry out lumbar disc surgery in most cases by means of the unilateral interlaminar approach.

Double-check Side of Lesion

Prior to induction of anesthesia, the patient is always asked to indicate the painful leg. Of course, the painful side is noted on the chart and the myelograms are also appropriately labeled. Because the patient in the prone position has his "sides reversed" the "wrong" or unaffected side is occasionally operated upon in lumbar disc surgery. Always guard against this error by remaining alert to this possibility.

Anesthesia

Many surgeons prefer the use of spinal anesthesia, employing a hypobaric solution; epidural anesthesia also has some advocates. Intravenous pentothal supplemented with nitrous oxide and oxygen given through endotracheal tube is the anesthesia of personal choice and probably utilized by the majority of clinics for lumbar disc surgery.

* Rupture of the Intervertebral Disc Without Involvement of the Spinal Canal. New England Surgical Society, Boston, September 30, 1933.

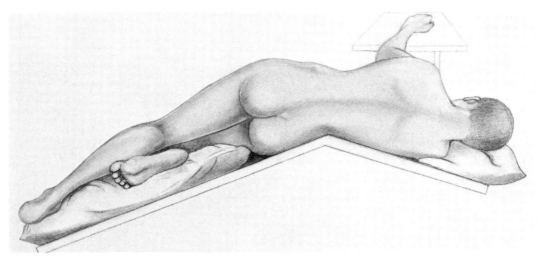

Fig. 6-30. Lateral position for lumbar disc surgery.

Position

A variety of positions have been used for operating upon patients with protruded lumbar discs.

Many surgeons favor the lateral position. The chief advantage of this position is considerable reduction of direct pressure on the abdomen or chest and hampering of respiratory excursions, since at least half of the chest wall is unencumbered in the lateral position, allowing free excursion of the upper half of the chest. As a result of decreased abdominal pressure, Batson's lumbar venous plexus is not engorged, resulting in less epidural bleeding. Also, this position does not allow blood to pool within the depths of the intervertebral space. The disadvantage of this position is some increased difficulty on the part of the assistant in holding the root retractor or performing other necessary functions. Those who are not familiar with this position may find it technically more difficult to carry out the paraspinal muscle dissection and interlaminar bony removal.

A knee-chest position is utilized by some surgeons, with the purpose of avoiding any pressure whatsoever on the abdomen and so decreasing epidural bleeding. One minor disadvantage of this position is the number of people required to place the patient in satisfactory position. A more objectionable

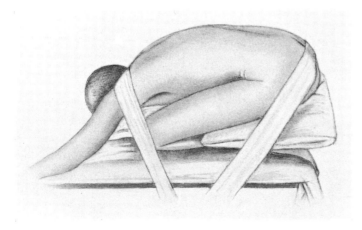

Fig. 6-31. Knee-chest position for lumbar disc surgery.

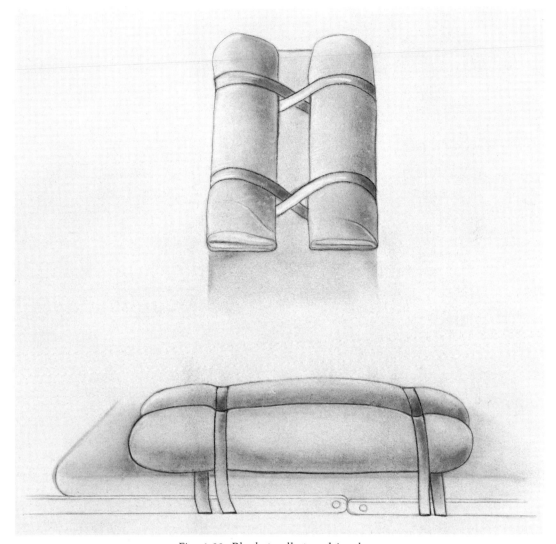

Fig. 6-32. Blanket rolls taped in place.

disadvantage is the frequent postoperative discomfort the patient suffers from stretching the hamstring muscles and from pressure lateral to the knee, resulting from this position under the total relaxation of general anesthesia.

The dangers of the acute hip and knee flexion associated with this position, exerting a tourniquet effect to the muscles of the lower extremities, must also be considered. Some surgeons are of the opinion that the resulting damage to muscles in the leg triggers the release of myoglobin. The myo-

globin in turn can overload the kidneys, while at the same time the degradation products of the muscle globulin seem to be renotoxic. An instructive case of renal failure, following a 4-hour spinal fusion performed in the knee-chest position attributed to this mechanism, was described by Dr. Keim and Dr. Weinstein.[12]

In the early and mid 1950s, a number of physicians advocated the sitting position, indicating that this position resulted in less hampering of respirations and was also associated with less epidural bleeding. Relatively

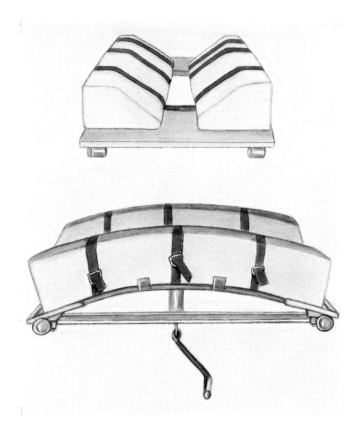

Fig. 6-33. Prone position frame.

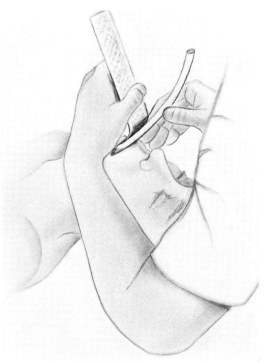

Fig. 6-34. Endotracheal anesthesia.

few clinics continue to utilize the sitting position.

My personal preference is the prone position, in which the patient is intubated on a litter, and after the endotracheal tube has been taped securely in place, the patient is rolled onto the operating table, which has previously been prepared either with blanket rolls or a "prone position frame."

A modification of the prone position is obtained by a 90° flexion of the hips and knees, with no effort to flex the lumbar spine itself. The hip flexion affords satisfactory flexion of the lumbar spine comparable to the other positions and may be associated with somewhat less abdominal pressure. To achieve this position, a minor adjustment of the operating table is accomplished by removal of the adjustable headrest and fitting it to the footrest so that it will provide adequate support for the legs.

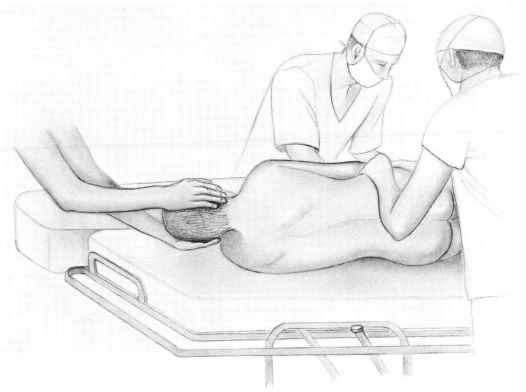

Fig. 6-35. Rolling intubated patient from litter to operating table.

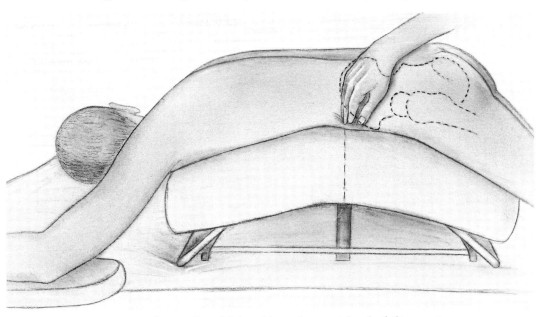

Fig. 6-36. Flexion "break" in table or frame at level of iliac crest.

Surface Landmarks

If a myelogram has been recently done, the lumbar puncture mark on the skin is used as a landmark for spinal level. For example, if the lumbar puncture needle is seen on the myelogram films to be at the L3–4 interspace, this will serve as an excellent surface guide for identification of the underlying vertebrae.

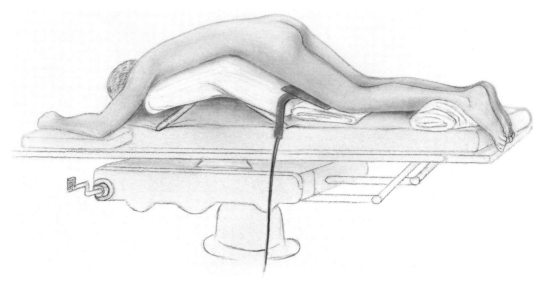

Fig. 6-37. Prone position.

If a myelogram has not been recently carried out, the first interspace at, or immediately below, the iliac crest can be considered L3–4; and using this as a starting site, one may count down to the involved interspace, scratching a "crosshatch" in the skin at that level with a sterile hypodermic needle subsequent to cleansing the skin with an alcohol sponge.

When utilizing surface guides, the elasticity of the skin must be recognized, particularly in obese patients. This elasticity may permit a surface marking to shift the extent of an interspace, with the distortion from the use of retractors and alterations in the degree of flexion during surgery.

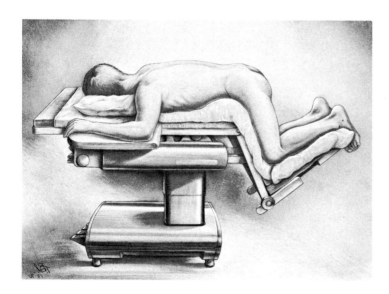

Fig. 6-38. Modified prone position.

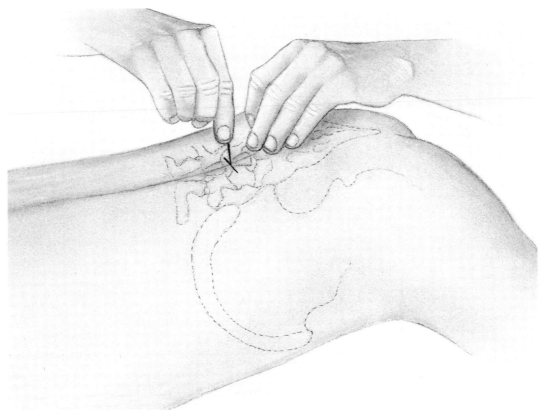

Fig. 6-39. The skin is scratched at the "involved" interspinous space.

Preparing the Skin and Draping

A variety of solutions and methods for preparing the skin surface prior to surgery are currently available. After the skin is prepared, sterile drapes can be applied in a variety of ways according to individual choice.

The draping technique of my preference is to place an adhesive transparent plastic covering sheet over the skin initially. A sterile sheet is placed above and below the previously made "crosshatch," which will be utilized as a point of reference in draping, a rectangularly perforated sheet placed overall, and the sheets then pushed up and down an appropriate distance and secured at four corners, using towel clips penetrating through the skin and adhesive plastic drape. The placement of the adhesive plastic drape initially and subsequent placement of the plain sheets and lap sheet is done to insure that no contamination will occur by moving a drape back and forth from a "nonprepped" area to the "prepped" area of proposed surgery. The Bovie cord is attached to a towel clip on the assistant's side and suction is

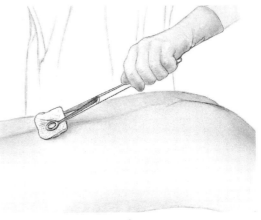

Fig. 6-40. Skin "prep."

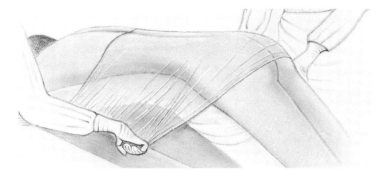

Fig. 6-41. Adhesive plastic skin covering sheet.

slipped through the handles of the towel clip on the surgeon's side.

Through the steri-drape, a double cross-hatch is placed at the involved interspace to be exposed, using the previously made needle scratch as a reference, and a single crosshatch an interspace above and below the involved interspace. If a single interspace is to be explored, there will be one double crosshatch and two single hatches above and below. If two interspaces are to be explored, two double crosshatches and a single above and below are made. The incision should extend a bit beyond the spinous processes of the vertebrae above and below surgery, since the self-retaining retractors will tend to shorten the incision length. For example, an L5–S1 disc should have an incision from L4 spinous process to the midsacrum. Prior to making the incision, palpate the spinous processes to be sure that the skin incision is made exactly in the midline. Mark only the upper and lower portions of the incision; if the entire incision is marked, one is apt to stray from the exact marking line and make a "double" incision.

Skin Incision

Guided by the preexisting marks, the initial incision should extend to the fat with the first stroke.

There are a variety of methods to control

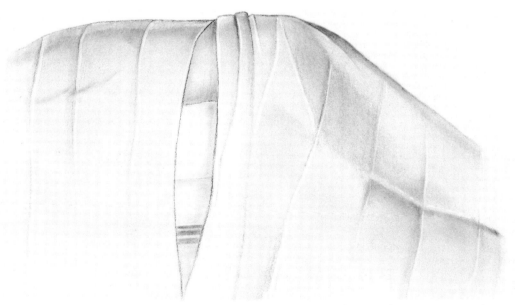

Fig. 6-42. A, Sheets above and below "crosshatch," which is used as a reference point in draping. B, Draped and clipped.

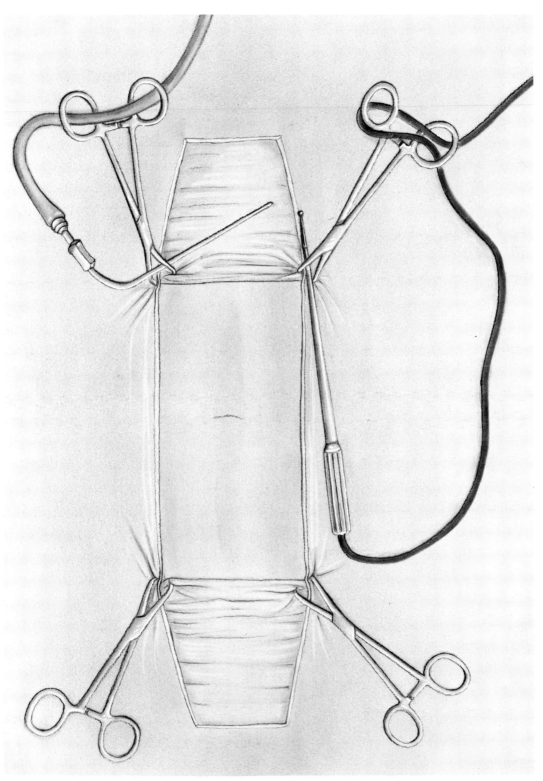

Fig. 6-42B.

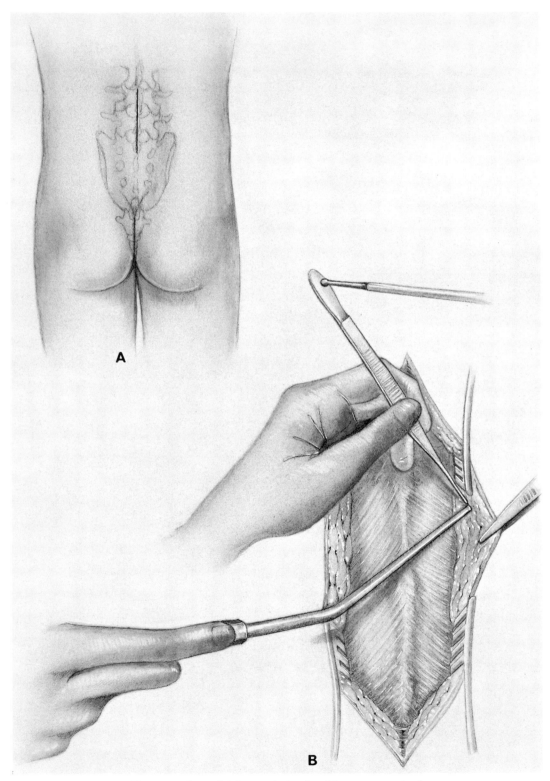

Fig. 6-43. Superficial vessels in the skin are cauterized.

skin bleeding, including Michel clips, Kolodney clamps and mosquitoes. The use of Weitlaner self-retaining retractors, which places the skin under tension, will stop most of the minor skin bleeding; the several remaining subcutaneous vessels are easily controlled by cautery. Blood vessel cauterization should not be performed with a hemostat, since it invariably results in considerable tissue destruction. When carried out near the surface of the skin, hemostat cauterization may result in a full thickness skin burn and the resulting skin slough or necrosis may eventuate into a wound infection. To properly control skin bleeding with a cautery, an assistant should use fine-toothed forceps to evert the skin edge, while the surgeon employs a sucker to locate the bleeding vessel and uses fine-tipped Cushing forceps to cau-

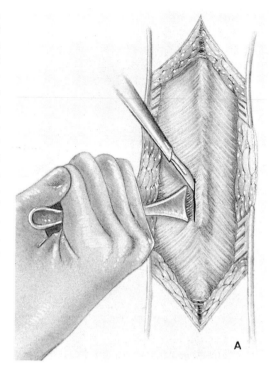

Fig. 6-44. A, B, Subperiosteal dissection technique.

A

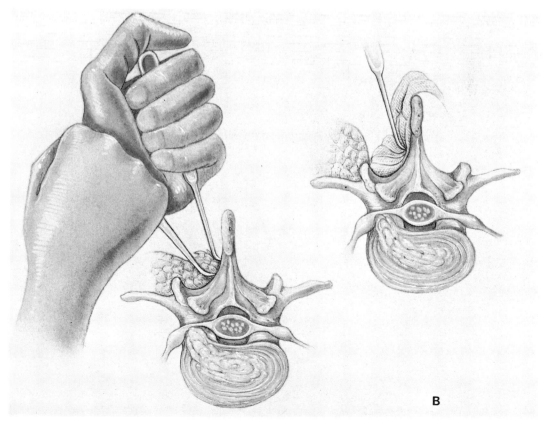

B

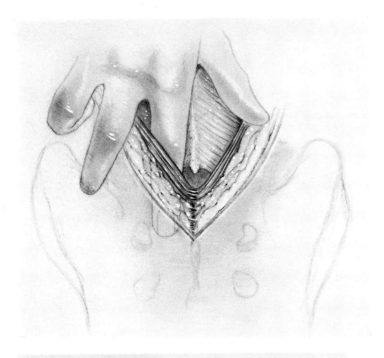

Fig. 6-45. Interspace localization, using the sacrum as the point of reference.

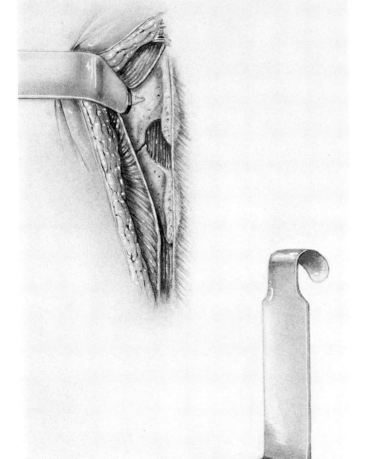

Fig. 6-46A.

Fig. 6-46. A, Taylor hemilaminectomy retractor; B, Hoen hemilaminectomy retractor; C, if the hemilaminectomy retractor blades are longer than necessary, the depth through which the surgeon must work is increased.

terize only the vessel, taking care to avoid
cautery spread to surrounding tissue.

A second knife ("clean knife") is used to
incise through fat to the fascia. If the patient
is extremely obese, the Weitlaner retractors
may have to be reset more deeply. Additional bleeding is controlled with the use of
the cautery. Do not be obsessive about
sweeping the fat cleanly away from the fascia, remember you are carrying out a surgical
procedure not an anatomical exposure. This
wasted step can only serve to increase the
blood loss, and even more serious, a false
space has been created, which may fill with
blood in the postoperative period.

Subperiosteal Dissection

A subperiosteal dissection is carried out
unilaterally, using bimanual periosteal elevator technique. The periosteal elevator is used
to retract the muscle from the spinous process. Then cut directly against the bone of the
spinous process and a second periosteal elevator is used to peel the fascia cleanly from
each spinous process and lamina without
penetrating muscle, which is the principal
source of bleeding. After the subperiosteal
dissection has been accomplished under
direct vision, a sponge extended to its full
length is used to strip the bone of any remaining fragments of muscle and fascia. As

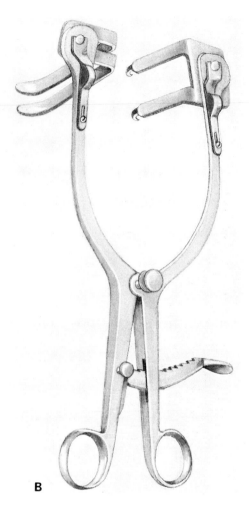

B

Fig. 6-46B.

Blades of suitable length

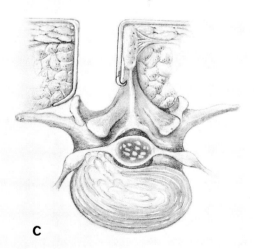

C

Blades too long

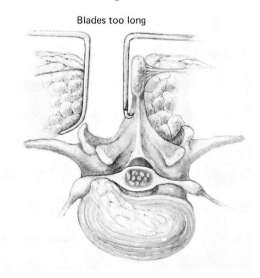

Fig. 6-46C.

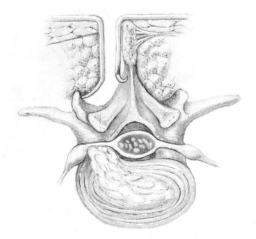

Fig. 6-47. Avoid impinging tip of muscle blade against articular facet.

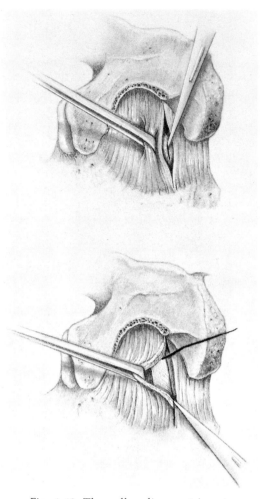

Fig. 6-49. The yellow ligament is cut.

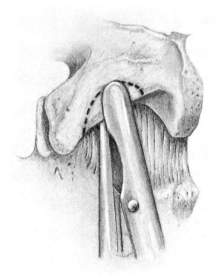

Fig. 6-48. The overhanging edge of the superior lamina is rongeured.

bone is cleaned with the sponge, allow it to accumulate within the incision to act as a tamponade, preventing muscle bleeding. Any bleeding occurring from the cut edge of the fascia is controlled with cautery before advancing to the next spinous process. The subperiosteal muscle dissection is continued until the laminae above and below the involved interspace are exposed. For example, an L4–5 disc requires an exposure of L3 to the upper edge of the sacrum. The sub-

periosteal muscle dissection is carried out laterally to expose the articulation between the superior and inferior articular processes.

After all surface bleeding has been controlled, remove sponges and localize the desired interspace by the time-honored method of palpating the sacrum and then counting up from it. Check this localization with plain spine x-rays to be sure that the patient does not have a lumbarized first sacral segment or sacralized fifth lumbar segment. Then correlate skeletal localization with the myelographic defect.

After being completely satisfied that proper localization has been established, place the hemilaminectomy retractors in po-

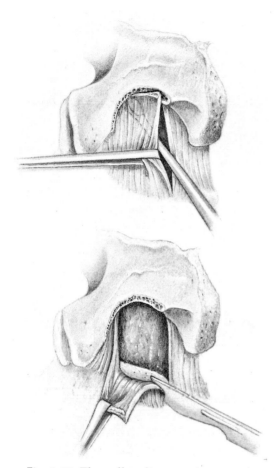

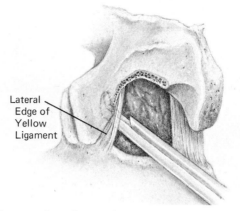

Fig. 6-51. In widening the interspace, do not mistake the rolled up lateral edge of yellow ligament for the root.

Fig. 6-50. The yellow ligament is curetted.

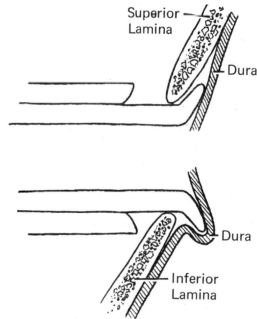

Fig. 6-52. The laminectomy punch with a 40° angled jaw is helpful when working on the superior lamina, but is not suited for the slope of the inferior lamina and may produce a dural tear.

sition. A variety of hemilaminectomy retractors are available, the simplest being the Taylor spinal retractor, consisting of a right-angled metal ribbon with a slightly hooked tip, which can be inserted laterally and cephalad to the articular facet. The great advantage of this retractor is its simplicity, with lack of any moving parts; the disadvantage is that it either has to be handheld by the assistant or tied to the base of the operating table and in some cases tied to the foot of the operator. Also, it has the unhappy propensity of slipping out of place, invariably during the worst possible moment of the procedure.

Most surgeons prefer a self-retaining hemilaminectomy retractor based on the many modifications of the Hoen hemilaminectomy retractor.

When positioning the hemilaminectomy retractors, use the shortest blades possible to achieve adequate exposure, so that the flange

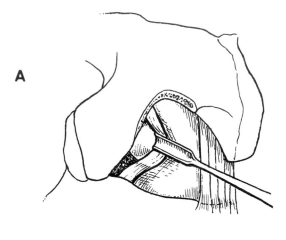

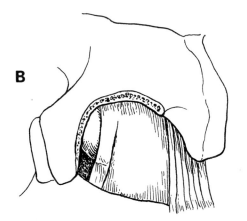

Fig. 6-53. A, Overstretched root and dural sac with an inadequate lateral bony exposure; B, very little root retraction is necessary with adequate lateral bony exposure.

of the blades will rest flush with the skin surface rather than projecting above the skin and increasing the depth through which the surgeon must work. The spinous process blade of the retractor should fit between the spinous interspaces with the hook or hooks embedded into the interspinous ligaments. The muscle blade should rise above the hump of the articular facet. An occasional error is to impinge the tip of the muscle blade against the facet, causing the exposure to be needlessly narrow. By placing the para-

spinal muscles under tension, the retractors will stop most muscle bleeding. After the retractors are in place and the exposure is deemed satisfactory, any remaining muscle bleeding is controlled with the use of the cautery.

Developing the Interspace

The laminae vary greatly in width and also in angulation and relative position to each other, so that occasionally the interlaminar space is sufficiently wide to permit exposure and removal of a protruding intervertebral disc without removal of any, or very little, bone. This widened interlaminar space is seen most commonly between the L5–S1 levels and much less frequently above that interspace.

When dealing with an interspace of normal dimensions, a duck-billed rongeur is used to remove the overhanging, inferior edge of the superior vertebrae. If working on the L5–S1 interspace, this would be the inferior edge of the L5 lamina. Bone wax is used to control all bone bleeding from the rongeured edge of the lamina. After the overhang of the superior lamina has been removed, an ample area of the ligamentum flavum is exposed to view. It is incised with a No. 11 blade on a long handle making a shallow incision in the ligamentum flavum; the edge of the incision is grasped with an Alyce forceps and gently tugged in order to spread the incision, allowing the No. 11 blade to carefully incise the entire thickness of the yellow ligament down to the epidural fat. After introducing a small moistened cotton patty beneath the ligamentum flavum to separate the dura from the ligamentum flavum, this incision is then extended from superior lamina to inferior lamina, taking care to insert merely the tip of the blade beneath the ligament to avoid accidentally cutting into the dura. A second Alyce is used to get a firmer grasp on the full thickness of yellow ligament, and a curette is introduced below the yellow ligament against the inferior surface of the superior vertebra, per-

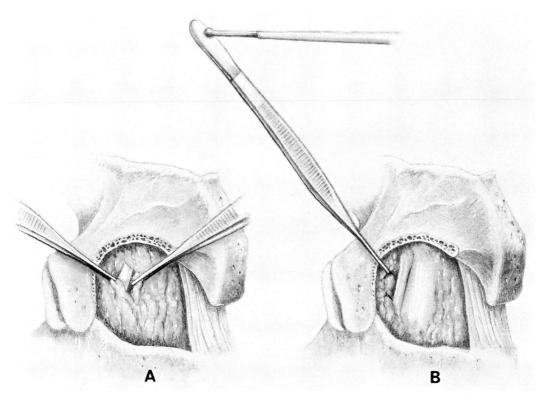

Fig. 6-54. A, Separation of epidural fat to expose dura and root; B, avoid cauterization of blood vessels within the epidural fat unless nerve root is completely exposed. Cauterization is best carried out when nerve root is visualized and out of cautery range.

mitting a flap of yellow ligament to be curetted laterally with the remaining attachment to the dorsal surface of the inferior lamina. This attachment can then safely be excised with scalpel or scissors. A Kerrison laminectomy punch with a 40° angled jaw is used to increase the size of the interspace. When introducing the Kerrison punch into the interspace, be sure to go below the yellow ligament as it sweeps up laterally. To mistake the lateral roll of yellow ligament for the nerve root can be a dangerous error, since in attempting to retract the root, one would actually be retracting a rolled sliver of ligamentum flavum and could potentially damage the root which is often underlying this site.

A thin edge of bone is removed from the superior edge of the inferior lamina using a laminectomy punch that is not angled downward. The 40° angled jaw is helpful in working on the superior lamina and laterally, but may produce a dural tear at the inferior lamina.

In carrying out a lateral bony exposure, a partial or complete removal of a facet may be expedient in approaching a foraminal disc and does not appear to result in postoperative weakness or pain in the spine.

Extension of the lateral exposure into the facet may be of value for 3 reasons:

1. Facilitation of satisfactory disc excision with less danger of "overstretching" the nerve root and dural sac as these structures are retracted medially. With an adequate lateral exposure, very little, if any, root retraction is necessary to afford good access to the disc.

2. With a satisfactory lateral exposure, a

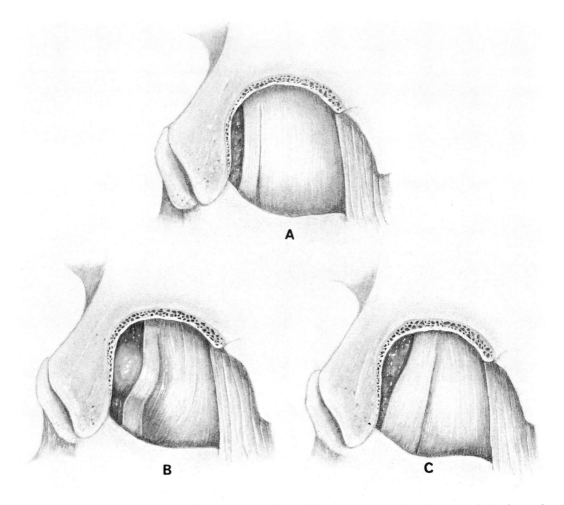

Fig. 6-55. The root may appear elevated or swollen indicating compression; A, normal; B, elevated; C, swollen.

partial foraminotomy is accomplished, providing more space for the involved root, which almost always manifests some degree of edema and swelling. Such reduction of root compression is associated with decreased postoperative pain.[15]

3. Years after surgery, hypertrophic osteoarthritic spurring, in association with postoperative epidural scarring, will be less likely to lead to root compression symptoms in the presence of a generous lateral exposure and foraminotomy.

Following adequate bony removal, the epidural fat is completely exposed to view. Use two Cushing forceps to separate the fat from the underlying dura and peel it laterally, exposing the nerve root. Only after exposure of the nerve root can blood vessels within the epidural fat be safely cauterized without danger of damage to the root by the cautery current.

Interlaminar Surgery

Although the interlaminar space is rather small, the minute anatomy of this area does vary considerably. It is always amazing to me to see how much can be hidden in this tiny

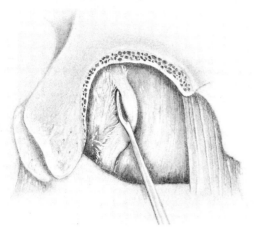

Fig. 6-56. Adhesions between nerve root and annulus in a patient with long-standing symptoms.

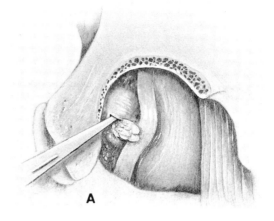

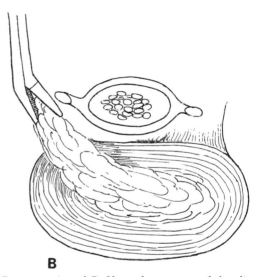

Fig. 6-57. A and B, If good exposure of the disc protrusion can be accomplished only by overstretching the root, attempt only a lateral partial exposure and disc excision.

space, and an orderly and systematic approach to this area is paramount to successful disc surgery.

Inspection. The field should be dry at this stage. If it is not possible to control the venous bleeding with the cautery, tucking small moist cotton patties under the superior and inferior laminae may be helpful. If bleeding remains a problem, decreasing lumbar flexion to a flatter prone position may alleviate abdominal pressure and so reduce engorgement of Batson's lumbar venous plexus. If this change in position is effective in controlling epidural venous bleeding, proceed with surgery in the flatter position.

Is the root elevated or is it flat? Does the root appear swollen or hyperemic, or is it of the same color as the rest of the dura?

In patients who have had long-standing symptoms, adhesions between the nerve root and the posterior longitudinal ligament are occasionally quite dense. Very careful dissection of the root and the dura may be necessary to allow free retraction and exposure of the protruding disc.

Root Tension. Using a narrow elevator, it should be possible to medially retract without resistance a root that is under no pressure. As a rule, the typical protruding disc will be quite apparent with retraction of the root medially. This manifests itself with slight elevation of the root, and upon retracting it medially one feels increased pressure. It is at this stage of the procedure that considerable care must be taken to avoid stretching a compromised root. When the disc protrusion is extensive, it is best not to retract the root too vigorously over such a high disc protrusion to avoid excessive root

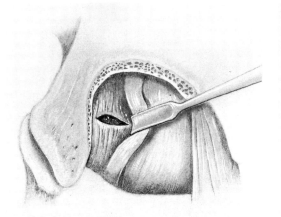

Fig. 6-58. After this partial excision has been accomplished, further root retraction is more easily accomplished over the "shell" of the protruded disc.

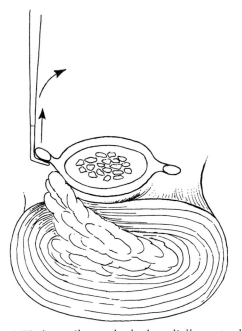

Fig. 6-59. An easily overlooked medially protruding disc. Exposure requires elevation of the root before medial retraction.

stretch. Avoid the human tendency to demonstrate, both to assistants and nurses, how large the protrusion is, for as they all gaze at this mound, the root is often being sorely stretched. It may be more desirous to only partially expose the edge of the protruding

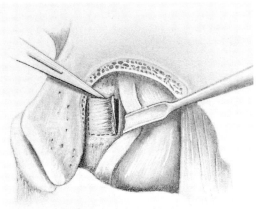

Fig. 6-60. Incision of rectangular window through the annulus fibrosus.

disc and begin the intervertebral disc excision by means of posterolateral approach before attempting to retract the root. After initially decompressing the disc posterolaterally, one can retract the root more medially over the "shell" of the protruded disc with less danger of stretching the root.

Sometimes a disc protrusion is a bit more medial and the nerve root does not appear elevated or under pressure. However, on attempting to retract the nerve root medially, an obstruction is encountered and the surgeon must take care to "lift" the root and dura to determine whether a medially protruding disc is present.

Intervertebral Disc Excision. With adequate retraction of the nerve root and dura medially, a No. 11 blade on a long handle is used to incise a rectangular window through the annulus fibrosus. This window extends from the most medial exposure of the annulus to the lateral limits of the bony exposure and comprises the entire width of the intervertebral disc, bounded by the bodies of the superior and inferior vertebrae. Through this opening, an adequate subtotal excision of disc contents can be accomplished with intervertebral disc rongeur forceps, followed by a curettage and removal of cartilaginous plates. Following such a removal of intervertebral disc material and

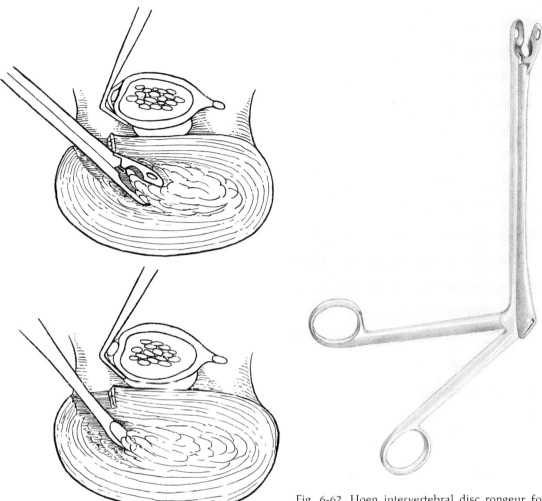

Fig. 6-61. Excision of disc contents.

Fig. 6-62. Hoen intervertebral disc rongeur forceps.

cartilaginous plates, the area of subtotal excision is replaced by firm fibrous tissue. It is generally accepted that some reduction of the intervertebral space will occur, yet when Foltz (*et al.*) checked postoperative patients a year after surgery no significant thinning was noted.[2] Possibly a year is too short a time for intervertebral narrowing to be visualized, but after a longer interval this change might be more apparent. This seems likely in view of the fact that patients with long-standing disc disease who have not had surgery will often demonstrate interspace narrowing.

A profusion of intervertebral disc rongeur forceps have been designed and modified by a host of surgeons. These variations of the forceps designed by Cushing (pituitary rongeurs) include: Love-Gruenwald, Spurling, Poppen, Cloward, Hoen, Oldberg, Raaf-Oldberg, Schlesinger, Mount, Selverstone, Spence, Voris, Louis, Takahashi, Wilde, Ferris-Smith, Farnum, Hartmann-Gruenwald. These modifications involve alterations in shaft length, type of grip, jaw shape, size and angulation.

My personal preference is the Hoen forceps, because its fenestrated jaws can grasp

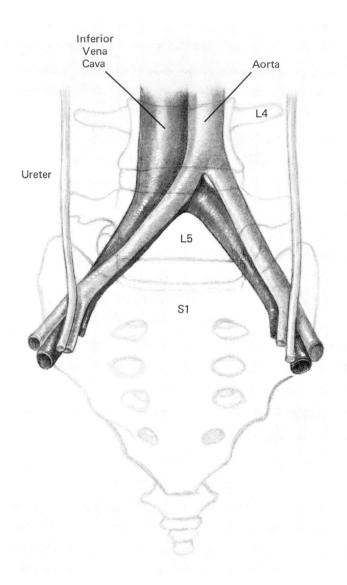

Inferior
Vena
Cava

Aorta

L4

Ureter

L5

S1

Fig. 6-63. The major vessels and ureters and their relationship to the anterior lumbar spine.

larger fragments of intervertebral disc material than is possible when the jaws are solid.

In using intervertebral disc rongeur forceps within the intervertebral space, great care is necessary to avoid instrument penetration through the anterior annulus fibrosus and the anterior longitudinal ligament. Such penetration is precarious and may be associated with laceration of one of the great vessels, located anterior to the vertebral bodies, lying within the prevertebral space. Experienced and competent lumbar disc surgeons have suffered this calamity; and when working deep within the intervertebral space, the surgeon must remain alert to the possibility of this mishap. Degenerative changes affecting an intervertebral disc are generalized and may cause softening of the anterior annular fibers and anterior longitudinal ligament, permitting inadvertent penetration by an instrument.[4]

Some years ago, this potential surgical catastrophe received nationwide publicity when it resulted in the death of a popular

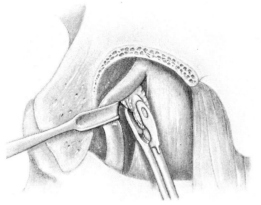

Fig. 6-64. This large free disc fragment between the nerve root and dural sac can easily be overlooked.

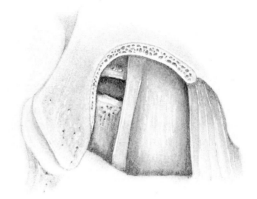

Fig. 6-66. "Free" nerve root following disc excision and foraminotomy.

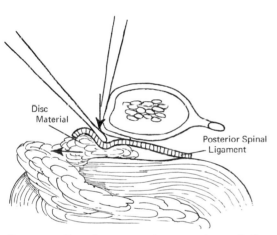

Fig. 6-65. Disc fragments that extrude medially beneath the posterior spinal ligament are easily overlooked, and once identified, not easily removed.

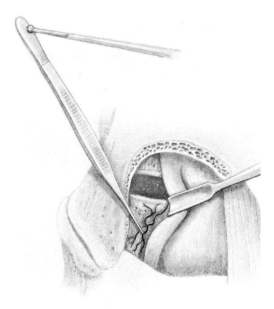

Fig. 6-67. Cautery of epidural vessels.

Hollywood actor, Jeff Chandler. The residents, in those days, mindful of the inherent danger, capriciously referred to the intervertebral space as "Chandler's canal."

Free Disc Fragments. Occasionally the protruded disc is in the "axilla" between the dural sac and the nerve root. A most meticulous dissection of this extruded fragment is necessary, with care used in grasping this fragment with an intervertebral disc rongeur forceps to avoid damage to the adjacent laterally displaced nerve root. It is occasionally difficult to recognize a completely free extruded fragment within the axilla. It may resemble epidural fat and in some cases, only the tip of the extruded fragment presents dorsally, with the bulk of this free fragment not visible and indenting the inferior portion of the dural sac medially. The surgeon, unaware of this large extrusion, may

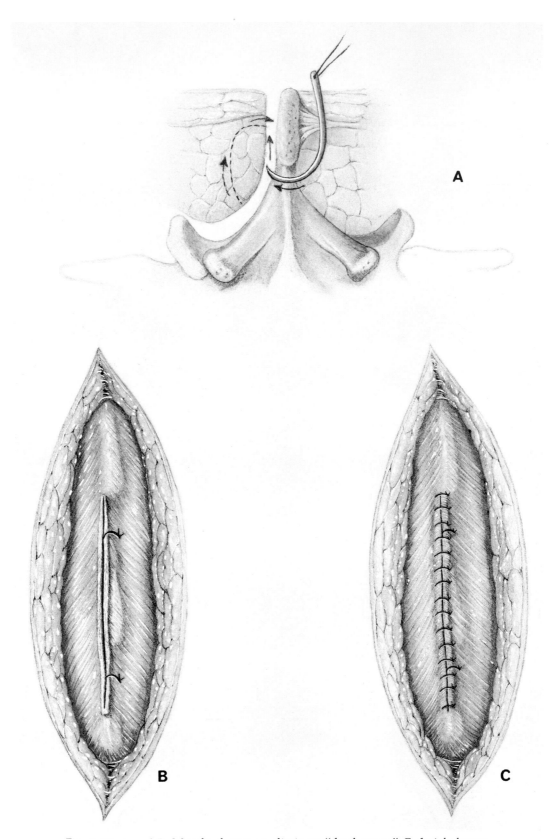

Fig. 6-68. A and B, Muscle closure to eliminate "dead space;" C, facial closure.

retract the nerve root and dural sac together with the free fragment medially, exposing the intervertebral disc. The disc protrusion will be excised and the interspace evacuated as thoroughly as possible by the usual methods, including curettage and the use of the intervertebral disc forceps; but the offending free fragment, causing root pressure, will be inadvertently left untouched. An indication that such a fragment is present may be the lack of free nerve root mobility, so that it cannot be easily retracted medially. When the nerve root is not free, further inspection is necessary.

A free disc fragment may extrude beneath the posterior spinal ligament and occasionally will produce a sizable mass capable of producing symptoms that will not be evident to casual inspection. Palpation over the posterior spinal ligament with a thin elevator will disclose this extrusion, and it can be "milked" laterally exposing sufficient disc tissue to grasp with the intervertebral disc forceps and removed.

Surgical Judgment. In those patients in whom there is no gross protrusion of the disc, but rather a slightly humped-up annulus, the surgeon must use judgment in deciding whether to excise the high annulus and curette the intervertebral disc space, or to be content with posterior bony decompression of the nerve root by means of a foraminotomy.

After the protruded intervertebral disc has been adequately excised, the operating room table, or spinal rest, is flattened so that the originally flexed position is now a relatively straight one. This change in position places the root under less tension, narrows the posterior intervertebral space and increases the depth between the skin surface and the interlaminar space. The interspace is then re-explored and occasionally several additional fragments of disc material can be removed, with the vertebral bodies closer together. At the termination of the procedure, the nerve root should be under no pressure whatsoever, either anteriorly from the intervertebral disc or from bony constriction within the

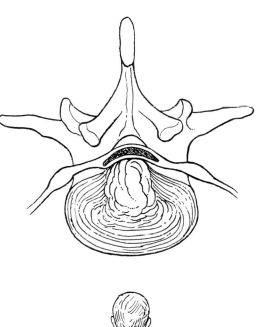

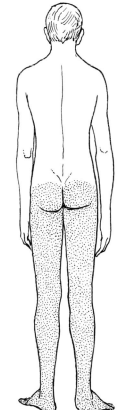

Fig. 6-69. Cauda equina syndrome.

intervertebral foramina, which should have been partially opened during the original bony dissection.

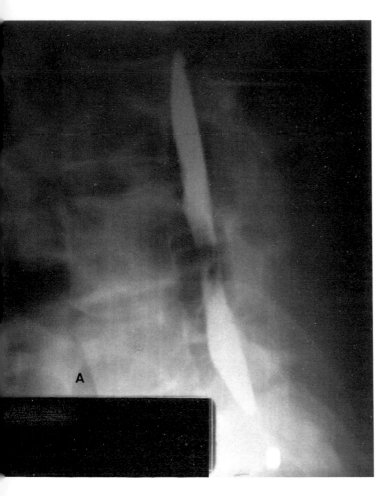

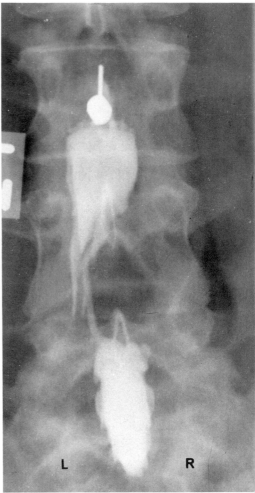

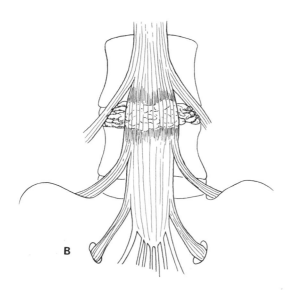

Fig. 6-70. This 39-year-old lady had a history of moderate low back pain and occasional right sciatica for several years. Because of an acute exacerbation of her symptoms, she was hospitalized 2 years previously and responded well to conservative treatment consisting of bed rest and traction. She was relatively pain free until she bent forward over a sink while brushing her teeth and appreciated a sudden excruciating low back pain extending into both lower extremities—the right more severe than the left. She was admitted with severe weakness of the left foot extensor muscles and slight weakness on the right. Because of inability to void, an indwelling Foley catheter was necessary. A, An emergency myelogram revealed an extensive defect at L4–5 level. B, Surgery performed on same day revealed massive extrusion of the intervertebral disc at the L4–5 level.

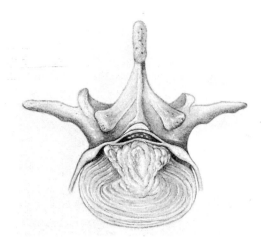

Fig. 6-71. Midline disc protrusion requiring transdural excision.

Bleeding from epidural veins should be carefully controlled before closure of the wound. Removing the lumbar flexion and placing the patient in a flat, prone position is helpful in relieving abdominal pressure and reducing lumbar venous engorgement; this change in position alone often controls venous epidural bleeding. This alteration of the table is advisable even if no epidural bleeding is encountered, since it does allow the surgeon to recheck for any retained fragments of disc and changes the minute anatomical relationships of the root and intervertebral space, affording additional inspection. Continued epidural bleeding is controlled with the use of electrocoagulation; and the use of the Malis bipolar coagulation forceps is of great help in preventing spread of the cautery current. Occasionally, a small pledget of Gelfoam is required to control bleeding.

Wound Closure. Suture material of personal preference is 2–0 chromic gut for muscle and fascia, 3–0 plain gut for subcutaneous, and 32 stainless steel wire for skin.

An important, but often overlooked, hemilaminectomy closure technique is elimination of the dead space, which may fill with clot contributing to postoperative discomfort. This is accomplished with two or three 2–0 chromic sutures passed through the interspinous ligaments to approximate the paraspinal muscles against the laminae and spinous processes.

VASCULAR AND VISCERAL INJURIES DURING DISC SURGERY

Most vascular injuries occur during excision of disc material, with the intervertebral disc forceps producing a laceration of one of the major vessels lying in the prevertebral space such as the aorta, inferior vena cava, or the iliac arteries or veins. Ordinarily, such a catastrophe is signaled by copious bleeding from the intervertebral space immediately after the introduction of an instrument deep within it. Occasionally, no such bleeding is recognized through the intervertebral space, all bleeding occurring anteriorly; during surgery, the patient will go into shock with sudden hypotension and a rapid thready pulse.[4] Occasionally, injury to an artery or a vein results in the formation of an arteriovenous fistula, which may not be noted for years after the original surgery. Sometimes, the first sign of such an injury is cardiac decompensation.[3,6,11]

As soon as such evidence of vascular injury is recognized, it must be understood that this is a serious surgical emergency which requires immediate action. The anesthesiologist is appraised of the situation and instructed to institute rapid blood transfusion in large volumes. The wound is packed with several large abdominal sponges and closed with a few deep sutures through skin and muscle. The patient is turned to the supine position; and if a general surgeon is available, he should proceed with the laparotomy. If not, the abdominal cavity must be opened by a midrectus incision. Occasionally, no evidence of bleeding is noted in the abdominal cavity, but a large hematoma can be visualized in the retroperitoneal space. The posterior peritoneum is then divided, and the hematoma is evacuated by means of suction. The site of bleeding can easily be determined, and vascular clamps are applied above and below that region. The lacerated vessel is repaired with vascular suture.

Occasionally, an abdominal viscus such as the ureter, the bladder, and the ileum is perforated.

OPERATIVE REPORT

When dictating the operative report, a detailed description of the significant operative findings is important. Too often, the operative note briefly states that a protruded disc was found and removed. Those subsequently reviewing the case are left to wonder whether there was an extrusion of the nucleus pulposus, a ruptured protruding annulus, a combination of both, or simply a high annulus.

POSTOPERATIVE MANAGEMENT

Immediately after lumbar disc surgery, postanesthesia care, including monitoring of vital signs and maintenance of an adequate airway, is best managed in the recovery room under direction of the anesthesiologist.

The following postoperative orders are routine:

1. Flat on back 4 hours, then assist patient to turn from side—back—side (alternating sides) every 2 hours. (Traditionally, all spine surgery patients are initially maintained flat and supine in the presumption that this position is associated with decreased venous epidural bleeding and the direct pressure upon the paraspinal muscles will tend to reduce bleeding from this source.)

2. Demerol, 100 milligrams, every 4 hours prn for pain.

3. Food and fluids by mouth as tolerated.

4. If patient is unable to urinate in the recumbent position, assist patient to sit up or stand while voiding. Insert Foley catheter if these efforts are unsuccessful. (The discomfort of standing on the day of surgery is best endured to avoid the potential complication of a urinary tract infection from the catheter. When a Foley catheter is used, a suitable antibiotic is administered.)

5. First postoperative day:
   a. Dangle 5 times
   b. Stand by side of bed once
   c. Assist to bathroom if he desires

6. Second postoperative day:
   Out of bed in chair.

7. Third postoperative day:
   Ambulatory.

8. One week:
   Sutures out.

Discharged the next day wearing nonreinforced lumbosacral support. (Although the patient is ambulated during the immediate postoperative interval without external support, the increased activities at home are tolerated more kindly with a light canvas support constructed without paravertebral steels.)

9. At home activities gradually and progressively increased
   Ride in car—2 weeks
   Drive car—4 weeks.

10. Return to work depends largely on the nature of the job.

Clerical and office work usually can be managed in 4 to 6 weeks.

Jobs involving heavy physical activities are best not attempted for 3 to 4 months.

CAUSE OF OPERATIVE FAILURE

Probably the most common cause of surgical failure is an error in judgment with regard to the indication for initial surgery. Was the lesion really a symptom-producing markedly protruding disc or merely a slightly protruding disc in association with a stenotic lumbar canal? Was a neoplasm overlooked? Were the symptoms primarily due to a lumbosacral strain associated with some slight irritation of the nerve root? If the preoperative symptoms persist after surgery, questions of this nature should be considered. Careful analysis may reveal that surgery was not in order or that a significantly altered surgical procedure was indicated.

Inadequate surgery is the second ranking cause of operative failure. Was the proper interspace explored? Was a fragment of extruded disc lying within the axilla between the root and the dural sac overlooked? Did the surgeon fail to identify either clinically or by myelography a second protruding disc? Was evacuation of the disc space inadequate with considerable disc material remaining causing persisting root pressure?

A most significant cause of persisting pain or even worsening pain following surgery is nerve root damage. This can be caused by excessive medial retraction of the root so that it is stretched or direct root trauma during the removal of intervertebral disc material with the root being contused, pinched or sometimes even badly torn. Damage to the nerve root from spread of the cautery current may also be the cause of persisting symptoms.

Common Causes of Postoperative Pain

1. Surgery not indicated initially.
2. Persisting nerve root pressure from inadequate disc excision or an overlooked second disc protrusion.
3. Radiculitis secondary to nerve root trauma.
4. Radiculitis secondary to postoperative scarring (intradural or extradural).

RESULTS OF INITIAL SURGERY

The results of initial surgery are classified, on the basis of pain relief and ability to perform physical activity, as satisfactory or unsatisfactory.

Included in the satisfactory classification are those who were advised to change from their physically demanding jobs to occupations that were less physically taxing and housewives who were placed on restrictions in their daily activities but were able to continue on this restricted basis in relative comfort.

Included in the unsatisfactory classification are patients who considered surgery "worthwhile" because it reduced the severity of pain, but were unable to work in relative comfort.

Satisfactory	928	93%
Unsatisfactory	72	7%

Secondary Gain and Unsatisfactory Results

Secondary Gain	38 patients out of 343	11%
No Secondary Gain	34 patients out of 657	5%

EXCEPTIONAL LUMBAR DISC PROBLEMS

Cauda Equina Syndrome

Massive extrusion of the intervertebral disc produces compression of the cauda equina with a complete block seen on the myelogram. This will result in severe signs and unmistakable symptoms. There may be impaired motor function in both lower extremities as well as widespread hypesthesia, extending from the buttocks down to the

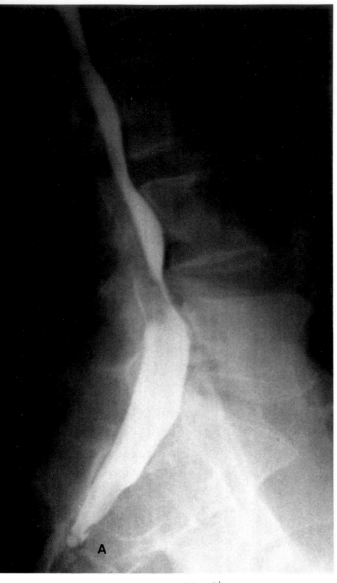

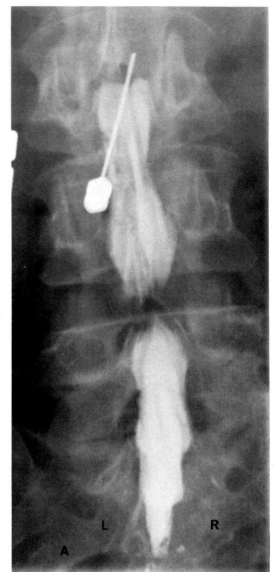

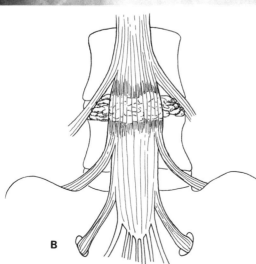

Fig. 6-72. A and B, This 67-year-old man presented with a long-standing history of low back pain extending into both posterior thighs. He experienced occasional tingling and numbness but no actual pain below the knees. Myelography revealed a midline intervertebral disc protrusion at the L4–5 interspace with considerable hypertrophy of the ligamentum flavum producing an annular constriction at the involved level. Because of the dorsal compression from the ligamentum flavum, a laminectomy of the fourth and fifth lumbar vertebrae was performed. The nerve roots and dural sac were so tightly stretched over the midline protrusion that a transdural excision was necessary.

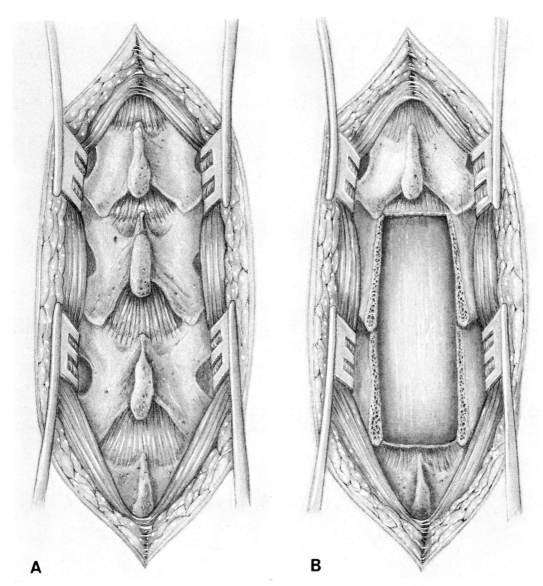

A   **B**

Fig. 6-73. A, Bony exposure; B, laminectomy of L4 and L5.

feet, in association with both bowel and bladder sphincter impairment. Such a condition is considered an emergency, and an expeditious myelogram is in order to confirm the clinical impression of cauda equina syndrome. This will reveal a complete block at the involved level. Prompt surgical intervention and decompression of this lesion is in order and delay of treatment in such instances is inadvisable and may add to the permanence of neurological deficit. In situations of such severe compression of the nerve roots, permanent changes may occur no matter how quickly decompression is performed; delay will only add to the deficit.

Surgical Technique for Massive Disc Protrusion and Cauda Equina Syndrome. When such a surgical emergency is present, it is best to carry out a most generous and complete laminectomy for several reasons. A more complete bilateral removal of the protruded disc can be accomplished with this generous exposure. Of even greater importance is the considerable edema and swelling

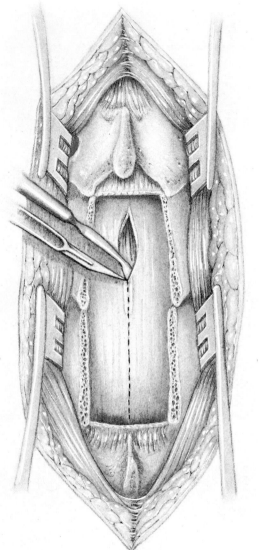

Fig. 6-74. Dural incision.

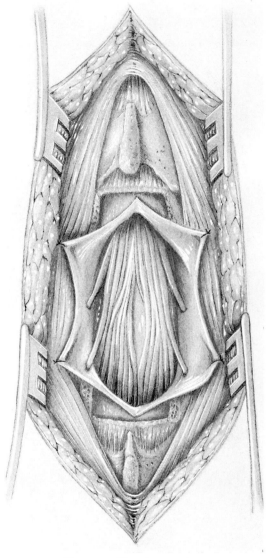

Fig. 6-75. Dural retraction.

of the nerve roots evoked by such a lesion. A major bony decompression is likely to result in a more prompt and more complete neurological recovery than would be the case if there remained bony compression overlying the site of cauda equina insult.

Transdural Excision of Midline Disc Extrusion

Indications. Occasionally a midline disc protrusion cannot be approached extra-

durally without undue retraction upon the nerve roots and dural sac. This lesion may be so extensive as to produce a cauda equina syndrome, but a less severe clinical picture occurs if the caudal roots are shifted laterally on either side of the mass. An unusually wide dural sac will permit such lateral root displacement, and attempts to forcibly retract the roots to enable an extradural disc excision may be associated with severe postoperative dysfunction. When this type of

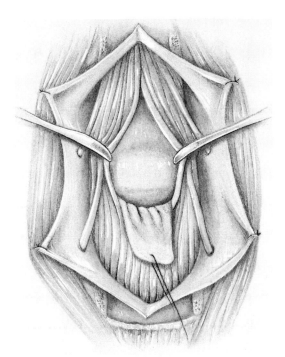

Fig. 6-76. Retraction of nerve roots.

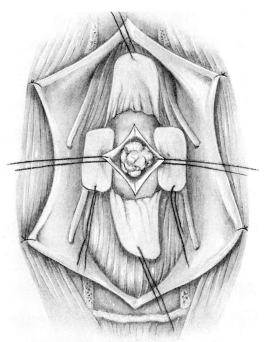

Fig. 6-77. Anterior dural incision.

lesion is encountered, a transdural disc excision is in order.

Technique. The surgery is performed with the patient in prone position but no effort is made to achieve lumbar flexion. Flexion is not particularly important in the transdural approach, and the decreased abdominal pressure resulting from the flatter position will be helpful in reducing epidural venous bleeding.

A bilateral subperiosteal muscle dissection is performed, exposing the spinous processes and laminae of two vertebrae above and below the involved interspace. A complete laminectomy of the two vertebrae adjacent to the lesion is performed, taking care to carry the exposure bilaterally to the facets. All bleeding from the bone edges is controlled with bone wax and epidural bleeding controlled with either the Malis bipolar coagulating forceps of small pledgets of Gelfoam. Have the operative field dry before opening the dura.

A No. 11 blade is used to make a small opening in the dura sufficient to permit introduction of a small grooved dural elevator, attempting to leave the arachnoid intact. The initial dural opening is made cephalad to, not over, the protrusion. The small grooved dural elevator with the No. 11 blade is used to extend the midline dural incision to the limits of the bony exposure.

Stay sutures are tied from the dural edge of the adjacent muscles to establish consistent dural retraction. If a small opening in the arachnoid was inadvertently made during the dural incision, place a small cotton patty over the rent while attaching the stay sutures; and in most cases this opening will seal off in a minute or two, eliminating the annoyance of cerebrospinal fluid drainage into the wound while retracting the dural edges.

After the dura is retracted, the nerve roots are carefully separated to either side of the protruding anterior dural mound and can usually be maintained in this position by cotton patties.

The exact center of the protruding disc, underlying the dura, can be established by gentle probing with a thin elevator. A one-

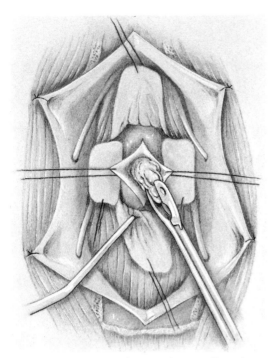

Fig. 6-78. Excision of protruding midline disc.

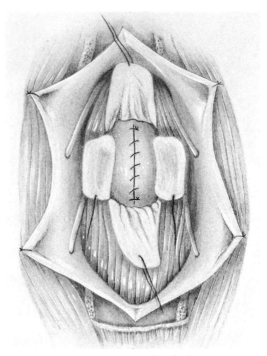

Fig. 6-79. Anterior dural closure.

centimeter incision is then made in the anterior dura and the dural edges retracted with stay sutures, which are attached to hemostats. Cotton patties can be placed between the anterior and posterior dural stay sutures to prevent the caudal nerve roots from slipping out of position and suffering damage.

The interspace now adequately exposed can be carefully incised with a No. 11 blade and the disc contents evacuated. Each insertion of an instrument into the interspace is performed only under complete vision to avoid danger of root trauma. Extravasation of blood and spinal fluid onto the operative field are controlled by indirect suction on a cotton patty, not direct suction, to avoid aspiration of a root into the suction tip.

Closure of the anterior and posterior dura is accomplished with interrupted 0000 black silk technique.

THE REPEAT OPERATIVE PROCEDURE

Indications for Repeat Surgery

Reoperation on an intervertebral disc space that has undergone previous surgery is technically more difficult to perform than a primary procedure. The normal tissue planes are usually obliterated by dense fibrous tissue extending from the skin down to the bony elements of the spine.

Of greater importance, both with regard to symptom production and operative difficulty, is the scar tissue enveloping the dural sac and nerve root. The patient who has persisting pain following lumbar disc surgery presents a problem to the physician involving all of the several factors that were weighed in the decision to operate initially, which are geometrically expanded by additional variables related to the previous surgery. Rarely are decisions involving this type of patient easily made.

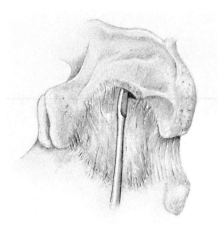

Fig. 6-80. Dissecting adherent dura from under-surface of the superior lamina.

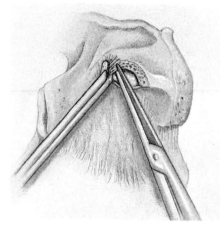

Fig. 6-81. Avoid tugging on epidural scar tissue.

The Four Questions. Four questions must be answered to properly evaluate such a clinical problem. The questions are naturally progressive with each succeeding question being based on a positive answer to the preceding question. A negative response to any of the first 3 questions eliminates the need to proceed with further consideration of additional surgery.

1. Was the original surgery indicated? Often, this is the most difficult question to answer. If the initial surgery was performed by another physician, a valid reconstruction of the original signs and symptoms may be based on the patient's deficient recollections. When the evaluating physician performed the initial surgery, it should be recalled that objectivity is not the most conspicuous human characteristic. It certainly "goes against the grain" for a surgeon to conclude that an operation he previously performed was not indicated.

If the physician comes to the conclusion that the initial surgery was not indicated, it is not likely that a "repeat performance" would serve a useful purpose. Only if, in retrospect, the original surgery was deemed warranted, can he proceed with the next logical question.

2. What went wrong? Was the original surgery the procedure of choice? Was it adequately or inadequately performed? Do the postoperative films indicate that the correct side and correct interspace were subjected to exploration or was a "site error" committed? Did irreversible nerve root damage occur from the original surgery, and is this the cause of persisting symptoms? Does the patient manifest symptoms of a mechanically unstable spine, and should a spinal fusion have been performed at the time of the original surgery? Should a spinal fusion be done now? If the answers to these questions enable one to explain the failure of the original surgery, we may proceed to the third question.

3. Is the patient's present dysfunction severe enough to warrant a repeat operation, in the knowledge that the repeat procedure is associated with a higher percentage of failure? An affirmative answer brings us to the last question.

4. What is the indicated surgical procedure? Repeat interlaminar exploration? Complete laminectomy? Fusion?

Technical Considerations in Repeat Spinal Surgery

The scarred paraspinal muscle is removed from the spinous processes and laminae in the same manner as in the primary proce-

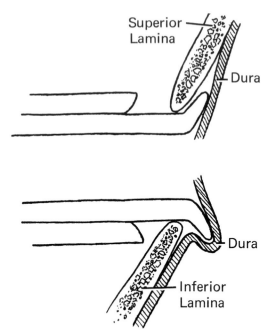

Fig. 6-82. The adherent dura covered by scar tissue is more easily damaged at the edge of the inferior lamina.

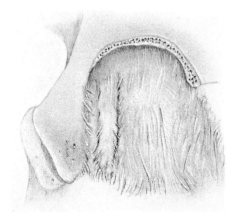

Fig. 6-83. The nerve root, surrounded by scar tissue, is more easily damaged at the edge of the inferior lamina.

dure, but the surgeon now must be much more careful to avoid injury to the dural sac and nerve roots by an instrument that may inadvertently slip between the widened interlaminar space at the site of the previous operative procedure. Scar tissue will be

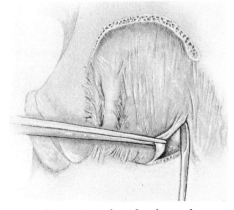

Fig. 6-84. Dissection of epidural scar from upper edge of inferior lamina. This dissection is continued medially until the superior lamina is reduced. The root is best exposed from the superior lamina downward.

tightly adherent to the dura and great care must be taken to avoid tearing the dura and arachnoid when sweeping the muscles laterally over the previously explored interspace. Once the muscle dissection has been satisfactorily accomplished, a new plane of cleavage must be established to allow adequate dissection of the dura and nerve root. The easiest way to start this dissection is to insert a thin elevator between the scar and the undersurface of the remaining lamina above. After a small area beneath the superior lamina has been freed, a 40°-angled small jawed laminectomy punch rongeur is introduced to bite a small rim of bone, exposing a zone of dura that has not previously been dissected. Once this first bite has been accomplished, the dura-scar dissection is carried a bit more laterally, allowing a second bite and cautiously proceeding until a thin rim of superior lamina has been completely removed. This dissection is best not hurried, and care is taken to avoid tugging on scar tissue which is adherent to the underlying dura and which may tear the dura and arachnoid. After this plane of cleavage has been carried laterally to the facet, it may be possible to separate the remaining dura from the overlying scar tissue.

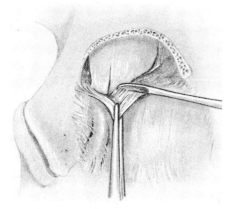

Fig. 6-85. Exposure of root encased in scar is best started at point of exit from dural sac rather than from a site where the root is free.

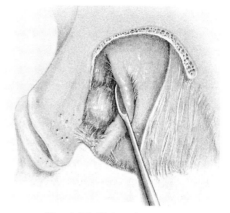

Fig. 6-86. Retracting root.

If the scar tissue is too dense and adherent despite this bony removal, it may be necessary to interrupt the dissection at the superior lamina and resume a similar dissection at the inferior lamina. This may be more technically difficult, since the superior edge of the inferior lamina dips downward, angled more anteriorly. The downward slope, in association with epidural scarring, creates a potential hazard of tearing the dura, which is increased by use of the 40°-angled jaw laminectomy punch. The danger to the root at this site is greater since dissection beneath the superior lamina exposes the origin of the nerve root as it separates from the dural sac, while the inferior lamina dissection exposes the free nerve root completely detached from the dura, making identification of the scar-encased root more difficult, giving rise to possible root damage. In the presence of dense adherent scar tissue, do not attempt to carry out the dissection laterally at the inferior lamina. The reason for developing the dura inferiorly is that it does provide an additional plane of cleavage between dura and scar tissue, and, in many cases, will allow the scar tissue to be more easily peeled away from the dura, so that the dissection can once more be carried out at the superior lamina. Use of the 40°-angled small jawed laminec-

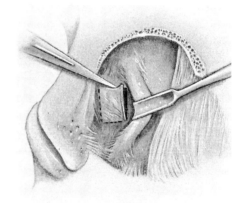

Fig. 6-87. Slab-shaped incision into recurrent disc.

tomy punch rongeur will achieve a more lateral bony exposure. Each time a bite of bone is taken, which carries with it scar tissue adherent to the underlying dura and root, refrain from tugging on the scar; instead use a Metzenbaum scissors to cut the bone fragment free. With careful dissection, the dura and root can eventually be adequately exposed and freed of most of the scar tissue. In some cases, it is necessary to perform a hemilaminectomy to develop a satisfactory scar-dural cleavage plane. Only after the dura and root are well identified can these structures be safely retracted medially, exposing the underlying intervertebral space.

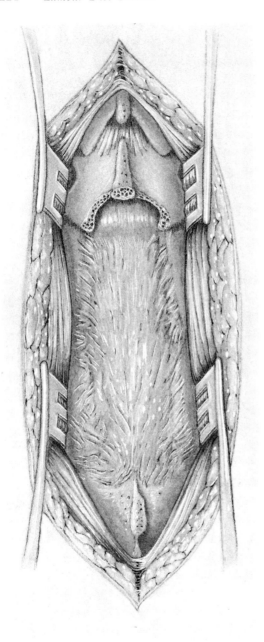

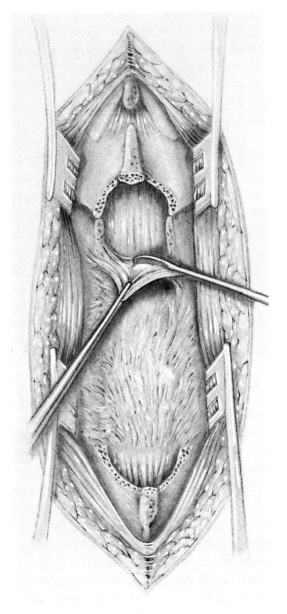

Fig. 6-88. Reexploration of complete laminectomy. The inferior edge of L3 lamina has been excised to expose unscarred dura.

Fig. 6-89. Plane of cleavage.

Previously explored intervertebral discs, in addition to recurrent annular protrusions, often manifest a significant mass of fibrous scar tissue, which in combination are capable of producing nerve root compression. At one time it was believed that painful root compression could occur solely from the development of epidural scar tissue. I have not observed this and am of the opinion that in addition to scar tissue, some degree of disc protrusion is necessary before root compression symptoms will develop. Such abnormal intervertebral discs should be reexplored, using a long-handled No. 11 blade to make a generous slab-shaped incision within the annulus, facilitating radical evacuation of old degenerated disc material, debris and cartilaginous plates. Following previous surgery it may be advisable to carry out a much wider, bony decompression, either a hemilaminectomy, or if the myelogram reveals considerable compression resulting from scar tissue, a complete bilateral wide laminectomy is in order.

Some years ago, in the face of myelographic evidence of adhesive arachnoiditis, it was considered advisable to open the dura and free up or "comb out" the nerve roots. This is often associated with increased nerve root pain and is seldom, if ever, helpful, possibly resulting in further scarring and potential root damage.

In some cases where the articular facets have been partially entered into by previous surgery, the articular capsules are stretched and dysfunctional. Resection of such abnormal capsules and facets may be symptom alleviating.

Reexploration Following Complete Laminectomy

In some instances it will be necessary to reexplore following a complete laminectomy. This presents much more difficulty because the scar tissue is intimately associated with a considerable area of dura, adding greatly to the possibility of a dural tear. In such a situation, the first step is a bilateral subperiosteal dissection of the intact vertebrae immediately above and below the laminectomy opening. After this has been accomplished, it is possible to approximate the depth of the dural sac between these two points; and working from intact bone and using meticulous dissection, the overlying scar tissue can be dissected free of the dura. Additional bony removal, at least a thin margin of untouched bone above and below the previous laminectomy, is most helpful in developing a plane of cleavage between the dura and the adherent scar tissue.

Results of Repeat Procedures

Of 146 patients requiring repeated spinal surgery, 31 manifested symptoms on the side opposite the original complaint; 8 manifested symptoms on the same side but developed disc disease at a different interspace from the original lesion, 107 manifested dysfunction related to the site of previous surgery. Of these 107, 14 were considered lumbar instability, with back pain absent and radicular symptoms, and had fusions with no interspace reexploration; 61 had interspace reexploration followed by fusion; and 32 had interspace reexploration not followed by fusion.

Of the 107 patients with dysfunction related to the site of previous surgery, 79 (74%) had satisfactory results, 28 (26%) unsatisfactory. Of the 31 with dysfunction on the side opposite the original complaint, 27 (87%) were satisfactory and 4 (13%) unsatisfactory.

REFERENCES

1. Andrew, J.: Sacralization: aetilogical factor in lumbar intervertebral disk lesions, and cause of misleading focal signs. Br. J. Surg. 42:304, 1954.
2. Foltz, E. L., Ward, A. A., Jr., and Knopp, M.: Intervertebral fusion following lumbar disk excision. J. Neurosurg. 13:469, 1956.
3. Fortune, C.: Arterio-venous fistula of left common iliac artery and vein. Med. J. Aust. 43:660, 1956.
4. Freeman, D. G.: Major vascular complications of lumbar disc surgery. Western J. Surg. 60:175, 1961.
5. Geiger, L. E.: Fusion of vertebrae following resection of intervertebral disc. J. Neurosurg. 18:79, 1961.
6. Glass, B. A., and Ilgenfritz, H. C.: Arteriovenous fistula secondary to operation for ruptured intervertebral disc. Ann. Surg. 140:122, 1954.
7. Goldner, J. L., McCollum, D. E., and Urbaniak, J. R.: Anterior disc excision and interbody spine fusion for chronic low back pain. American Academy of Orthopedic Surgeons, Symposium on the Spine. St. Louis, C. V. Mosby, 1969.

8. Harman, P.: Anterior extraperitoneal disc excision and vertebral body fusion. Clin. Orthop., *18*:169, 1961.

9. Hasner, E., Jacobsen, H. H., Schalimtzek, M., and Snorrason, E.: Lumbosacral transitional vertebrae. A clinical and roentgenological study of 400 cases of low back pain. Acta Radiol. *39*:225, 1953.

10. Hoover, N. W.: Indications for fusion at time of removal of intervertebral disc. J. Bone Joint Surg., *50A*:189–193, 1968.

11. Horton, R. E.: Arteriovenous fistula following operation for prolapsed intervertebral disk. Br. J. Surg. *49*:77, 1961.

12. Keim, H. A., and Weinstein, J. D.: Acute renal failure—a complication of spine fusion in the tuck position. J. Bone Joint Surg. *52A*: 1248, 1970.

13. Moore, C. A., and Cohen, A.: Combined arterial, venous, and ureteral injury complicating lumbar disk surgery. Amer. J. Surg. *115*:574, 1968.

14. Rolander, D.: Motion of the lumbar spine with special reference to the stabilizing effect of posterior fusion. Acta. Orthop. Scand. Suppl. 90 (1966).

15. Shenkin, H. A., and Haft, H.: Foraminotomy in the surgical treatment of herniated lumbar disks. Surgery *60*:274, 1966.

16. Speed, K.: Spondylolisthesis: Treatment by anterior bone graft. Arch. Surg., *37*:175, 1938.

17. Stewart, D. Y.: The anterior disc excision and interbody fusion approach to the problem of degenerative disc disease of the lower lumbar spinal segments. New York, J. Med., *61*:3252, 1961.

7

The Cloward Technique *

REMOVAL OF DISC

Introduction

Operative Technique

  Position and Anesthesia
  Skin Incision
  Fascia and Muscles
  Ligamentum Flavum and Laminae
  Disc Removal

Discussion

  Transverse Skin Incision
  Ligamentum Flavum
  Use of Chisel and Hammer
  Articular Facets
  Disc Removal
  Intrathecal Cortisone

Conclusion

POSTERIOR LUMBAR INTERBODY FUSION

Introduction

Disc Removal

Bone Grafts

Bone Grafting

Wound Closure

Postoperative Care

Discussion

Conclusion

*Text and illustrations adapted from monographs originally published by Codman & Shurtleff, Inc., Randolph, Mass.

7

The Cloward Technique

BY RALPH B. CLOWARD, M.D., F.A.C.S.

REMOVAL OF DISC

INTRODUCTION

The surgical technique for removal of ruptured lumbar intervertebral discs has changed very little since it was introduced by Mixter and Barr in 1934.[8] Protrusion of the nucleus pulposus or rupture and intraspinal herniation of fragments of the annulus fibrosus occur most often in a posterolateral position causing unilateral nerve root compression. A unilateral operation, either a hemilaminectomy or an interlaminal approach, is employed to remove the lesion from the spinal canal.

The technique of the interlaminar operation used by most neurosurgeons (Spurling,[12] Semmes,[11] Raaf[10]) consists of a vertical midline skin incision, unilateral stripping of lumbosacral fascia and muscles and exposure of spines and lamina on the side of the lesion. Part of the ligamentum flavum is removed, a notch is made in one or both margins of the laminae with a rongeur or Kerrison punch, creating an oval opening into the spinal canal usually about 1.0 to 1.5 cm. in diameter directly over or medial to the nerve root. A narrow blade is inserted and the nerve root is forcibly retracted medially to expose the intervertebral disc. Bleeding from epidural veins in this area is often troublesome but must be controlled before the disc lesion can be visualized, located and removed.

The technical difficulties and surgical failures encountered with this operation can be partially attributed to an inadequate exposure of the spinal canal. The small opening precludes extensive exploration above and below and medial to the nerve root necessary to locate and remove multiple and elusive disc fragments. Forceful manual retraction of the nerve root is required to arrest bleeding and to visualize and remove the disc fragments. This may account for postoperative pain and neurological deficits. Yet it is not unusual to hear surgeons boast of "taking out a disc in 20 minutes without even removing any bone."

A different surgical technique is described for removal of a ruptured lumbar intervertebral disc. By making an ample interlaminal opening into the spinal canal the problems of exposure of the lesion, control of hemorrhage and damage to the nerve roots are mostly eliminated while actually reducing overall operative time. This technique has been used by the author for over 29 years.[2]

The operation utilizes a transverse skin incision and a wide bilateral stripping and retraction of fascia and muscles. The ligamentum flavum is not removed but detached and reflected medially in a flap. Bone is removed only from the margins of the lamina and the articular facets. A complete laminectomy is never done except for spondylolis-

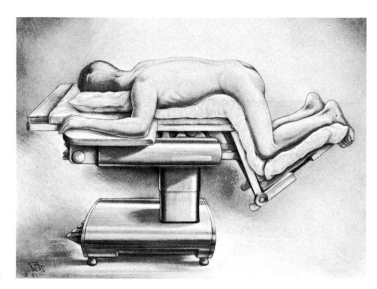

Fig. 7-1.

thesis when the separate neural arch is disarticulated and removed.[5] Using a "Vertebra Spreader," an interlaminar exposure is developed two to three times larger than that obtained by the "standard" technique. The advantages are obvious.

OPERATIVE TECHNIQUE

Position and Anesthesia

The patient is placed in the kneeling position over the lower end of the operating table. A vertically placed sponge rubber roll beneath each ilium prevents pressure on the abdomen (Fig. 7-1). General endotracheal anesthesia is used. After antiseptic preparation of the skin, ½ percent Xylocaine with adrenalin and Wydase* is infiltrated intracutaneously in the line of the incision, and 50 cc. of this solution injected bilaterally into the paravertebral lumbar muscles will prevent muscle bleeding.

Skin Incision

An 8 cm. transverse skin incision is made over the lesion (Fig. 7-2; L4-5). Bleeding from skin is arrested by fixing a towel to the skin with multiple small towel clips or skin clips

*Trademark of Wyeth Co.

placed 1 cm. apart. Skin bleeders are never cauterized. The skin and subcutaneous fat is undermined and retracted vertically with an Adson retractor (Fig. 7-3).

Fascia and Muscles

A midline incision the desired length is made with a scalpel through lumbo-sacral

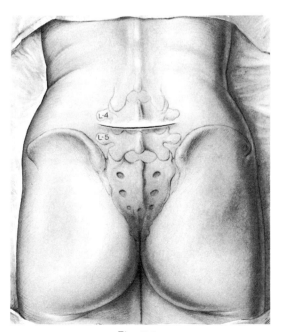

Fig. 7-2.

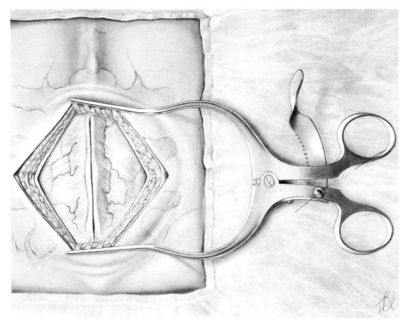

Fig. 7-3. Adson self-retaining 8-inch cerebellar retractor (8″).

fascia and muscle attachments to the tip of the spinous processes. Using two large sharp periosteal elevators, the muscles are stripped subperiosteally laterally beyond the capsule of the articular facets. The blades of the self-retaining laminectomy retractor are inserted on each side. The new retractor handle with a ratchet opening is attached and opened, giving a wide bilateral exposure of the entire lamina (Fig. 7-4). About 1 cm. of the adjacent margins of the spinous processes and the interspinous ligament is removed with a rongeur and the raw bone surfaces waxed.

Ligamentum Flavum and Laminae

On the side of the lesion a narrow, full curved sharp periosteal elevator is worked deep beneath the upper laminae to release the attachments of the ligamentum flavum from its lower margin and anterior surface (Fig. 7-5). Using a chisel 6 mm. wide, the lower $\frac{1}{3}$ of this lamina (about $\frac{1}{2}$ to 1 cm.) is removed from the base of the spinous process laterally to include the lower $\frac{1}{3}$ of the superior articular facet (Fig. 7-6). The

bone edges are waxed. On the opposite side of the spine the ligament is partially detached from each laminar margin with the narrow elevator, sufficient to permit insertion of the tips of the new vertebra spreader beneath the margins of the lamina. By turning the thumb screw the spreader widens the interlaminal opening putting the ligamentum flavum on a stretch. The upper fibers of the ligament still attached to the lamina are carefully divided with a No. 11 scalpel blade as far lateral as possible (Fig. 7-7), then the ligament attachments to the lower lamina are cut, being careful not to puncture or incise the dura or epidural veins which lie immediately beneath (Fig. 7-8). A small grooved director or a patty beneath the ligament may be used here. The incision is continued laterally, follows the laminal edge and then superiorly along the medial margin of the inferior facet until it meets the lateral cut of the upper incision. A heavy silk retention suture is passed through the lateral edge of the ligament and the flap of ligament reflected medially and secured to the laminectomy retractor on the opposite side (Fig. 7-9); 1

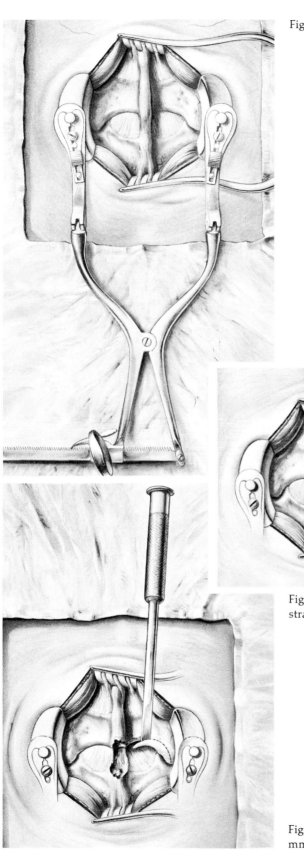

Fig. 7-4. Cloward lumbar lamina retractor.

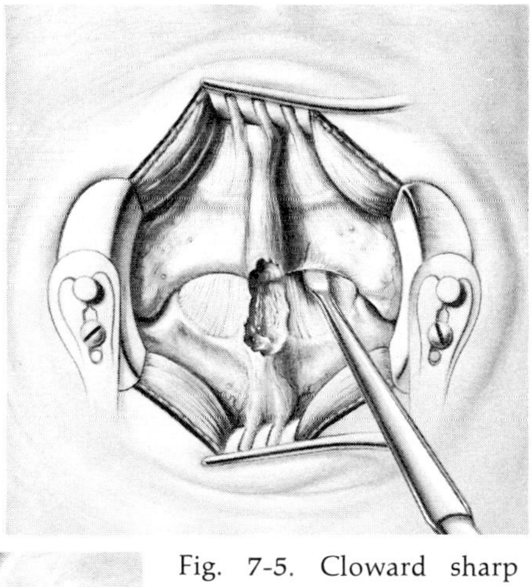

Fig. 7-5. Cloward sharp periosteal elevator, straight (8").

Fig. 7-6. Cloward spinal fusion chisel, straight (6 mm. wide, 9½" long).

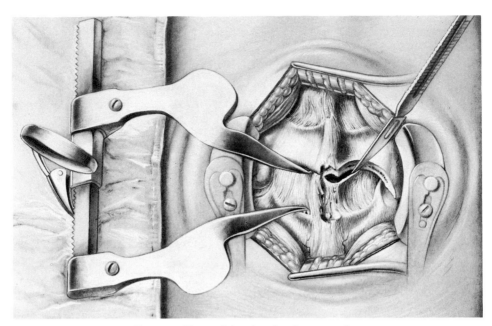

Fig. 7-7. Cloward lumbar lamina spreader.

cm. of the margin of the lower lamina is removed with the narrow chisel, as above, from the base of the spinous process to the facet. This bone is usually thin compared to the upper lamina so chiseling is done carefully and with a prying action and the bone removed with a heavy disc rongeur. The chisel is next placed in a vertical position about 3 mm. lateral to the medial margin of the lower facet cutting this overhanging edge (Fig. 7-10). A second bone cut is made parallel and lateral to the first and then a third

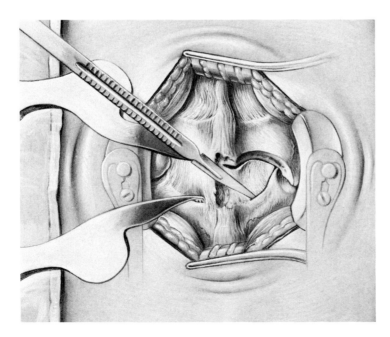

Fig. 7-8.

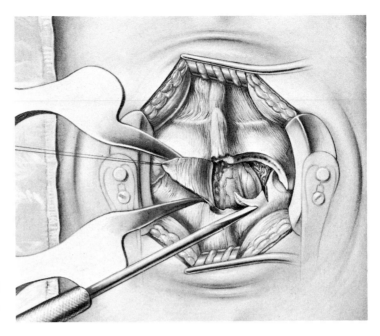

Fig. 7-9. Cloward intervertebral disc rongeur (4 mm. × 8 mm., shaft length 6½″).

lateral to it, each 3 mm. wide. These 3 bone slices are grasped with a disc rongeur and removed. Bleeding from bone margins is arrested with wax and from epidural veins with Gelfoam* and thrombin and packed with a cottonoid† pattie.

* Trademark of Upjohn.
† Trademark of Codman & Shurtleff, Inc.

Removal of the medial half of the inferior facet will expose 1 cm. or more of the spinal canal lateral to the nerve root. This area is filled with epidural fat and veins. These are separated from the lateral margin of the nerve root and dural sac and the latter gently retracted medially with a flexible retractor blade held manually or by a self-retaining

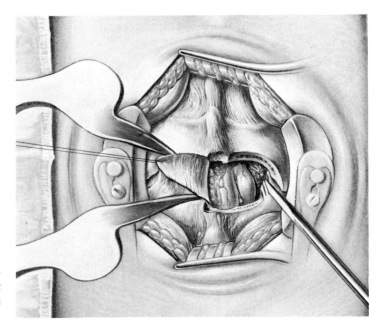

Fig. 7-10. Cloward intervertebral disc rongeur, straight (4 mm. × 10 mm., shaft length 6½″).

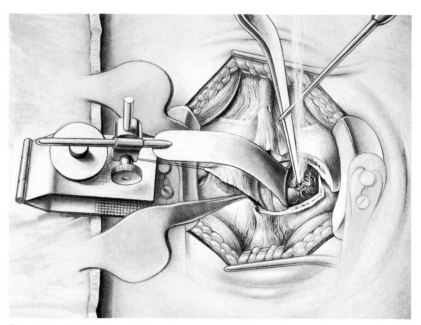

Fig. 7-11. (*Left*) Cloward dural retractor, self-retaining with two malleable blades, $\frac{5}{16}$″ and $\frac{1}{2}$″ wide (blade length 4″; blade and shaft length $8\frac{1}{4}$″). This instrument can be attached to any laminectomy retractor. The blade is engaged beneath the nerve root and dura, which structures are retracted medially to the desired position and held in place by the turn of a screw. (*Center*) Cloward flexible nerve root retractor. ($8\frac{1}{2}$″). (*Right*) D'Errico dressing forceps, bayonet shape ($8\frac{3}{4}$″).

retractor.[1] The veins and fat are grasped with tissue forceps and obliterated with the electro-coagulator, using the cutting current at a low setting (Fig. 7-11). A broad self-retaining retractor blade with a "shoe" tip is placed under the nerve root and dural sac, gently retracted to the midline, and secured in this position to the clamp on the laminectomy retractor. This eliminates strong manual retraction of the nerve root and possible trauma to it yet gives a wide exposure of the spinal canal. All vessels lateral and anterior to the dura are methodically cauterized under direct vision with little or no blood loss. The charred tissue is clipped with scissors and removed with a disc rongeur. Venous bleeding under the upper lamina beyond the surgeon's vision is "packed off" with Gelfoam and thrombin and a string-patty. Bone bleeding from the posterior surface of the vertebral body is burned with the cutting current. With the anterior wall of the spinal canal completely dry and widely exposed, the operative attack on the intervertebral disc is more easily and effectively accomplished.

Disc Removal

From this point on the surgical treatment of the disc lesion will differ with the surgeon's discretion. One of three operative procedures used are: (a) only the mass of disc which protrudes or has sequestrated in the spinal canal is removed: (Fig. 7-13) (b) the posterior fibers of the annulus fibrosus are incised and the interior of the disc is curretted, usually removing remnants of the nucleus pulposus and any loose fragments of the annulus: or (c) an interbody fusion is done by removing the entire disc, including the cartilage plates and the cortex of the adjacent vertebral bodies and inserting four

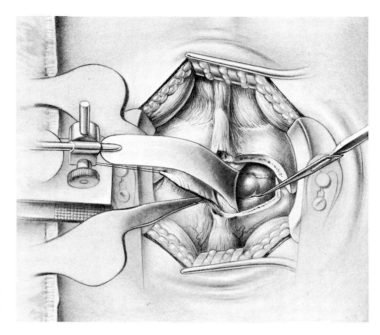

Fig. 7-12. (*Top left*) Spinal fusion curette, angled, No. 0. (*Bottom left*) Spinal fusion curette, angled, No. 1. (*Right*) Spinal fusion curette, angled, No. 2.

large blocks of bone into the intervertebral space. The latter technique is used by the author. (See pp. 227–236.) Prior to the wound closure a No. 22 spinal needle is inserted through the dura in the midline and 4 cc. of cerebrospinal fluid aspirated into a syringe.

This is used to dissolve 50 mg. of pure powdered prednisolone (Meticortelone)* which is reinjected intrathecally. *Closure:* Interrupted No. 0 chromic catgut sutures in the

*Trademark of Schering.

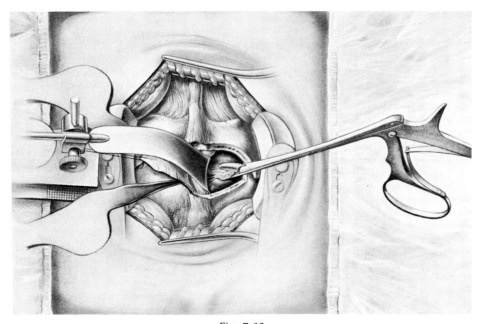

Fig. 7-13.

lumbar muscles and fascia and No. 00 in the subcutaneous layer are used to close the wound. The skin is held together with Steritapes.* If an interbody fusion is performed a rubber tissue (Penrose) drain is always used.

DISCUSSION

The reasons for radical departure in operative technique from that almost universally used requires further explanation.

Transverse Skin Incision

This was first used by the author in the late 40's for lumbar disc surgery when bone for the interbody fusion was removed from the patient's ilium.[2] Both operations were done through a single transverse incision. A wider lateral exposure for the skin wound, being made parallel to the lumbar operation was possible and the normal skin lines, heals better with less scar.

Ligamentum Flavum

Almost all "disc" surgeons remove this ligament. The defect resulting from its removal fills with dense scar tissue which may encompass and possibly compress the dural sac and nerve roots. If the entire ligament is preserved, by separating its attachments from the lamina and reflecting in a flap, a larger opening into the spinal canal is obtained and the replaced flap protects the dura and prevents scarring (Fig. 7-14).

Use of Chisel and Hammer

Spinal rongeurs, including the Leksell and the Kerrison have been the standard instruments used by neurosurgeons for laminectomy or laminotomy. The operative technique described here recommends the use of a narrow, sharp chisel and hammer. The rongeurs may be used to remove part of the laminal edge, but the hard bone of the facet must be removed with a chisel or air drill. When the surgeons become accustomed to

*Trademark of 3 M.

Fig. 7-14.

the use of the hammer and chisel technique to contour the interlaminar exposure, as well as the bed for the intervertebral grafts for interbody fusion, he will find that it can be done more effectively than using rongeurs or other instruments.

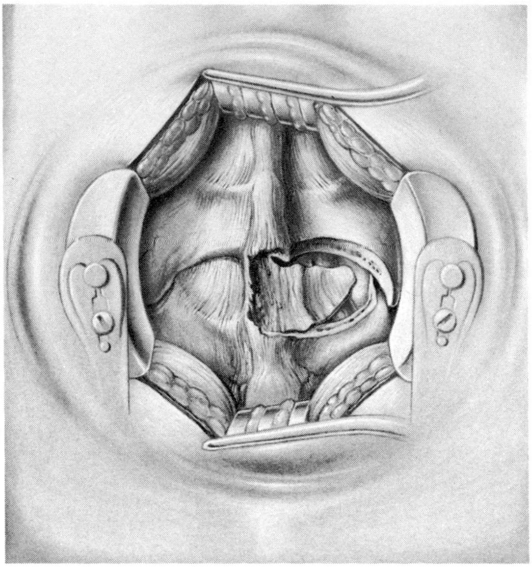

Articular Facets

It is the recommendation of most orthopaedic surgeons to leave the articular facets of the lumbar spine intact in lumbar disc surgery. Removal of all or any part of these vertebral elements is not advised for two reasons: (a) they are considered important major elements in the articulation of the vertebral joint, and (b) they must be preserved as an essential bony surface to be used in posterior spinal fusion operations (Hibbs, Albee). The reluctance to remove a part of the articular facets is one reason for failure to obtain an adequate lateral exposure in the spinal canal for effective surgery. In the author's experience, the advantages from removing a part of the articular facets far outweigh the disadvantages.

Disc Removal

Once the ruptured and symptomatic lumbar disc is diagnosed and exposed at operation, its removal may be "simple" or "radical." Either the intraspinal mass is simply removed (Fig. 7-10) or, in addition, the intervertebral space is opened and a portion of its contents evacuated. The reasons given to justify the latter procedure are based on a false assumption that the persistent low back pain which frequently follows the simple disc removal is caused by disc substance remaining in the intervertebral space. Patients are often subjected to repeat operations for removal of "more of the disc." The same theory is used to explain the recent use of protolytic enzymes to "remove the disc" chemically.[7]

The author's experience has shown that the persistent disabling pain following rupture and loss of the supporting function of the intervertebral disc is caused by movement of the abnormal painful joint, as well as from retained disc substance.[5] This pain can most effectively be cured by total disc removal followed by interbody fusion. This arrests joint movement and relieves the back pain.

Intrathecal Cortisone

The routine use of intrathecal cortisone after lumbar disc operations has been used since 1964. Its effectiveness was verified by a series of patients who showed marked reduction in the degree of postoperative pain. The effect of removing operative (traumatic) edema of the nerve roots and cauda equina is suggested by the infrequent occurrence of bladder dysfunction and sensory and/or motor impairment in the lower extremities. Finally, the prevention of postoperative arachnoiditis by the fibrolytic action of the prednisolone is presumed.

CONCLUSION

The surgical technique used by the author for exposure of ruptured intervertebral discs is described. Poor results following some lumbar disc operations are attributed to faulty technique and inadequate surgical exposure. Other causes and their correction are discussed.

POSTERIOR LUMBAR INTERBODY FUSION (P.L.I.F.)

INTRODUCTION

In the treatment of lesions of the lumbar intervertebral disc, the question as to whether the patient should or should not be treated by a spinal fusion operation always arises. There is no unanimity of thought among neurosurgeons and orthopaedic surgeons and one of the founding fathers of lumbar disc surgery, when asked this question replied: "If an operative procedure can be devised which will give satisfactory fusion as well as satisfactory removal and without lengthening the convalescent period, then I will concur with the idea of a fusion as part of the original operation."[6] These criteria laid down by Dr. Mixter are fully met by the operation of posterior lumbar interbody fusion. This operation was originated by the author and has been used for 29 years in the treatment of over 2000 patients with lumbar

disc disease.[2,3,9] A complete cure rate of approximately 96 percent has been accomplished.

The operative technique of P.L.I.F. is not difficult for the average disc surgeon to learn. However, there are three necessary prerequisites for the success of this operation.

1. The surgeon must be motivated to spend the time at the operating table to properly perform and complete the operation.

2. He must have available and be properly trained to use the special instruments designed for and required to do this operation.

3. He should have a bone bank with adequate supply of good quality bone to use as bone grafts.[4]

If these criteria are met, most lumbar disc operations will be gratifyingly successful.

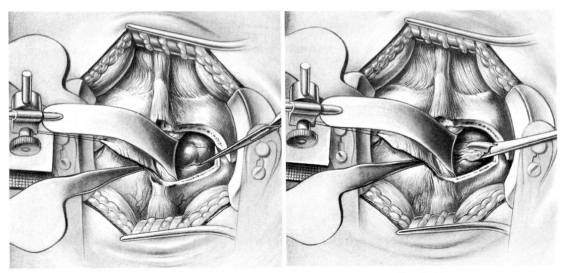

Fig. 7-15.   Fig. 7-16.

DISC REMOVAL

Exposure of the anterior wall of the spinal canal and the posterior surface of the intervertebral disc by an interlamina approach has been described (pp. 219–226). Special instruments are used to prepare a wide exposure of spinal canal to retract the nerve root and dural sac and to eradicate epidural vessels in preparation for removal of the disc.

A long scalpel handle with No. 11 Bard Parker blade is used to cut out the posterior half of the disc. A vertical incision is made in the disc in the midline beneath the retracted dura and nerve root. Then horizontal incisions are made following the margins of the adjacent vertebral bodies extending as far lateral as possible, usually beyond the pedicle of the lower vertebra (Fig. 7-15). The incised disc is withdrawn with a large disc rongeur giving an opening into the intervertebral space through which the remainder of the disc is removed (Fig. 7-16).

The bony ledge or "shelf" of the posterior superior margin of the **lower** vertebral body which overhangs the interspace is removed (Fig. 7-18B). This bone margin is first cut vertically in the midline beneath the dural sac with a 7 mm. osteotome (Fig. 7-17A). Then the second cut is made as far lateral

as possible, usually into the base of the pedicle (Fig. 7-17B). A wide osteotome (10 mms.) connects these two cuts with a transverse one about 3 to 5 mms. behind the margin of the vertebra (Fig. 7-18A). The osteotome is hammered straight down passing through bone and cartilage and into the intervertebral space (Fig. 7-18B). Removal of this wedge of bone gives a wide opening into the interspace (Fig. 7-18C). A strip of Gelfoam soaked in thrombin is packed over the bleeding surface of the vertebral body. This immediately arrests bone bleeding which may be brisk. The cartilagenous plate remaining on this vertebral body and on the entire plate of the upper one is stripped free with a long curved thin osteotome used as a manual elevator. Half of the interspace is thus cleaned of all soft tissue down to the anterior longitudinal ligament using a large disc rongeur, an English rongeur and a ring currette.

The cortical surfaces of the vertebral bodies are methodically removed using an 8 mm. curved or straight osteotome and hammer (Fig. 7-19A). The cartilage plates may be removed with the bone. Repeated curls are made using a prying action until the vertebral bodies are completely decorticated (Fig. 7-19B). The cortex removal is extended medially beneath the dural sac and laterally

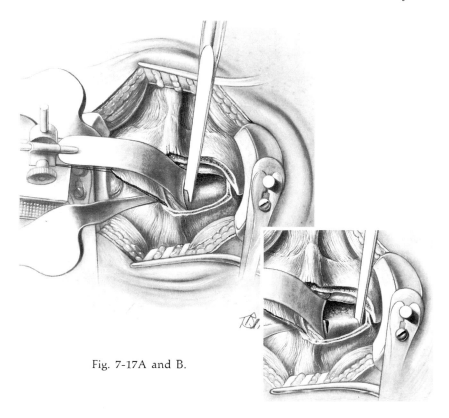

Fig. 7-17A and B.

Fig. 7-18A, B and C.

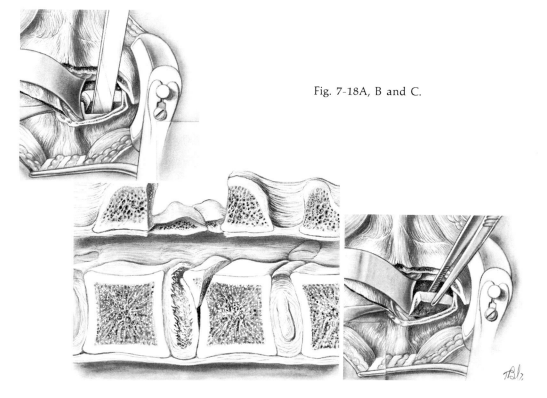

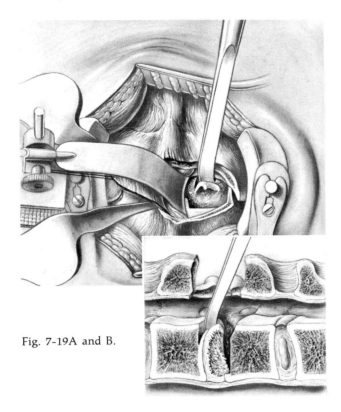

Fig. 7-19A and B.

to or beyond the vertebral pedicle. This will prepare a wide space for larger and more bone grafts.

BONE GRAFTS

If bone is to be obtained from the patient, it is advisable to remove the grafts the day before the spinal fusion. The best donor site is the left posterior ilium. With the patient in the prone position, a transverse skin incision is made parallel to and below the iliac crest from the posterior superior iliac spine to the cluneal nerves. These large sensory nerves which cross the ilium from above downward about 6 to 8 centimeters lateral to the midline, should be carefully dissected out and protected from injury to prevent painful postoperative neuromata from developing at the donor site.

The gluteal muscles are stripped subperiosteally from the posterior surface of the ilium and retracted using one long and one short self-retaining retractor blade. With a wide thin blade straight osteotome five parallel vertical cuts are made about $1\frac{1}{2}$ centimeters apart, starting at the iliac crest and driving downward approximately 3 centimeters (Fig. 7-20A). These cuts are connected at their base by a transverse cut made with a wide-curved osteotome driven inward to the inner table of the ilium. The three medial bone plugs thus outlined are removed by chiseling from above downward with a wide-curved osteotome, getting as thick a graft as possible, but leaving the inner table of the ilium intact (Fig. 7-20B). The fourth graft, most lateral, is removed full thickness of the ilium. Thus, three grafts will have cortex on one side and one will have double cortex. The raw exposed bony surface of the ilium is covered with bone wax to arrest all bleeding. The wound is closed in layers with a rubber tissue drain in place. The bone grafts are placed in a sterile jar containing

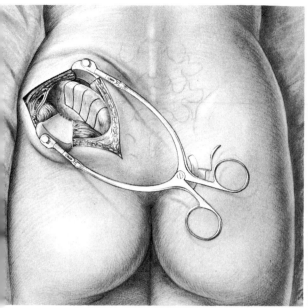
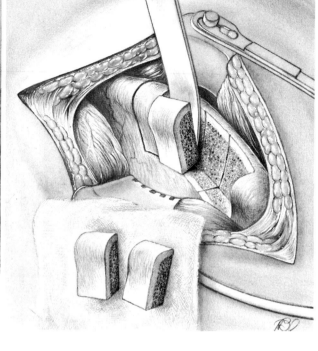

Fig. 7-20A and B.

streptomycin solution sealed and kept in a deep freeze until used.

The bone grafts preferred for this operation are obtained from the bone bank.[6]

These grafts or "plugs" are cut full thickness, 1 x 3 cm., from an ilium which has been removed from a fresh cadaver under sterile conditions, cultured and preserved by freezing (Fig. 7-20B). The grafts are prepared at the operating table by thoroughly washing with saline solution to remove fat and plasma from cancellous bone and placing in a solution of streptomycin until used.

BONE GRAFTING

A depth gauge is dropped into the prepared intervertebral space to measure its depth. A bone graft is trimmed with the air drill and rongeur to the proper size, slightly wider than the prepared interspace and 3 mms. shorter than the measured depth so the graft can be recessed below the anterior wall of the spinal canal. Several turns are made

on the thumb screw of the interlaminar spreader to widen the intervertebral space for insertion of the large bone graft. The graft is grasped with a tooth forceps and its lower end inserted into the center of the prepared disc space. The bone graft impactors are available in various sizes and shapes depending on the contour and the consistency of bone on the upper end of the bone graft. If the graft has cortex on the end, an oval or round impactor with a sharp pin is used (Fig. 7-23A). This prevents it from slipping as the graft is driven into the interspace. If the graft has no cortex on its upper end, the impactor with a broad base and lip is used to prevent the graft from breaking or crumbling with hard pounding (Fig. 7-21A). An attempt is made to drive the bone graft in a perpendicular direction so that its cancellous surface will be parallel to the vertical walls of the interspace (Fig. 7-21B). If the thickness of the bone graft is much less than the width of the prepared hemi-interspace, to prevent the graft from twisting or rotating

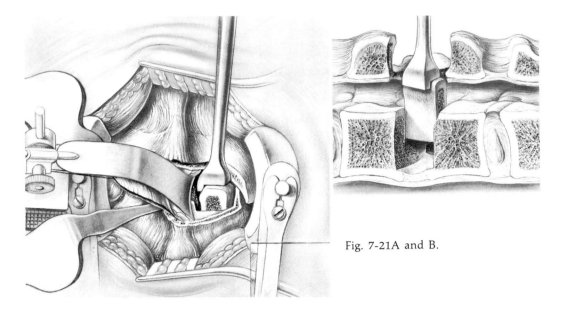

Fig. 7-21A and B.

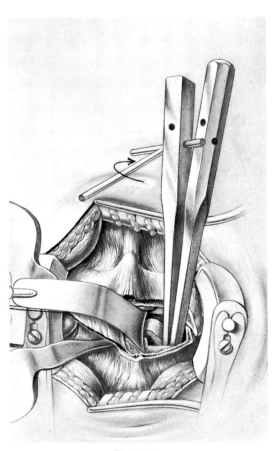

Fig. 7-22.

a "puka" chisel may be placed on one or both sides of the graft for vertical support.

The next step is to move the first bone graft medially to enlarge the opening lateral to it for insertion of the second or third graft. This is accomplished by using the two "puka" chisels. These instruments have heavy, flat, dull blades with holes perforating the handle. They are inserted or driven vertically into the interspace lateral to the bone graft. The T-shaped handle is inserted into a hole of the medial chisel to make a prying, twisting action against the lateral chisel. This will "walk" the bone graft toward the midline (Fig. 7-22).

The second "plug" is trimmed to fit the opening, thus prepared and impacted into the interspace (Fig. 7-23B). If this graft does not fill the space, the "puka" chisels are again used to crowd this graft medially and prepare a space for a third graft. Bleeding from epidural veins may result from jarring the spine when the grafts are impacted, this is arrested with Gelfoam and packing. Bleeding from the cancellous bone of the vertebral bodies is arrested by the compression force of the bone grafts. The bone margin of the vertebral bodies not covered by the bone graft is waxed.

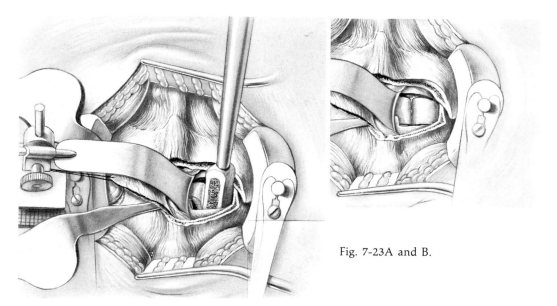

Fig. 7-23A and B.

The self-retaining retractor blade is removed from the nerve root and dural sac and these structures permitted to return to their normal position. The space lateral to the nerve root is filled with a large strip of Gelfoam and the flap of ligamentum flavum replaced over the dura and nerve root. This half of the wound is then packed off with a gauze sponge.

On the opposite side of the spine, a similar operative procedure is carried out. The vertebra spreader is not required to increase the width of the intervertebral space, since this has been accomplished by the inserted bone grafts. However, the spreader may be used to widen the interlaminar space. The intervertebral space on this side is prepared in the same manner, removing disc, cartilage and cortical end-plates. The first bone graft is moved forcibly toward the midline until it is in close proximity to the medial graft inserted from the other side (Fig. 7-24A). After the final graft is impacted, the instruments and all sponges and Gelfoam are removed from the spinal canal (Fig. 7-24B).

The two flaps of ligamentum flavum are elevated and the nerve roots and dural sac are gently compressed to the midline with a bayonet forcep to allow inspection of the entire grafted area (Fig. 7-25A). This is done to assure that all grafts are equally recessed and that there is ample space between the anterior surface of the nerve roots and dural sac and bone grafts.

Prior to the closure of the wound a No. 25 lumbar puncture needle is inserted through the dura in the midline beneath the upper spinous process and 3 cc. of clear cerebrospinal fluid removed. This is used to dissolve 50 mg. of pure powdered prednisolone (Meticortelone) which is reinjected intrathecally.

WOUND CLOSURE

Flaps of the ligamentum flavum are replaced over the dural sac and nerve roots (Fig. 7-25C). The open space lateral to the roots is filled with a strip of thrombin-soaked Gelfoam. A long strip of gauze is packed over the lamina and interlaminar space and the blades of the self-retaining laminectomy retractor are removed. An Addison retractor is placed in the lumbar fascia and retracted. The large paravertebral muscles which bulge into the field are closed with No. 0 chromic catgut sutures, using a very large full curved cutting needle which is passed around the

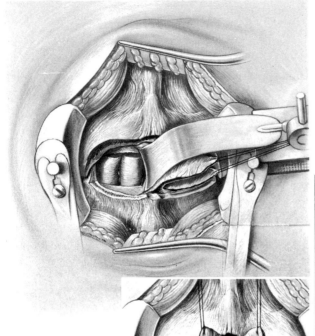

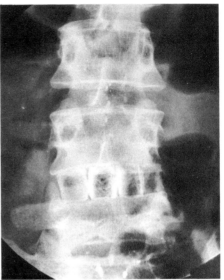

Fig. 7-24A, B and C.

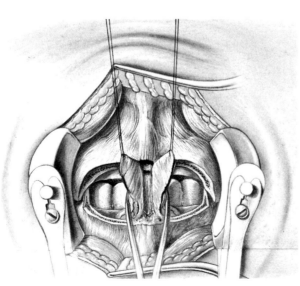

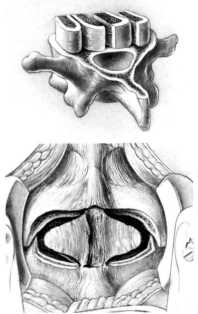

Fig. 7-25A, B and C.

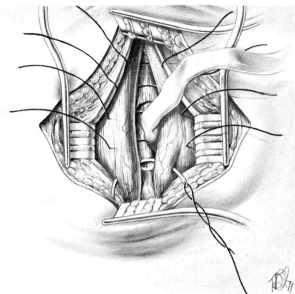

Fig. 7-26.

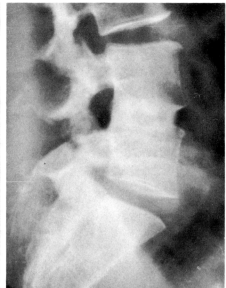

Fig. 7-27.

muscle belly on each side (Fig. 7-26). These sutures are tied loosely to approximate the muscle layer. The deep gauze sponge is removed and a wide rubber tissue drain or a Hemovac tube is inserted down to the lamina before the muscle sutures are tied. The lumbosacral fascia is closed snugly with interrupted silk or nylon sutures, No. 00 catgut is used for the subcutaneous layer. This latter stitch is placed as close to the dermis as possible and inverted with the knot down, giving an excellent skin closure. Steri-tapes on the skin complete the closure. A very small safety pin is placed in the drain to prevent it from slipping beneath the skin. A loose dressing is applied.

POSTOPERATIVE CARE

The patient is placed on his back on a firm mattress. Following recovery from the anesthesia he may move himself in bed for comfort. A Foley catheter may be required within the first 8 hours if the patient does not void voluntarily. The patient is relatively free of pain (cortisone) with infrequent requests for morphine. The suction drainage tube or the Penrose drain is discontinued and removed in 24 hours, depending on the amount of

postoperative oozing. The patient is permitted to sit on the side of the bed or stand at the bedside on the third postoperative day. The following day he may walk to the toilet and ambulate as desired thereafter, gradually increasing activity. Most patients are able to leave the hospital on the seventh day. Postoperative x-rays of the lumbosacral spine are obtained prior to discharge. No corsets, braces, belts or casts are used. The patient is encouraged to bend and stretch his back muscles after the tenth postoperative day. By continuing these exercises, the patient is assured a flexible painless back. Follow-up x-ray will show a good interbody fusion in three to four months.

DISCUSSION

Fusion of the vertebral bodies by the posterior approach through the spinal canal (P.L.I.F.) is a superior method of fusion for the lumbar spine. It has many advantages over other types of spinal fusion currently in use either by the anterior or posterior approach. These are listed as follows:

1. P.L.I.F. permits visualization and removal of disc fragments protruding into or invading the spinal canal, causing compres-

sion of the nerve root and/or the cauda equina.

2. Posterior marginal osteophytes frequently associated with adhesive attachments to the nerve roots can be removed.

3. Ankylosis of the vertebra is more rapid than other types of spinal fusion because:

(a) the bone grafts are placed at right angles to the weight-bearing axis of the spine.

(b) the vertebral joint is mechanically fixed at operation eliminating the need for external support or braces.

(c) compression of the bone grafts against the raw surface of the vertebral bodies is conducive to early vascularization and rapid fusion.

4. Morbidity of the operation is lower. Limited exposure of the spine preserves muscle and ligament attachments.

5. Recovery is rapid. The patient walks on third or fourth postoperative day and leaves the hospital in one week. Active flexion exercises of back muscles are begun 10 days following operation and continued thereafter.

6. The percentage of complete cures without disability is higher due to

(a) infrequency of nerve root and cauda equina scarring, which may cause persistent postoperative pain;

(b) minimal stiffness of lumbar muscles due to fibrosis and shortening, which frequently follows long periods of immobilization;

(c) low rate of pseudoarthrosis (less than 5%)

CONCLUSION

The surgical technique of posterior lumbar interbody fusion is described and its advantages discussed. This operation may be difficult for the beginner. The superior results obtained compared to other spinal fusion methods justify the time required to learn this technique and to perform the operation.

REFERENCES

1. Cloward, R. B.: Creation and Operation of a Bone Bank. J. Neurosurg. 23:682–688. 1970.
2. Cloward, R. B.: The Degenerated Lumbar Discs. Treatment by Vertebral Body Fusion. J. of I. C. S. 22:375–386. Oct. 1954.
3. Cloward, R. B.: Lesions of the Intervertebral Discs and Their Treatment by Interbody fusion methods. (The painful disc) Clin. Orthop. 27:51–77. 1963.
4. Cloward, R. B.: A Self-Retaining spinal dura retractor. J. Neurosurg. 9:230–232, 1952.
5. Cloward, R. B.: The Treatment of Ruptured Lumbar Intervertebral Discs by Vertebral Body Fusion. I. Indications, Operative Techniques and After Care. J. Neurosurg. 10:154–168. 1953.
6. Cloward, R. B.: Vertebral Body Fusion for Ruptured Lumbar Discs. Roentgenographic Study. Ann. Surg. 90:969–976. 1955.
7. Flor, L. T.: Clinical Use of Chymopapin in Lumbar and Dorsal Disc Lesions. An End-result study. Clin. Orthopd. 67:81–87, Nov.–Dec. 1969.
8. Mixter, W. J.: Symposium on Intervertebral Discs and Sciatic Pain. (Discussion) J. Bone & Joint Surg. 29:468. 1947.
9. Mixter, W. J. and Barr, J. S.: Rupture of the Intervertebral Disk with involvement of the spinal canal. New Eng. J. Med. 211:210, 1934.
10. Raaf, John: Removal of Protruded Lumbar Intervertebral Discs. J. Neurosurg. 32:604, 1970.
11. Semmes, R. E.: Ruptured Lumbar Intervertebral Discs: Their Recognition and Surgical Relief. Clin. Neurosurg. 8:78–92, 1960.
12. Spurling, R. Glen: Lesions of the Lumbar Intervertebral Disc. Chas. C Thomas. Springfield, Ill. 1953, pp. 95–99.

8
Analgesic Blocks

Lumbar Epidural Block

Site of Injection
Position
Technique

Caudal Block

Sacral Canal
Sacral Hiatus
Technique
Complications

Paravertebral Block

Indications
Technique

8

Analgesic Blocks

Occasionally, the use of analgesic blocks is helpful in managing the patient with severe low back and sciatic pain. These blocks are often reserved for persons who were not responsive to previous surgery and in whom it was felt that further surgery was best deferred. Generally, the purpose is to provide temporary relief of pain, but when a combination of local anesthesia and corticosteroid is used, a long-term beneficial effect may be achieved.

LUMBAR EPIDURAL BLOCK

The lumbar epidural block, a form of peripheral nerve block is accomplished by introducing the anesthetic agent into the peridural or the epidural space. Although the anesthetic drug is deposited into the extradural space, the site of drug action is more peripheral, since in most instances the drug solution must spread out into the intervertebral foramina before the spinal nerve sheath is sufficiently permeable.

Site of Injection

When this technique is used for patients who have never previously had surgery, the injection is carried out in the low lumbar region as close as possible to the site of suspected dysfunction. However, most of these blocks are performed on patients who have had previous low back surgery and continue to manifest symptoms. With these patients it is well to carry out the block away from the site of the original incision for two reasons: (1) If the needle is inserted into the dense scar, it will not be possible to recognize the various tissue levels which the bevel of the needle is penetrating, and this may lead to an inadvertent puncture of the dura; (2) because the dura is usually quite adherent to the overlying laminae following surgery, an adequate epidural space is eradicated, making it impossible to successfully carry out an injection at that site. Since most lumbar laminectomy scars extend over the sacrum, the postoperative peridural injection is best performed at either the L1-2 or L2-3 levels.

Position

The lateral recumbent position is preferred. When performing a lumbar puncture for myelography, the sitting position is advantageous because it creates increased hydrostatic pressure within the caudal sac, making it easier for the spinal needle to cleanly penetrate the distended dura and arachnoid. Since our objectives are to avoid penetrating the dura and to place the bevel of the needle in the extradural space, it is advantageous to have as little distention of the caudal sac as possible. For this reason the lateral recumbent position is advantageous. Since the injected medication will spread to some extent on the basis of gravity flow, the patient is instructed to lie on the painful side so that the involved nerve roots will be lowermost and affected by the medication to the greatest extent. It is important that the patient be well flexed with the thighs upon the abdomen, because it is felt that flexion increases the "negative pressure" within the

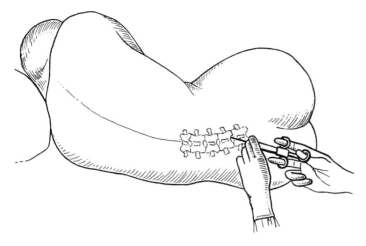

Fig. 8-1. Technique of introducing needle into epidural space.

peridural space allowing easier identification when the needle bevel reaches this level.

Technique

A 25-gauge hypodermic needle is used to make a local anesthesia wheal over the desired interspace, and a 20-gauge, short beveled spinal needle is introduced between the spinous processes. After penetrating the interspinous ligament, the stylet is removed and the needle connected to a 10 cc. "three-ringed" syringe that is half filled with air. Using gentle pressure on the plunger of the syringe, a small amount of air is injected as the needle is slowly advanced toward the extradural space. The entrance of the bevel of the needle into this space is signaled by a sudden absence of any resistance to injection of the air; and as a result, the syringe is usually emptied into the peridural space.

This air injection often causes discomfort or paresthesia in the low back.

It is necessary to carefully observe the hub of the needle for a minute or two to be sure that no cerebrospinal fluid drainage is present as a result of partial penetration of the dura. Gentle aspiration of the needle is now attempted, with great care being taken not to dislodge or move the needle in any way. If spinal fluid is obtained the block is terminated, since dural puncture is a contraindication to epidural block. If blood is aspirated, the stylet is reinserted, and after a 3- to 5-minute wait for coagulation to occur, aspiration is reattempted. If the second aspiration is negative, the block may be done, but at frequent intervals aspiration with the injecting syringe is carried out. After the satisfactory position of the needle has been established, 6 cc. of 1 percent Xylocaine,

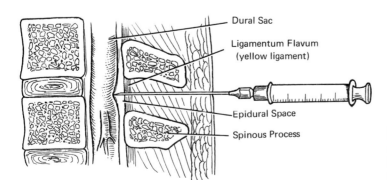

Dural Sac

Ligamentum Flavum (yellow ligament)

Epidural Space

Spinous Process

Fig. 8-2. The "potential" epidural space is in part created by needle pressure upon the nondistended dura.

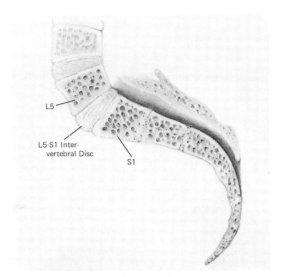

L5

L5-S1 Inter-
vertebral Disc

S1

Fig. 8-3. Lateral view of sacral canal.

specifically prepared for spinal anesthesia without fixatives, is slowly injected. The needle is left in place and the stylet inserted. A mixture of 75 to 100 milligrams of prednisolone acetate suspension is prepared with normal saline to a total volume of 8 cc. After several minutes, some degree of anesthesia is appreciated as a result of the Xylocaine injection, and the patient's discomfort is reduced. The prednisolone acetate suspension mixture is then injected and the needle withdrawn. Some physicians feel that in addition to the effects of the medication there is a possible neurolysis effect by "mechanically breaking up adhesions."

Following the injection the patient is placed in a hospital bed with his head slightly elevated and knees flexed. After approximately half an hour, he is allowed to leave in a wheelchair and can be driven home but must rest in bed for at least 2 hours. If a patient has no one to drive him home, he must remain in the hospital for 2 or 3 hours.

The 2 major complications of epidural block are inadvertent injection of the local anesthesia into either the subarachnoid space or into a blood vessel. If this occurs, the patient should be immediately given artificial respiration, intubated as quickly as possible and placed in a respirator. Oxygen, vaso-

pressor drugs and intravenous fluids are in order. After these basic supportive measures have been instituted, if the inadvertent injection was into the subarachnoid space, a lumbar puncture is performed and large volumes of cerebrospinal fluid are immediately withdrawn in the hope of removing as much of the drug as possible from the subarachnoid space. If these measures are instituted in time, the spinal anesthetic effect will eventually recede, spontaneous respirations will resume and the blood pressure improve.

The epidural block is technically less difficult to perform and is associated with somewhat less discomfort than the caudal block. Some are of the opinion that more effective pain relief is obtained with the epidural block. Occasionally, for technical reasons such as extensive scarring, or the personal preference of the injector, the caudal block is used.

CAUDAL BLOCK

The caudal block is a form of peridural analgesia or anesthesia performed by injecting the solution into the caudal or sacral canal through the sacral hiatus.

Because the injection is performed into the sacral canal, the normal anatomy of the sacrum and the sacral canal and the anomalies of this structure should be known. Many of these anomalies present unfavorable conditions both for needle insertion and also for the satisfactory dispersion of the injected solution.

Sacral Canal

The sacral canal is merely the sacral prolongation of the vertebral canal. Viewed laterally its longitudinal axis is curved like the sacrum with anterior concavity. The anterior floor of the canal is formed by the fused vertebral bodies and the overlying posterior longitudinal ligament. The lateral boundaries are formed by the sacral pedicles and the intervertebral foramina. The posterior roof is formed by the fused laminae. Occasionally, as a result of the transverse ridges found

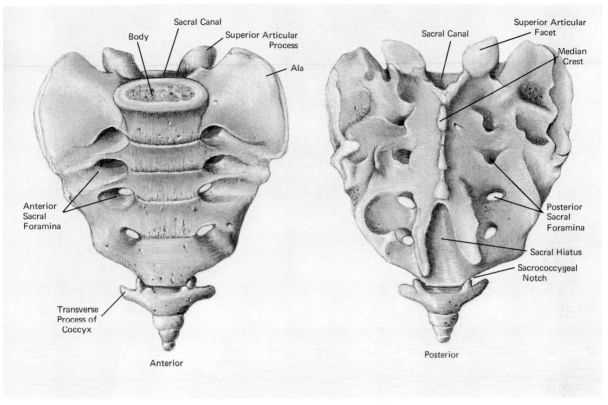

Fig. 8-4. Anterior and posterior views of sacrum.

between the fused sacral vertebrae, the anterior floor is so irregular as to prevent the needle from advancing cephalad during caudal injection.

A continuation of the caudal sac extends from the lumbar region into the upper segments of the sacral canal. Generally, the terminal end of the caudal sac extends no further than the second sacral vertebra. This is far from an absolute rule, however, as is apparent to those who review lumbar myelograms which demonstrate the considerable variability of the end of the dural sac in relationship to the sacrum. This anatomical variability is of considerable technical importance in the performance of a caudal block, which is based on installation of solution into the peridural space but not the subarachnoid space. The length of the sacral canal varies from 7 to 9 centimeters and the distance between the apex of the sacral

hiatus and the end of the dural sac exhibits even greater variation—from 2 to 7 centimeters with an average of 4.5 centimeters. When performing a caudal block on patients who have had previous myelography, it is most helpful to review the films, since this will give a clear indication regarding the exact termination of the caudal sac in relationship to the sacral canal.

When the caudal sac terminates, it ends in a dural strand called the filum terminale which passes through the sacral canal and fuses to the periosteum of the dorsal surface of the coccyx. The sacral nerve roots are surrounded by sleeve-like extensions from the caudal sac and these dural prolongations are variable in their extent, in some cases reaching below the caudal end of the dura. This anatomical variation, usually revealed by the myelogram, is also of practical importance in considering a caudal block. In addi-

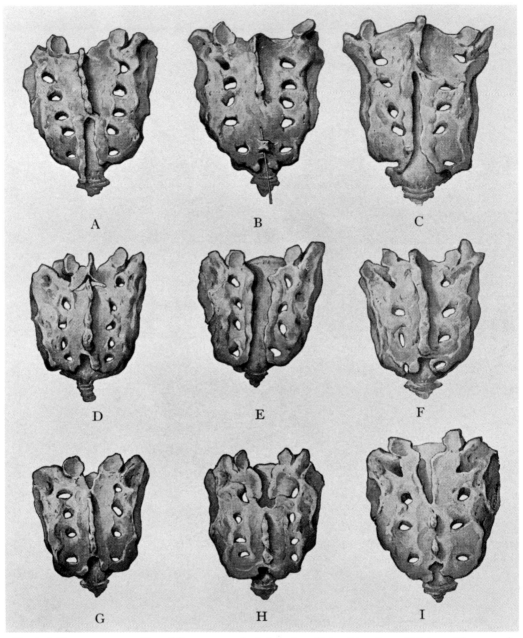

Fig. 8-5. Common anomalies of the sacrum: A; deformity of lateral borders of hiatus with upward extension; B; fairly normal hiatus but with an additional foramen in a sacral spinous process through which the needle has been inserted; C; hiatus extending upward to the level of the body of the first sacral vertebra; D; deformity of the sacrum resulting from injury; E; open sacral canal; F; flattened anteroposterior diameter of canal; G, H, I; failure of fusion of lamina of the first sacral vertebra. (M. Williamson.)

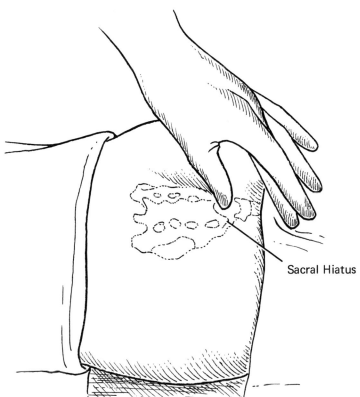

Sacral Hiatus

Fig. 8-6. Locating the sacral hiatus.

tion to nerve roots and their enveloping membranes, the sacral canal contains blood vessels, fat, loose areolar tissue and lymphatics. The blood vessels are primarily veins and are most prevalent along the anterior lateral aspect of the canal similar to the lumbar epidural vessels.

Sacral Hiatus

The caudal portion of the sacral canal terminates as an inverted U-shaped or V-shaped opening on the dorsum of the sacrum called the sacral hiatus. Its formation is due to a fusion failure of the last one or two (fourth and fifth) sacral laminae. It is about 5 centimeters above the tip of the coccyx and is usually a centimeter or two above the upper limit of the gluteal crease. Two bony prominences on either side of the sacral hiatus are valuable as landmarks when performing a caudal block and are referred to as the sacral cornua. Completely covering

the sacral hiatus is the posterior sacrococcygeal ligament, which actually forms the caudal end of the vertebral canal. Superficial to this ligament lie the subcutaneous tissues and skin.

Technique

The patient is placed in the prone position with 2 pillows beneath the pubis to make the lower portion of the sacrum more prominent. The sacral hiatus is palpated by running the finger up and down from the midline of the sacrum down to the gluteal crease and palpating a slight depression just above the inverted U-shaped crease. Further identification is obtained by palpating the lateral walls of this hiatus, the so-called sacral cornua. Another confirmation of position is to palpate the tip of the coccyx and then proceed cephalad approximately 5 centimeters again ending at the slight depression just above the gluteal crease.

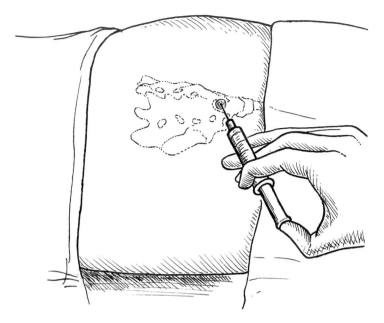

Fig. 8-7. Local anesthetic wheal over sacral hiatus.

Little difficulty is encountered in identification of the sacral hiatus in thin patients; but if a patient is obese, difficulties may arise. Occasionally, the knee-chest position in obese patients is helpful.

After establishing the location of the sacral hiatus, the hair overlying this site is shaved and the area cleansed with antiseptic solution and draped with a sterile towel. A local anesthetic skin wheal is made over the sacral hiatus with a 25-gauge hypodermic needle; the needle is introduced deeper to infiltrate the subcutaneous tissues and the sacrococcygeal ligament. The 25-gauge needle is temporarily allowed to remain in place as a landmark. A 20-gauge lumbar puncture needle with stylet in place, maintained perpendicular to the skin, is then introduced directly through the center of the sacral hiatus going through the skin and subcutaneous tissues. As the needle penetrates the sacrococcygeal ligament, it is met with firm resistance which suddenly subsides. The bevel of the needle will then encounter bony resistance, indicating that it has impinged upon the body of the fourth sacral vertebra. At this point, the needle is withdrawn slightly and the shaft is depressed; the needle is then advanced 2 or 3 centimeters, bringing the

bevel to the level of the third vertebra. Because of a high transverse ridge between the last 2 sacral vertebrae, the needle is occasionally obstructed before it can be adequately introduced into the sacral canal. If this occurs, the shaft and hub of the needle are depressed further, causing the bevel to move upward so that, hopefully, it will be able to glide over this bony ridge. In some instances either the sacral canal is so small or the obstructing ridge is so great that the needle cannot be further advanced. If such be the case, an attempt can be made to inject the solution without further needle advancement.

At this point it is most important to be sure that the needle is neither in the subarachnoid space nor in a blood vessel. Careful aspiration of the needle is done at least 3 or 4 times and before each aspiration $\frac{1}{2}$ cc. of air is injected through the needle to be sure that it is not obstructed by fat or areolar tissue. If spinal fluid is obtained the block is terminated, since dural puncture is a contraindication to caudal block. If blood is aspirated, the needle is moved back by half a centimeter, the stylet reinserted and after a 3- to 5-minute wait for coagulation to occur, aspiration is reattempted.

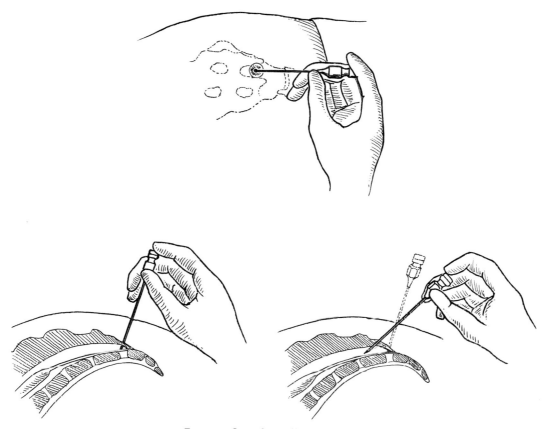

Fig. 8-8. Spinal needle placement.

After being satisfied that the needle is neither in a blood vessel nor in the subarachnoid space, 8 cc. of 1 percent Xylocaine without fixative specifically prepared for spinal anesthesia are initially injected. The needle is left in place with the stylet inserted. During this injection, it is well to place the hand over the sacrum to be sure that a subcutaneous injection is not being made directly over the sacrum. Occasionally, marked resistance to injection is encountered, usually indicating that the point of the needle has embedded into the periosteum. In such a case, a slight withdrawal of the needle is usually helpful. After injection of the anesthetic solution, the patient may note reduction of discomfort in 5 or 10 minutes. One hundred milligrams of prednisolone acetate suspension is diluted to 12 cc. making a total of 20 cc. of medication injected.

The level achieved by a caudal block primarily depends upon the volume of solution used. Other factors are speed of injection and the position of the patient. The more rapid the injection, the higher the level; a patient in head down position may obtain anesthesia or analgesia reaching 1 or 2 segments higher.

Some anesthesiologists feel that in addition to relieving pain, a measure of therapeutic effect may be achieved in the use of the caudal block by mechanically relieving "nerve root adhesions" within the spinal and sacral canal.

Complications

The major complication of caudal block is inadvertent injection of the local anesthesia, either into the subarachnoid space or into a blood vessel. If this occurs, the patient

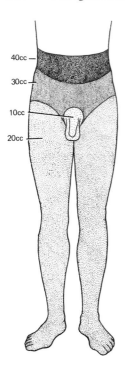
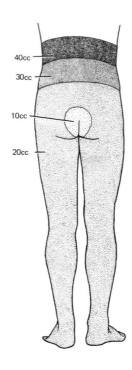

Fig. 8-9. Amounts of anesthetic solution necessary for various levels of anesthesia.

should be immediately given artificial respiration, intubated as quickly as possible and placed on a respirator. Oxygen, vasopressor drugs and intravenous fluids are in order. After these basic supportive measures have been instituted, and if the inadvertent injection was into the subarachnoid space, a lumbar puncture is performed and large volumes of cerebrospinal fluid immediately withdrawn, in the hope of removing as much of the drug from the subarachnoid space as possible. If these measures are instituted in time, the spinal anesthetic effect will eventually recede, spontaneous respirations will resume and the blood pressure improve. The patient will invariably have a severe postspinal headache resulting from the withdrawal of spinal fluid.

If the inadvertent injection was intravascular it may be associated with convulsions, which must be treated by intravenous anticonvulsant medication, or with cardiorespiratory collapse, which is treated by vasopressor drugs, intubation, artificial respiration and general supportive management.

Another complication of caudal block may be hypotension which is due to paralysis of the sympathetic vasoconstrictors. This complication usually occurs only if the block is quite extensive and is prevented by vasopressor medication prior to the injection.

PARAVERTEBRAL BLOCK

Indications

The paravertebral block can be also applied as a diagnostic aid in determining whether a specific root is the source of pain. When a dorsal rhizotomy is contemplated for surgical relief of pain, it can be employed in the form of a short-term presurgical therapeutic trial.

Since the L5 and S1 nerve roots are the 2 most commonly involved roots, the technique of injecting these nerves will be discussed.

Technique

The patient is positioned on the x-ray table in a prone position with either 2 pillows or a large foam rubber sponge beneath the abdomen to achieve some degree of lumbar

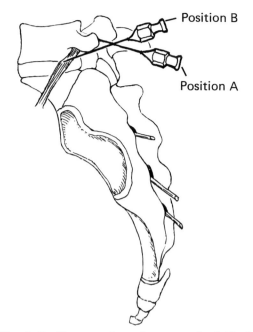

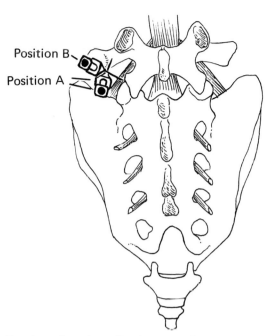

Fig. 8-10. Cross-section of paravertebral block.

Fig. 8-11. Spinal needle placement for paravertebral block.

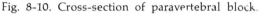

flexion. What is estimated as the L5-S1 interspace is identified using x-ray guidance. A 25-gauge hypodermic needle is used to place a local anesthesia skin wheal 4 centimeters lateral to the L5 spinous process, and again x-ray guidance is used to check the accurate position of this hypodermic needle. An 8 centimeter 22-gauge needle with a depth marker is introduced in a direction perpendicular to the skin and advanced until its point impinges upon the L5 lumbar vertebra transverse process, a depth between 4 to 6 centimeters. The depth guide on the needle is then placed 3 centimeters from the skin, the needle withdrawn until its point is in the subcutaneous tissue and then redirected slightly more medially and caudally so that it will pass inferior to the transverse process toward the intervertebral foramen and the exiting L5 nerve root. The needle is advanced very slowly and as soon as paresthesia is produced by the needle striking the L5 nerve root its progress is immediately stopped. At this point, the needle is aspirated for either spinal fluid or blood; and if the aspiration

is negative, 3 to 5 cc. of 1 percent Xylocaine are injected into the nerve root. Do not inject the anesthetic solution until a recheck x-ray is taken.

After having performed the paravertebral L5 root block, we can now prepare to do the transsacral (paravertebral sacral) block. The sacral hiatus and cornu are identified and a line drawn between the sacral cornu on the side of the block and the previously inserted L5 root block needle. The first posterior sacral foramen is located approximately 4 centimeters caudad from this needle on the previously drawn line. The 8 centimeter, 22-gauge needle is introduced through the wheal in a slightly medial direction so that the roof of the sacrum is contacted. After this bony impingement has occurred, the depth marker is placed 1.5 centimeters from the skin, the needle slightly withdrawn and re-inserted in a more perpendicular fashion. As the needle contacts the first sacral foramen, penetration of the ligament covering the foramen will produce a slight sensation of resistance which immediately disappears.

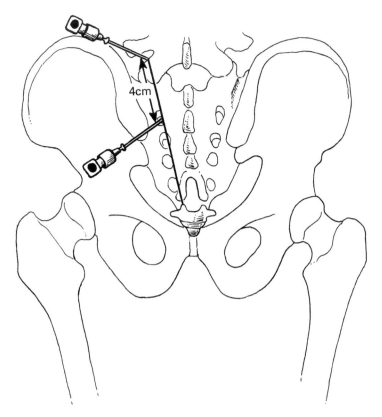

4cm

Fig. 8-12. Localization of first sacral foramen.

The needle is advanced until paresthesia is experienced by the patient or until the depth marker is flush with the skin. If no paresthesia is appreciated, and an x-ray check indicates the needle within the first sacral foramen, 5 cc. of 1 percent Xylocaine can be injected.

Complications of the paravertebral block are similar to those discussed under caudal block, but generally of a lesser magnitude.

9
Posterior Lumbar Rhizotomy

THE PATIENT SELECTION

Posterior lumbar rhizotomy has been employed for many years in patients who have continued to complain of radicular pain after low back surgery. One or another surgeon who would utilize this technique might derive an occasional good result with the procedure and then, because of several less than satisfactory results, would give it up. Although this operation has a use, its application is best limited to a specific type of problem. This is the patient who, subsequent to multiple surgical procedures designed to alleviate nerve root pressure, continues to manifest nerve root pain. The results are best when the pain is confined to a single root, although in certain instances sensory rhizotomies of the L5 and S1 roots are helpful. If the pain syndrome includes low back discomfort in addition to radicular symptoms, the likelihood of success for this procedure is poor.

Prior to consideration of a dorsal rhizotomy, a diagnostic paravertebral block, using x-ray guidance for needle placement, should be performed. Only after obtaining pain relief with anesthetic blockade of the suspected nerve root should posterior lumbar rhizotomy be considered. See section on analgesic blocks (pp. 246–248).

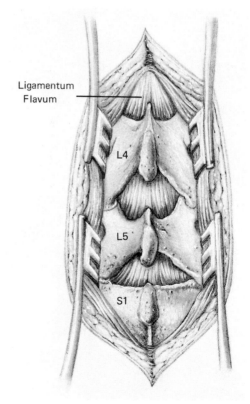

Fig. 9-1. Exposure of spines and laminae.

249

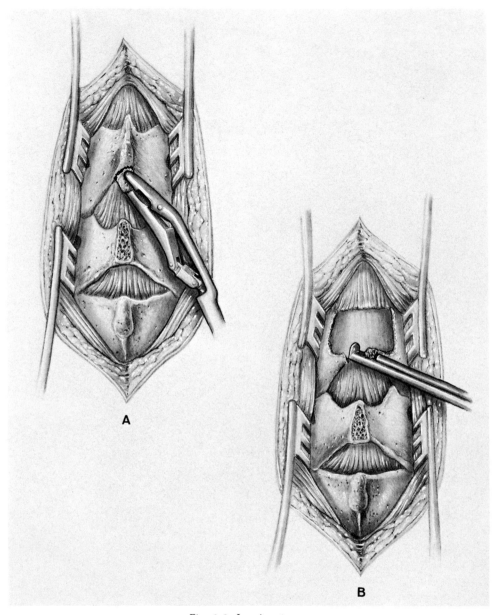

Fig. 9-2. Laminectomy.

PROCEDURE

Under general anesthesia with the patient in prone position, a bilateral subperiosteal muscle dissection is performed exposing the spines and laminae above and below the nerve root to be sectioned. If the S1 dorsal root is to be sectioned, a laminectomy of L5 and the superior margin of S1 must be accomplished; for the fifth lumbar dorsal root, a laminectomy of L4 and the superior portion of L5. The dura is opened in the midline and

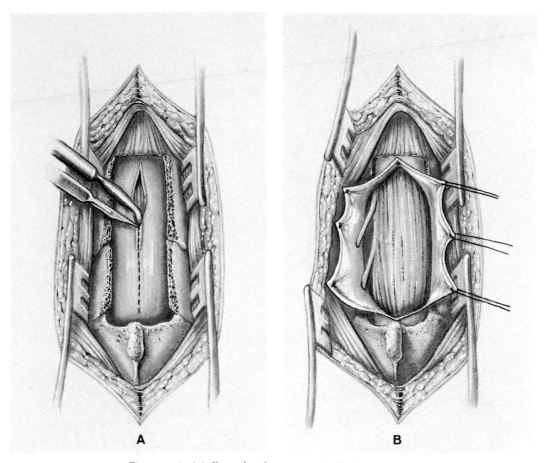

Fig. 9-3. A, Midline dural incision; B, dural retraction.

the edge on the side of the proposed root section is retracted by sewing to the paraspinal muscles. Identification of the specific root is vital to the procedure and is best done by tracing the combined motor and sensory root to its dural exit. Only after this has been clearly demonstrated should separation of the motor and sensory rootlets be carried out. Magnifying loops are helpful in identifying and separating the motor from the sensory rootlets. Oftentimes, there are 2 sensory rootlets and 1 motor root. Identification is best done with a nerve stimulator. A small silver clip can be placed on either side of the sensory roots to be sectioned, and they are then cut with fine scissors.

Dr. R. K. Jones has devised what he describes as a "provisional" posterior rhizotomy. When surgery is undertaken to relieve persistent lower extremity pain, particularly in recurrent disc disease, if obvious pathology, such as a recurrent disc protrusion, is encountered and excised, one hesitates to section the involved posterior root with the hope that the removal of the offending pathology will result in the relief of pain. To obviate the necessity for cutting a posterior root when it is not necessary, Dr. Jones places an absorbable No. 3-0 catgut suture around the posterior root and brings both ends of this suture out through the skin incision including it in the wound dressings. If

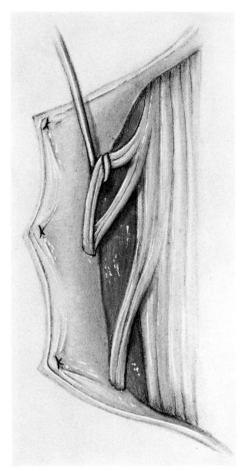

Fig. 9-4. Separation of motor and sensory rootlets.

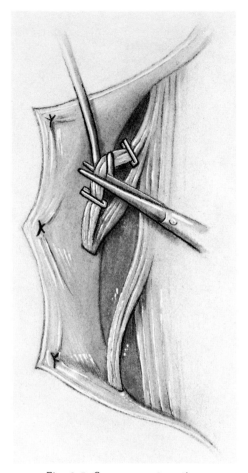

Fig. 9-5. Sensory root section.

the radicular pain in the first 4 or 5 postoperative days is noted to be persistent and unrelieved, the suture is withdrawn and the rhizotomy accomplished. If after that period of time the patient was satisfied with the relief of the radicular pain, the suture is cut flush with the skin and left to dissolve. In carrying out this procedure, Dr. Jones exposes the root by carrying out a generous hemilaminectomy and foraminotomy exposing the dural root sleeve; an incision is made in the dural sleeve and the dorsal roots identified and separated by means of this minute dural exposure.

The sensory deficit following section of one root is often quite minimal and in some cases equivocal. Following the section of the L5 and S1 roots, there is greater sensory dysfunction, particularly with regard to position sense. For the first 4 to 6 months the patient must wear an ankle and foot brace to facilitate ambulation and weight-bearing in the presence of such significant sensory loss around the ankle and foot. After 6 months, this loss is to some degree compensated and this appliance can often be discarded.

This procedure should not be recom-

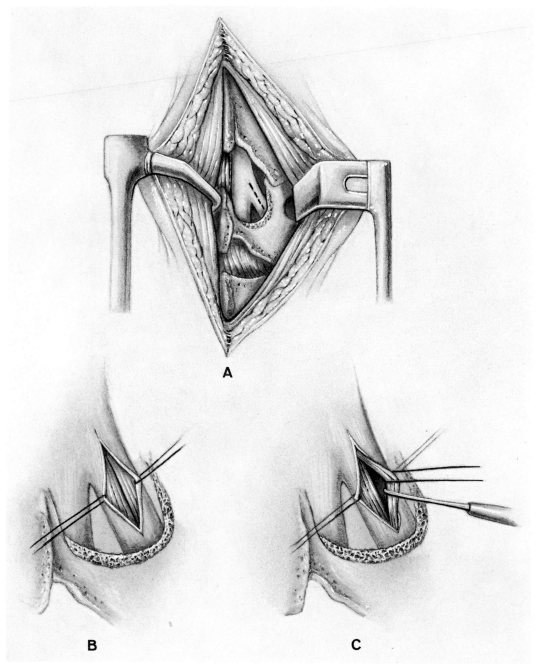

Fig. 9-6. A, Incision into dural root sleeve; B, identification of dorsal rootlets; C, suture around sensory rootlets.

mended lightly. If there is any suspicion that the patient's symptoms are nonorganic, or if there is a question regarding secondary gain, or if the physician is uncertain in his mind regarding the anatomical limitations of the dysfunction, it should be deferred. Even when all of the indications are clear, the results are occasionally less than desirable.

10
Stenotic Lumbar Spinal Canal Syndrome

STENOTIC LUMBAR SPINAL CANAL

Historical Data
Cervical Versus Lumbar Spinal
  Canal Stenosis
Anatomical Characteristics
Radiographic Characteristics

Lumbar Mobility
Clinical Characteristics
Plain X-ray Changes
Myelography

LUMBAR SPONDYLOSIS AND THE STENOTIC LUMBAR SPINAL CANAL

Lumbar Disc Dynasty

Pathology of Lumbar Spondylosis

**Progressive Development of
Lumbar Spondylosis**

Degeneration of the Nucleus Pulposus
Degeneration of the Annulus Fibrosis
Fibrosis
Complete Fibrous Ankylosis of the
  Intervertebral Joint

X-ray Changes

**Lumbar Spondylosis with Spinal Cord of
Normal Dimensions**

History
Examination

**Lumbar Spondylosis with Stenotic Lumbar
Spinal Canal**

History
Examination
Treatment

Impacted Spinous Processes

ACHONDROPLASIA AND THE STENOTIC LUMBAR SPINAL CANAL

Abnormalities of the Spine
Spinal Degenerative Changes
Achondroplastic Dogs

Myelogram
Treatment

PAGET'S DISEASE OF THE LUMBAR SPINE (OSTEITIS DEFORMANS)

Pathology
Microscopic Changes
X-ray Changes
Myelogram

Signs and Symptoms
Laboratory Findings
Diagnosis
Treatment

10
Stenotic Lumbar Spinal Canal Syndrome

STENOTIC LUMBAR SPINAL CANAL

In the past 4 years the concept of the "stenotic lumbar canal" has received increasing emphasis. Among the physicians most responsible for redirecting our attention to this syndrome is George Ehni of Baylor University College of Medicine in Houston, Texas, who has redefined this clinical entity with specific signs and symptoms separating the stenotic lumbar spinal canal from other conditions affecting the lumbar spine. His important 5-part article, was originally presented as part of a panel discussion he chaired on "syndromes of the small lumbar spinal canal" at a meeting of the Southern Neurosurgical Society, New Orleans, Louisiana on February 17, 1968.[7]

Historical Data

In a case report[16] published in 1900, a patient was described with lumbosacral pain who walked in a stooped forward position. A laminectomy was carried out and apparently was helpful in relieving some of the symptoms. At the time of surgery Dr. Gerster, the surgeon, noted unusual heaviness of the laminae and thickness of the periosteum but found no evidence of mass or infection. This early case report was followed by others of a similar nature in which laminectomy was found to be helpful. The explanation in most cases indicated hypertrophic osteoarthritic changes in addition to hypertrophy of the yellow ligament causing compression of the nerve roots of the cauda equina. Included in these early papers was one written by Charles Elsberg.[8] In his paper, which was a review of 60 laminectomies for various spinal dysfunctions, he mentioned several patients with "symptoms very much like those of tumor of the cauda equina, although nothing is found at the operation that can be relieved by surgical means. All of the patients improved very much after the operation, and the result can only be ascribed to the laminectomy." Throughout the subsequent years this entity has been recalled to our attention by a number of authors in various ways. In 1947, M. A. Sarpyener discussed "congenital stricture of the spinal canal."[18] H. Verbiest has written on this subject from 1949 to the present[25,26,27]; J. A. Epstein and his associates have written several papers describing nerve root compression caused by narrowing of the lumbar spinal canal.[9] From 1965 on, increasing numbers of papers have been written discussing this entity.

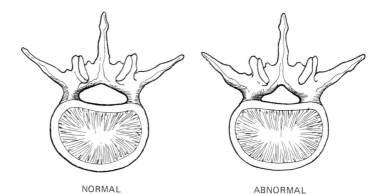

NORMAL   ABNORMAL

Fig. 10-1. Anatomical differences between the normal and stenotic lumbar spinal canal.

Cervical Versus Lumbar Spinal Canal Stenosis

In the past two decades encroachment upon the cervical spine resulting from a stenotic cervical spinal canal has been generally accepted as a recognizable clinical entity. A number of patients whose neurological symptoms initially led to a diagnosis of multiple sclerosis, amyotrophic lateral sclerosis, or other neurological degenerative disease, were found to have spondylotic encroachment upon the cervical cord documented by cervical myelography. Great attention is paid to cervical spine x-rays, and in some x-ray departments, A-P and lateral measurements of the cervical spinal canals are now routinely done.

The diameters of the lumbar spinal canal have not received similar attention, primarily because they do not seem to be clinically important and because of the technical difficulty of measuring x-rays of the lumbar spine in comparison with the cervical region. In the cervical area, the lateral films permit fairly accurate measurement of canal depth, because the highest point of the laminal arch and the dorsum of the vertebral body are quite easily identified but these landmarks are not so easily identified in the lumbar region. Unless the need is emphasized for x-rays of the lumbar region, this technical difficulty will cause radiologists and clinicians alike to skirt the problem. Improved radiographic techniques to more clearly deliniate this entity have been described.

Anatomical Characteristics

1. More acute angle between the right and left halves of the laminae.
2. Decreased pedicle length.

Radiographic Characteristics

1. Clinically the A-P dimension is most important with the so-called "shallow canal." In many cases the side-to-side diameters of the canal are also limited, but this is usually not delineated by a diminution in the interpedicular measurements, which usually remain normal and are seldom helpful in determining the size of a spinal canal.
2. Measurements on conventionally made lateral lumbar x-rays reveal the bodies to measure from 42 to 45 mm. and the normal canal about one half that, from 21 to 23 mm. Measurements of the canal below 19 mm. are suspicious and some lumbar canals are as shallow as 15 mm.

Lumbar Mobility

In patients with stenotic lumbar canal, any changes which further decrease the space within this canal are more likely to produce symptoms than would be the case in a normal-size spinal canal. Movements of the lumbar spine will cause minor changes of the structures within the canal and when the spinal canal is of normal size and configuration, these changes are of no clinical significance. However, in the case of a small lumbar spinal canal, such changes may be symptom producing.

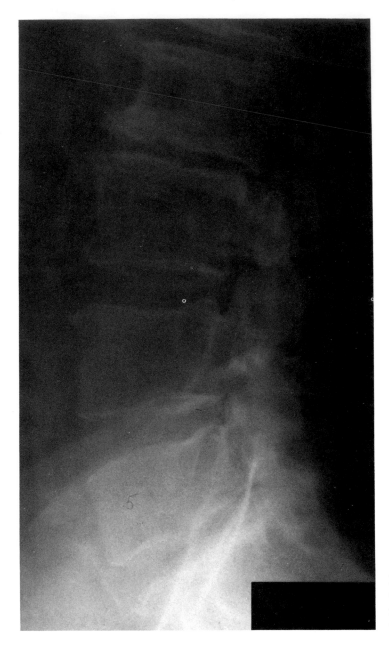

Fig. 10-2. Compare this stenotic lumbar spinal canal with normal sized spinal canal Figure 2-21B, page 53.

Flexion of the lumbar spine produces:

1. Decrease in intraspinal protrusion of lumbar intervertebral disc.

2. Slight decrease in the length of the anterior wall of the spinal canal.

3. Significant increase in length of the posterior wall of the spinal canal.

4. Stretching and decreased bulge of the yellow ligaments within the spinal canal.

5. Stretching and decreased cross-sectional area of nerve roots.

The overall effect of spinal flexion is to produce a general increase in spinal canal volume and decreased nerve root bulk.

Extension of the lumbar spine produces:

1. Bulging of intervertebral discs into the spinal canal.

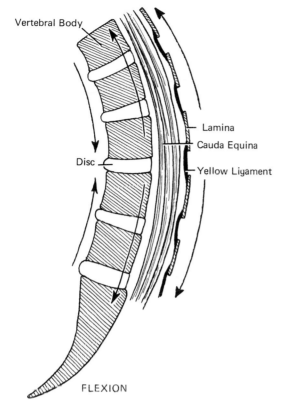

Vertebral Body

Disc

Lamina
Cauda Equina
Yellow Ligament

FLEXION

Fig. 10-3. Increased spinal canal volume and decreased nerve root (cauda equina) bulk with flexion.

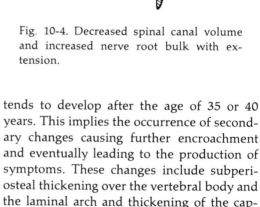

Vertebral Body

Disc

Yellow Ligament
Cauda Equina
Lamina

Extension

Fig. 10-4. Decreased spinal canal volume and increased nerve root bulk with extension.

2. Slight increase of anterior canal length.

3. Moderate decrease of posterior canal length.

4. Enfolding and protrusion of yellow ligaments into the spinal canal.

5. Relaxation and increase in cross-sectional diameter of nerve roots.

It can be seen that spinal extension produces an overall decrease in the volume of the lumbar spinal canal and increased nerve root bulk.

Clinical Characteristics

It must be recognized that coexistence of the stenotic lumbar spinal canal with either the herniated lumbar disc or lumbar spondylosis is extremely common. It is also clear that a congenitally stenotic lumbar spinal canal that is present from birth is not usually associated with symptoms in early life, but tends to develop after the age of 35 or 40 years. This implies the occurrence of secondary changes causing further encroachment and eventually leading to the production of symptoms. These changes include subperiosteal thickening over the vertebral body and the laminal arch and thickening of the capsular ligaments and the ligamentum flavum.

The stenotic lumbar spinal canal syndrome has certain of the following clinical characteristics which allow us to distinguish this condition from spondylosis or lumbar disc disease in a canal of normal size.

1. Patients often have multiple root involvements with a greatly increased frequency of bilateral leg pain. In lumbar disc disease it is usually possible to identify a "single root lesion" with the examination pointing to one specific root. In the stenotic lumbar spinal canal syndrome, 2 and some-

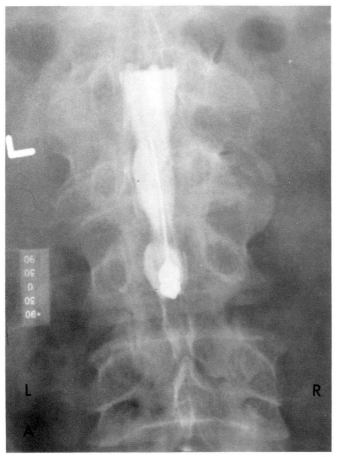
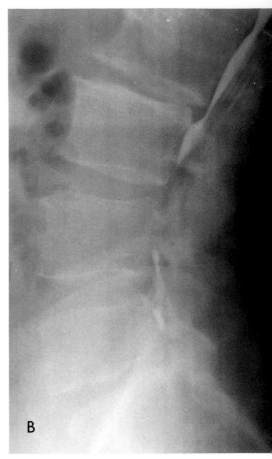

Fig. 10-5. A and B, Myelographic demonstration of stenotic lumbar spinal canal. Six cc. of Pantopaque were injected through the lumbar puncture needle, inserted at the L1–2 interspace; the free flow of dye column cranially; block is at midportion of L3.

times 3 roots on the same or both sides may be involved.

2. The position of maximum comfort differs considerably in this syndrome from a typical herniated lumbar disc picture. Most lumbar disc patients are improved with bed rest and are reasonably comfortable when lying flat. But in the small lumbar spinal canal syndrome, often the only position of comfort is with the hospital bed angulated in such a fashion that the patient's head is elevated from 40° to 60° and the hips and knees are flexed allowing lumbar flexion to occur. In many instances the patient may be completely relaxed after 24 to 48 hours of this position and be in no discomfort whatsoever. If the bed is then flattened out, so that the position of lumbar flexion is changed to a slight lumbar lordosis, the pain may immediately and promptly recur to almost its original severity. This is a fairly reliable clinical sign that we are dealing with a stenotic spinal canal.

3. The patient often is unable to walk with comfort unless he bends forward, producing a reversal and flexion of the normal lordotic curve.

4. On examination it is noted that straight leg raising is often much less painful than might be expected, despite the fact that the patient may have pain radiating down one or both legs; forward bending, which ordinarily causes considerable discomfort in lumbar disc disease, is not at all painful and may actually ease the pain.

See Figures 10-3 and 10-4.

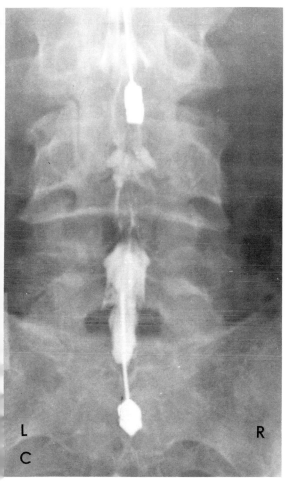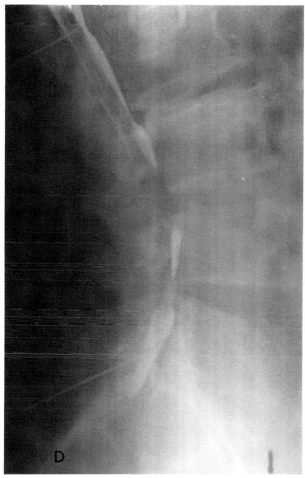

Fig. 10-5. C and D, Three cc. of Pantopaque were injected through the second lumbar puncture needle injected at L5–S1 interspace; the dye column is blocked at the L4–5 level. The lateral view reveals no evidence of disc herniation at L1–2, L2–3, L4–5, L5–S1; L3–4 is not adequately visualized.

Plain X-ray Changes

1. Flattening of the lumbar lordotic curve.
2. Slight spondylolisthesis of L4 on L5 without a pars defect.
3. Increased density of facets.
4. Hypertrophic osteoarthritic spurs and interspace narrowing. This finding must be given increased clinical significance. In a normal-size spinal canal a considerable amount of arthrosis may be well tolerated, but with the preexistence of a stenotic canal such changes may cause symptoms. In this regard one must look for facet enlargement, heaviness of laminae and spondylolisthesis. Narrowing or vertebral malalignment at the L5–S1 interspace in association with a steno-

tic lumbar canal is less likely to be symptom producing than even a slight L4–5 spondylolisthesis. This is because there is a great deal more space between the neural elements and the bone at the L5–S1 level and considerable hypertrophic spurring can exist at that site without compromising the nerve roots. However, at the L4–5 level the roots are normally more snugly enclosed within their bony boundaries, so that a minimal "offset" may be symptom producing.

Myelography

The myelogram is frequently misinterpreted in this condition. Because the roots are compressed against each other and not freely floating, as is the case when the spinal canal is of normal size, introduction of the myelographic spinal puncture needle is often painful and may be associated with slow cerebrospinal fluid flow. The myelographer may feel that technical deficiencies on his part are producing both the pain and sluggish passage of Pantopaque. In many cases the interpretation of the myelogram is erroneous and may be mislabeled as a subdural injection or adhesive arachnoiditis. It is most disturbing for me to review old myelograms that I had originally interpreted as either "technically inadequate" or diagnosed as adhesive arachnoiditis when actually they were diagnostic of a stenotic lumbar spinal canal, the symptoms in retrospect fitting this syndrome quite well. One must always consider a needle that is properly placed and in the midline but is pain producing, as being in a pathologic process.

LUMBAR SPONDYLOSIS AND THE STENOTIC LUMBAR SPINAL CANAL

Lumbar spondylosis is a condition in which there is a progressive degeneration of the intervertebral disc leading to changes of the adjacent vertebrae and ligaments. Although it is also called hypertrophic arthritis, osteoarthritis and lumbar spondylitis, the term spondylosis is considered preferable, since the condition is a degenerative rather than an inflammatory one. For the past 20 years this term was utilized primarily in relation to the cervical spine and was generally accepted as meaning a generalized deterioration of the cervical intervertebral disc and its associated ligamentous and osseous structures. Cervical spondylosis implies an accumulation of degenerative changes in the cervical spine resulting in narrowing of the vertebral canal, and associated with cervical cord compression, nerve root compression and in many cases vertebral artery compression resulting in a vertebrobasilar ischemia.

Using the term lumbar spondylosis invites the clinician to recognize that degenerative changes can occur in the lumbar spine as well as in the cervical spine and that these changes will also produce diminution and narrowing of the spinal canal, creating specific clinical symptoms.

This condition has been confused with other disorders capable of producing low back and sciatic pain such as disc herniation, lumbosacral strain, adhesive arachnoiditis, neoplasm and functional backache. Some of the unsatisfactory responses and disap-

pointments resulting from treatment can be avoided if this entity is recognized and appropriately treated.

It is important to distinguish between the relatively benign and often inconsequential symptoms of lumbar spondylosis in the normal canal and the severe encroachment produced by a similar degree of spondylosis in a stenotic canal, which may result in multilevel interferences with cauda equina function requiring surgical decompression of several levels.

LUMBAR DISC DYNASTY

The chief hindrance to recognition of the importance of lumbar spondylosis is the domination of lumbar disc disease. Beginning in the mid-1930's, the term lumbar disc disease assumed considerable popularity and was utilized to explain low back pain with radiation into one or both lower extremities. As the neurosurgeons and orthopaedic surgeons who practiced lumbar disc surgery became technically proficient, a large group of successfully treated patients gave increased authority to this entity, leading to a sort of mental despotism so that any lumbar sciatic pain syndrome was essentially considered a "disc problem." Such a patient was identified as a herniated lumbar disc suspect, and efforts in investigation and management were directed toward that specific entity. If the usual course of conservative management did not alleviate the pain, a myelogram would be performed to "verify the existence of a herniated lumbar disc." When such a lesion was disclosed by myelography, interlaminar excision of the symptom-producing fragment of extruded disc was often followed by an excellent clinical improvement.

However, a number of myelograms reveal some constriction of the dural sac with a slightly protruding intervertebral disc in the lower lumbar region. On the basis of persisting symptoms and an equivocal myelogram many of these patients are subjected to interlaminar explorations, in the course of which a firm, slightly protruding intervertebral disc is violated and excised. Occasionally, because no significant disc protrusion is visualized at surgery, a "negative exploration" results. Included in this sizable group of patients are many cases of lumbar spondylosis in association with a stenotic lumbar spinal canal; and as a result of such inappropriate management they do not fare well.

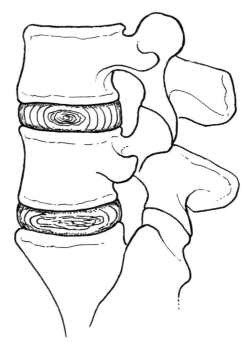

Fig. 10-6. Degeneration of the nucleus pulposus.

PATHOLOGY OF LUMBAR SPONDYLOSIS

Whenever we attempt to understand what produces degenerative changes within an anatomical structure, we must have an appreciation of its primary functions. Although we are using the term lumbar spondylosis to emphasize the similarities involving degenerative changes of the cervical and lumbar spines, the significant differences in function between these two areas must be recognized. The *cervical spine* is structured primarily for mobility and secondarily for weight bearing while the *lumbar spine* is structured primarily for weight-bearing with mobility being of secondary importance. These differences would imply that degenerative changes involving the lumbar spine arise primarily from the stresses of weight bearing and to a lesser extent from mobility, whereas the opposite is true in the cervical region.

Spondylitic changes of the lumbar spine involve narrowing of the intervertebral disc spaces, lipping and osteophyte formation around the margins of contiguous vertebral bodies, which may occur anteriorly or laterally but also often occur posteriorly. In addition, hypertrophic changes involving the posterior intervertebral joints are present affecting the joint capsules and ligaments which become swollen. This is usually seen as a multilevel process, symmetrical bilaterally, with hypertrophy of the laminae, facets and usually the yellow ligaments.

PROGRESSIVE DEVELOPMENT OF LUMBAR SPONDYLOSIS[3]

Degeneration of the Nucleus Pulposus

Exactly why this occurs in some persons and not in others is an issue that is not completely settled. It is generally felt that the intrinsic tissue strength of the nucleus pulposus in association with the stress of weight bearing and the deteriorative changes of aging are the determining factors. The nucleus pulposus softens, disintegrates and eventually becomes fragmented.

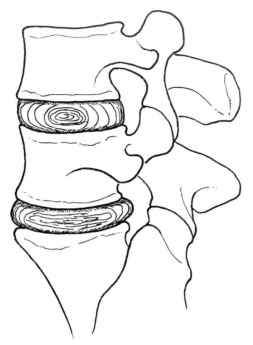

Fig. 10-7. Degeneration of the annulus fibrosus.

Degeneration of the Annulus Fibrosus

As the nucleus pulposus degenerates, it can no longer function as a semi-incompressible fulcrum for intervertebral movement and is unable to distribute pressure equally over the annulus and vertebral end-plates. This degeneration subjects the annulus to increased compression which, because of the normal lumbar lordosis, falls mainly in its posterior portion. As noted above, it is weight-bearing or compression which is a major factor in producing degenerative changes. The abnormal and constant pressure often leads to fissuring of the posterior portion of the annulus fibrosus, the fissures usually occurring within a relatively small area and often unilateral.[14] The most common site of annular fissure is at the site where it is least reinforced by the posterior longitudinal ligament. At this stage in the degenerative process the nucleus pulposus develops a degree of fibrosis somewhat in excess of the normal state of fibrosis seen in the normal aging process. It is also at this

phase of degeneration that a divarication occurs and one of two separate and distinct moieties (disc herniation or spondylosis) will develop.

Herniation of the Nucleus Pulposus. In less than 20 percent of patients with weakening or tearing of the fibers of the annulus fibrosis, a large fragment of disc material will completely extrude through this opening in the annulus producing a mass effect large enough to cause nerve root compression. In such an instance, the symptoms are those of a herniated lumbar disc.

Spondylosis. In most cases, despite the stress placed on the annulus fibrosus, no complete rupture occurs. The annulus becomes softer and weaker, but never completely loses its integrity, so that it contains the disc contents within its bounds. If such a situation occurs, the disc becomes anatomically fixed but functionally impaired and no actual nuclear tissue displacement has occurred to cause nerve root compression. In some instances a minimal disruption of the annular fibers occurs with weakening and a slight protrusion. Although there is some increased bulge of the intervertebral disc into the spinal canal, it is relatively minimal and fibrosis subsequently occurs with the eventual disc protrusion becoming quite fibrous and stable in its consistency and mobility.

Fibrosis

Fibrosis is associated with decreased tissue bulk and loss of sponginess and elasticity. The tissue of the annulus fibrosus shrinks and becomes increasingly fibrous. Decreased elasticity will produce sclerotic changes in the vertebral bodies with sclerotic bone replacing the cartilaginous end-plates and new bone formation around the periphery of the contiguous vertebral surfaces. The intervertebral space narrows as a result of increased fibrosis and loss of tissue mass within the intervertebral disc. The posterior diarthrodial joints become involved as a result of the loss of the normal nuclear fulcrum for movement which, in combination with a

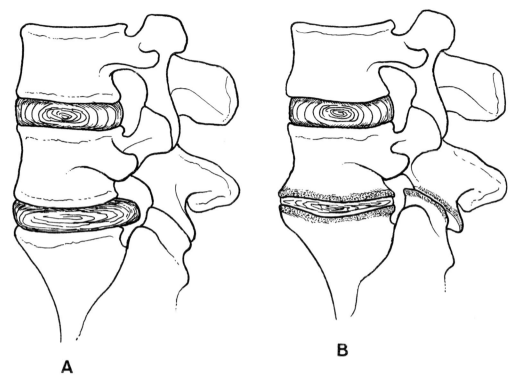

A   **B**

Fig. 10-8. A, Herniation of the nucleus pulposus; B, spondylosis.

decrease in the intervertebral space, alters
the planes of the articular surfaces of the
diarthrodial joints so that they are no longer
congruous, subjecting the joints to abnormal
stresses and strains. Such stresses are productive of degenerative arthritis, including
narrowing of the posterior diarthrodial joint
spaces, subchondral sclerosis, peripheral new
bone formation and periarticular fibrosis.

Complete Fibrous Ankylosis of the Intervertebral Joint

In rare cases if the ankylosis becomes
completely stable with no movement whatsoever, the patient's low back symptoms may
improve. However, such changes take many
years and in most instances involve more
than one interspace, each of which is undergoing degenerative changes at a different
stage. When improvement occurs, it is very
gradual over a time span of many years.

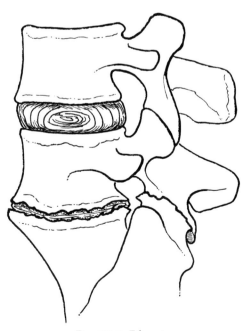

Fig. 10-9. Fibrosis.

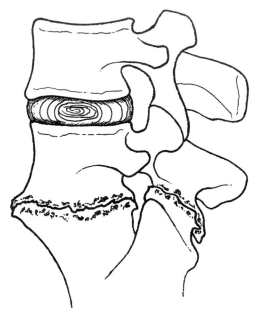

Fig. 10-10. Complete fibrous ankylosis of the intervertebral joint.

X-RAY CHANGES

Lumbar spondylosis is radiographically apparent. Plain x-rays of the lumbar spine reveal changes which are usually generalized throughout most of the lumbar spine and almost invariably involve the L3-4, L4-5, and L5-S1 interspaces. It is rare to see one interspace grossly affected with the rest not involved. Osteophyte formations often occur anteriorly or laterally but they may occur posteriorly. In addition, hypertrophic changes involving the posterior intervertebral joints are present, involving the joint capsules and ligaments which become hypertrophied with facet enlargement and heaviness of laminae.

Extensive x-ray evidence of lumbar spondylosis may be seen as an incidental finding in a patient who gives no history of significant low back or sciatic discomfort. In association with a stenotic lumbar spinal canal such findings are of clinical importance.

The myelogram may reveal invaginated yellow ligaments and moderate multilevel bulging of discs which in a constricted spinal canal are capable of producing pressure on the cauda equina from all sides.

LUMBAR SPONDYLOSIS WITH SPINAL CORD OF NORMAL DIMENSIONS

History

Most patients with lumbar spondylosis are older than those with primary lumbar disc lesions. A chief symptom is low back pain, often described as aching, and usually is both generalized and specific, involves certain areas of point tenderness. Activity, as a rule, worsens the discomfort; rest eases it. The pain experienced with lumbar spondylosis differs from that of lumbar disc disease in that it produces a more constant unrelenting discomfort with relatively low peaks of pain, never quite as severe or as crippling as lumbar disc disease and without the pain-free remissions. Sciatic pain is rare and when present is less acute or specific and more generalized, involving one or both lower extremities and more than one root within the distribution of the pain.

Examination

Examination of the low back reveals moderate paraspinal muscle spasm in the lumbar region with some limitation of mobility of the lumbar spine in most movements. Extension is usually a bit more restricted than flexion. There is invariably some flattening of the normal lumbar lordosis. Usually moderate paraspinal muscle spasm is elicited. As a rule, straight leg raising is not as painful as with lumbar disc disease. Occasional sensory, motor and reflex changes are elicited, but they are not frequent nor are they as specific as those seen in lumbar disc disease. The mechanism of nerve root symptoms is twofold. Lipping of the posterior portions of the vertebral bodies may cause root compression identical to the soft disc protrusion. In addition, the posterior intervertebral joint involvement, including the joint capsules and ligaments, develops hypertrophy of these structures in the area of the intervertebral foramina productive of nerve root compression and irritation. Anatomically, the size of the foramina becomes progressively decreased going downward in the lumbar region from 1 to 5, and the size of the nerve root increases a bit from above downward so that the lower lumbar roots are most likely to be affected by these changes. It is probably this generalized hypertrophy in the posterior joints that gives rise to the generalized, nonspecific pain seen with lumbar spondylosis.

LUMBAR SPONDYLOSIS WITH STENOTIC LUMBAR SPINAL CANAL

History

The patient has a long history of intermittent low back pain often related to specific positions and activities. He frequently is unable to sleep in a prone position, which would tend to increase the lumbar lordosis, but finds it necessary to sleep on his side with hips and knees flexed in the fetal position, assuring substantial lumbar flexion. Since prolonged car driving is often associated with considerable discomfort, he may achieve more comfort in moving the car seat as far forward as possible, requiring increased flexion of the hips and knees and providing increased lumbar lordosis. In addition to low back pain, nerve root symptoms often occur which may be monoradicular, less commonly involving compression of several roots or even the entire cauda equina. Occasionally, pain is only a minor complaint with some patients presenting with predominantly motor weakness.

A history of neurological deficit being produced during anesthesia while in a position of lumbar hyperextension, is occasionally elicited. Normally, patients with lumbar spondylosis in association with a stenotic lumbar spinal canal manifest protective pain mechanisms which will restrict excessive lumbar extension. Under anesthesia, these protective mechanisms are lost, making it possible to obtain extreme extension with the potential of cauda equina compression.

A number of case reports exist in the literature attesting to serious neurological dysfunction involving the cauda equina following extension of the lumbar spine, with or without anesthesia. One of the earliest reports documenting such a phenomenon was by Goldthwaite in 1911, whose 39-year-old patient with hypertrophic arthritis of the lumbar spine complained of low back pain for 7 years. Right-sided sacroiliac joint displacement had been diagnosed and "replaced" under anesthesia. However, intermittent pain persisted until one day, upon getting out of a hot tub, the patient was unable to assume an erect posture, and remained in a stooped forward position and complained of intense bilateral leg pains. He received another sacroiliac joint "adjustment" under ether anesthesia which did not relieve his pain. A decision was made to encase the patient in a body cast and he was placed supine on an orthopaedic frame for cast application. Just as his lumbar spine was extended, he complained for a moment of intense pain, after which he relaxed. Moments later his legs were found to be numb with rapid progressive worsening of his neurological status to sphincter incontinence and complete motor and sensory paralysis of the lower extremities. This neurological picture was reversible and function returned to a considerable extent when he was placed on his side in bed, but when placed in the supine position he worsened. Following an interval of supine recumbency, he developed persisting motor, sensory and sphincter paralysis associated with "explosive" cutting pains in the legs, feet and rectum. This state continued for 6 weeks until a lumbar laminectomy was performed by Dr. Harvey Cushing who found nothing other than narrowing of the bony canal at the lumbosacral level. Gradual improvement reportedly followed the surgery. In a 5-year-period Dr. George Ehni encountered 6 instances of cauda equina palsy following anesthesia, with the patient in increased lumbar extension. A number of additional episodes of sphincter dysfunction and motor and sensory disturbances in the lower extremities have followed anesthesia (for abdominal, pelvic, or chest surgery) and have been reported mainly as presumed complications of spinal anesthesia. The various explanations, including root trauma from the lumbar puncture needle, neurolytic effects or occult actions of the anesthetic agent, inadvertent introduction of chemical contaminants and infection are some of the factors mentioned. In retrospect, a certain number of these problems may have resulted from acute compression of the cauda equina by hyperextension of the lumbar spine while the patient was under anesthesia.

Occasionally, a history of intermittent claudication, similar in certain respects to the vascular occlusive syndrome produced by painful contraction of anoxic muscle, is due to spondylitic changes affecting the cauda equina. Both types of intermittent claudication produce signs and symptoms that appear after the patient has walked a predictable distance, and they disappear when he has rested. There are certain differentiating characteristics that will enable the clinician to establish a proper diagnosis.

The pain of anoxic muscle contractions characteristically occurs in the calves, and is the principal symptom associated with arterial insufficiency. Pain in cauda equina claudication may be absent but when present it has distinctly paresthetic qualities described as numbness, coldness or burning. The location of the pain is in the lumbosacral or sciatic distribution.

Sensory deficits in arterial insufficiency are rare and when seen are peripheral, involving toes and feet. In cauda equina claudication numbness and paresthesias beginning in the lumbar region and buttocks may remain confined to these areas, but often descend in the distribution of the lower lumbar and sacral dermatomes or may begin in the feet and ascend to the buttocks. Such a sensory "march" is common. Motor deficits are rare in arterial insufficiency, although during muscle anoxia the calf muscles often cramp and become tight. In cauda equina claudica-

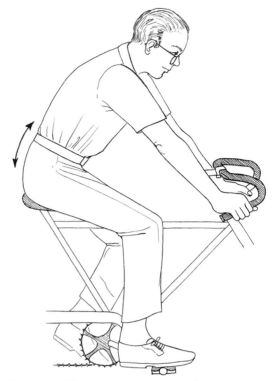

Fig. 10-11. The stationary exercise bicycle, available in most departments of physical medicine, is most helpful in differentiating vascular from cauda equina claudication. The patient with cauda equina claudication can pedal "endlessly" in a lumbar flexed position, but the vascular occlusive patient will develop painful muscle ischemia in a short time.

tion, sensory symptoms precede motor dysfunction causing the patient to stop walking; if, however, he continues walking beyond the appearance of discomfort or paresthesias, the legs may become weak to the point of collapse.

Examination

The physical examination in lumbar spondylosis with a stenotic lumbar spinal canal is often surprisingly unrevealing, despite intermittent cauda equina compression symptoms that are often severe. If a patient is examined immediately after such an episode, sensory deficits and loss of reflexes may be noted that will subside as the patient's symptoms disappear.

The diagnosis is tentatively made by careful examination and measurements of the lumbar spine films and confirmed by myelography.

Treatment

The symptoms of lumbar spondylosis in the presence of a spinal canal of normal dimensions are almost always nonsurgical.

A combination of medications and exercise, as well as alteration in the mode of daily living, is usually adequate. A low back support is rarely necessary. (See Conservative Treatment, p. 95.)

The treatment of spondylosis in the presence of a stenotic spinal canal is a generous decompressive laminectomy.

IMPACTED SPINOUS PROCESSES

An unusual source of osteoligamentous spinal pain is occasionally encountered when long-standing increased lumbar lordosis produces impaction or "kissing" of two of the spinous processes of the lumbar spine. This can occur at any lumbar level and the site of impaction is generally the site of maximal pain.

The exact cause of the pain is uncertain, with speculation that a traumatic neuritis of a branch of the posterior primary division of the spinal nerve which supplies the interspinous ligament and the surrounding soft tissues occurs.[28]

Digital pressure between the spinous processes with the patient standing elicits pain; such tenderness is increased in hyperextension and decreased during flexion. Occasionally, a small cystlike mass can be palpated during hyperextension that disappears on flexion.

The pain is frequently related to position, with lumbar flexion often affording relief.

Radiographically, lateral films of the lumbar spine will reveal a weight-bearing pseudoarthrosis between two lumbar spinous processes with contact sclerosis and some-

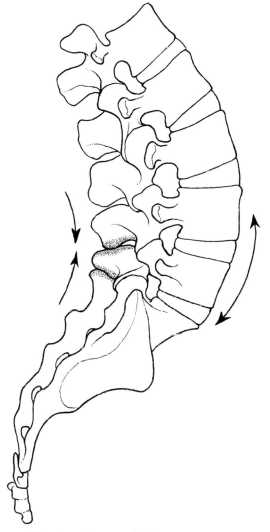

Fig. 10-12. Impacted spinous processes.

times visible "crumbling" at the point of contact.

If the pain is due to this condition, infiltration of the involved interspinous ligament with 1 or 2 cc. of 1 percent lidocaine will alleviate the pain. If relief is obtained with the local anesthetic, the needle should be allowed to remain in place and then be utilized for a methylprednisolone acetate injection. This may provide temporary improvement but an exercise and postural correction program must be instituted for eventual improvement of the lumbar lordosis.

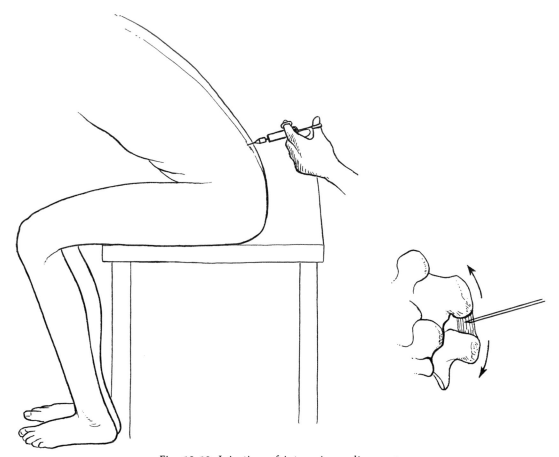

Fig. 10-13. Injection of interspinous ligament.

ACHONDROPLASIA AND THE STENOTIC LUMBAR SPINAL CANAL

The achondroplastic dwarf has been recognized as a distinct physical entity for centuries. There are many historical drawings and documents describing the typical physiognomy—large head, prominent forehead, extremely short arms and legs. Achondroplasia is a disease of unknown etiology which relates to a dysfunction involving endochondral ossification. The condition is familial and occurs not only in humans but, by selective breeding, can be developed in animals. The dachshund and bassett hound, French bulldog and the Pekingese are examples of achondroplastic dwarf forms created in dogs through selective breeding.

Abnormalities of the Spine

Many physicians are under the impression that from a neurological point of view achondroplasia is consistent with a normal life. However, abnormalities of the spine are a regular occurrence in this condition and in addition to the well-recognized increased lumbar lordosis, there are also changes produced in the individual vertebrae as well. There is a decrease in the height of the individual vertebral bodies and it is this that accounts for the relative shortness of the entire spine. The pedicles are extremely short, particularly in the thoracic and lumbar region, resulting from premature synostosis of the ossification centers of the vertebral body with those of the laminae, so that the laminae are almost in contact with the dorsum of the vertebral bodies. This results in a diminution of the A-P diameter of the spinal canal. In addition to the A-P diameter, there are changes in the transverse diameters of the lumbar vertebral bodies. Normally, the transverse diameters of the lumbar vertebrae increase slightly as we go caudal, so that the fifth vertebra is the widest of the lumbar vertebrae. In achondroplastic dwarfism there is a progressive terminal lumbar stenosis which is exactly opposite to that seen in the normal state. The vertebral canal is not only narrowed in the A-P diameter but tapers progressively downward, narrowing also in the transverse diameter in the lower lumbar region.[5] The spinal cord, cauda equina and conus medullaris are normal in width so that these changes in the size and configuration of the bony spine subject the neural elements to constriction.

Spinal Degenerative Changes

It is rare for neurological changes in the thoracic or lumbar region to occur in childhood or early adulthood. However, since the spinal cord, cauda equina and conus medullaris are normal in width, these elements fit very snugly into the small, bony canal and any encroachment on the lumen of the spinal canal or the intervertebral foramina has a constricting effect upon the cord and the spinal nerve roots.

The dorsolumbar segment of the achondroplastic spine is often unstable and may develop a dorsal kyphosis with large osteoarthritic spurs as well as changes involving the articular processes. By the time an achondroplastic dwarf becomes an adult, his spinal canal is further compromised by marginal hypertrophic osteoarthritic spurring of the vertebral bodies and occasionally by protrusion of intervertebral discs.[6]

Signs and Symptoms. Degenerative changes of the lower lumbar region will cause low back pain and lower extremity paresthesia, particularly on standing. Motor dysfunction in the lower extremities, such as foot drop, may occur. If the compression is in the thoracolumbar region, a spastic paraparesis may develop with bladder and bowel disturbances. Usually such changes occur after the age of 40. Both the conus medullaris and the cauda equina also may be severely constricted after the age of 40 when osteoarthritic spurs and degenerative changes in the intervertebral discs develop; all of these further encroaching upon the very snug spinal canal.[28]

Achondroplastic Dogs

The changes that are seen in human achondroplastic dwarfs are also seen in breeds of dogs that are typically achondroplastic. These dogs show an increased incidence of disc degeneration and will occasionally develop paraplegia with remissions and exacerbations. The highest incidence of disc protrusion in dogs is at the thoracolumbar interspace (the nineteenth interspace). The analogy between these occurrences and human achrondroplasia is striking.[14]

Myelogram

As in all stenotic lumbar spinal canal syndromes, attempts at performing a lumbar puncture are often unsuccessful. Even though the puncture has been performed properly and the Pantopaque successfully deposited in the subarachnoid space, the space is often so narrow that free flow of the contrast material is not possible. The Pantopaque often puddles at each of the concavities of the bodies of the lumbar vertebrae, resulting in an erroneous interpretation of the myelogram as being technically unsatisfactory and labeled as a subdural or extradural injection. Because of this, it may be necessary to introduce the Pantopaque from above, either by a cisternal puncture or through the lateral approach between C1 and C2.

Treatment

The treatment of this condition is decompressive laminectomy. In some patients the changes found at surgery are so severe that despite adequate decompression, no clinical improvement will occur. In the face of such severe cauda equina constriction, favorable results will be derived from surgery only in the early stages of compression. A laminectomy should not only be wide but also extensive, involving at least 2 laminae above the site of the block and 2 below. In many cases a laminectomy of the entire lumbar spine and the first 1 or 2 thoracic laminae is necessary. If there is a protruded intervertebral disc, this should be excised at the time of the laminectomy.[1]

PAGET'S DISEASE OF THE LUMBAR SPINE (OSTEITIS DEFORMANS)

Sir James Paget, the English surgeon who first described this disease as a clinical entity in 1877, believed the bony changes were related to an inflammatory process. Because the chief clinical manifestation was the deforming nature of bony changes, he called the disease "osteitis deformans."[16] This condition, particularly in its milder forms, is fairly common, affecting approximately 3 percent of all persons over 40 years of age. It is a generalized disease but it often affects the spine and may particularly involve the lumbar region producing lumbar and sciatic pain. The cause and mechanism of Paget's disease are unknown.

Pathology

The changes of Paget's disease are the result of a combination of both destructive and reparative processes. These changes are slowly progressive, starting in a solitary site and gradually extending to involve larger areas and more bones. The bones most commonly involved are the tibia, femur, pelvis, vertebrae and skull. Aside from the skull, the greatest incidence is in bones subjected to the most weight-bearing stress.

During the early and most active phase, resorption exceeds deposition. Deossification first occurs along the cortical surfaces, causing the bone to weaken and distort under pressure. Such distortion produces microfractures (infractions) of the cortex. Cortical demineralization is widely disseminated in patchy areas.

The osteolytic phase is followed by an osteosclerotic phase in which, in an attempt to repair the spongelike, weakened and deformed bone, the balance swings in favor of deposition. Osteoblastic proliferation within the remaining cortex produces some bony replacement.

In response to the bony distortion and resulting cortical infractions, the periosteum lays down new bone to strengthen the weakened bone. This periosteal osteogenesis is additive, causing widening of the bone as a whole without decreasing the medullary volume. This added bone is very primitive.

The involved areas of bone are extremely vascular and may even exhibit arteriovenous shunts.

Microscopic Changes

In normal bone, the outermost layer of the osteone (haversian canal with its lamellae) takes the hematoxylin stain more readily than surrounding tissue. When cut in cross-section, the result is a heavy blue line, called "the cement line," demarcating one osteone from its neighbor.

In Paget's disease, portions of osteones are irregularly eroded and to these areas of erosion, osteoblasts reparatively apply new osteoid in an erratic fashion. When cut in cross-section an irregular mosaic pattern is seen. This typical mosaic pattern of alternating mature and immature bone, which was first described by Schmorl, is characteristic of fully developed Paget's disease.[19]

X-ray Changes

In general the x-ray changes reflect osteolysis and excessive repair, either alone or in combination, resulting in areas of radiolucency and opacity.

Initially during the osteolytic phase there is a demineralizing process which causes skeletal radiolucency, deformity and a coarsening and prominence of the larger trabeculae in the line of weight bearing. The coarse trabeculations in affected vertebral bodies tend to be horizontal and accentuate the margins of the body. Compression fractures are not uncommon and result in narrowing of the vertebral body anteriorly.

As the disease progresses, areas of density appear which may eventually overshadow the surrounding normal bone, resulting occasionally in almost homogenous opacity of a vertebral body.

Oblique views may reveal narrowing of the intervertebral foramina, resulting from bony thickening of the foraminal boundaries.

Convex masses of partially calcified osteoid tissue frequently project beyond the vertebral bodies and displace the paraspinal shadow. These changes are seen best in the thoracic area.

Myelogram

The myelogram reveals multilevel vertebral encroachment with narrowing of the subarachnoid space. There is usually bilateral and often anterior compression. Occasionally, the body of the vertebra is so distorted that the resulting deformity produces a marked angulation and dorsal displacement of the Pantopaque column best seen on the cross-table lateral view. In some instances this dorsal displacement is extensive enough to produce a complete block.

The intervertebral discs remain intact and the deformity is almost always centered over the midportion of the vertebral body rather than the disc.

Signs and Symptoms

Frequently, Paget's disease is limited to a solitary bone (monostatic osteitis deformans), is noted as an incidental x-ray finding and may remain asymptomatic throughout life. Those cases that are symptomatic usually are polyostatic (numerous bones are affected).

The characteristic clinical picture of mature Paget's disease is striking. Collapse of the anterior portions of the vertebral bodies causes a typical kyphosis of the thoracic spine which thrusts the head forward and downward. The femurs bend outward, producing bowing and accentuating the deformity by an outward and forward bowing of the tibias. The stature is shortened by these lower extremity curvatures. Softening of the sacrum and the iliac bones, in association with a coxa vara from softening of the femoral necks, results in a waddling gait. In severe cases, the ribs and sternum are involved, causing lateral flattening and increased antero-posterior diameter of the thorax. This thoracic deformity, together with the kyphosis, interferes with normal respiratory excursions and is often associated with dyspnea. The forward curvature of the spine causes the abdomen to protrude. The calvarium is much enlarged.

Despite the rather unique and grotesque characteristics of this disease, the onset is so insidious that both the patient and associates who observe him at close intervals do not usually become aware of the changes until the condition is far advanced. The patient may first be aware of this condition when his hat seems too small. As a rule, the gradually increasing disabilities and deformities are attributed to old age, and may be overlooked by family and physicians alike.

Periosteal bone formation may impinge upon the foramina of emerging cranial and spinal nerves and interfere with motor and sensory nerve function and may also produce pain.

Cardiac output is considerably elevated and the impaired respiratory excursions may add to the increased work load of the heart. Cardiovascular disease is the most common cause of death in advanced generalized Paget's disease.

Laboratory Findings

The serum alkaline phosphate is always markedly elevated when the disease is disseminated but may be within normal limits when the disease is localized. Serum calcium is rarely elevated and serum phosphorus levels remain normal. Anemia is uncommon, despite considerable fibrosis in medullary hematopoietic areas.

Diagnosis

Patients suffering from Paget's disease involving the lumbar spine complain of pain in the low back area, the pain varying in intensity and character from a dull soreness to a most intense paroxysm. Some degree of pain is invariably present and, although activities such as heavy lifting, stooping and bending tend to aggravate the pain somewhat, rest will not relieve the pain. In many cases, periods of prolonged immobility are associated with increased pain described as "severe stiffness of my back." The pain is frequently worse at night, preventing sleep. Unilateral or bilateral nerve root irritation is occasionally present. The root symptoms are presumed secondary to narrowing of the intervertebral foramina from subperiosteal deposition of bone. Although the back pain is usually constant, the nerve root pain is generally intermittent, frequently related to activity and often eased with rest.

The localized periostitis over the anterior tibial areas produces exquisite pain which is aggravated by pressure over the affected bone. Severe and persisting cramps in both lower extremities are common. The anterior-tibial pain and calf cramps occasionally may be mistaken for root compression symptoms.

I have treated two patients with spinal cord compression secondary to Paget's disease of the spine, both of which involved the thoracic cord. Although osteitis deformans involves the lumbar spine more frequently than the dorsal spine, when cord compression occurs as the result of this condition it almost always develops in the dorsal region.[15,20] The probable explanation for this predilection is that the smallest cross-sectional area of the spinal canal is in the thoracic region; therefore, any thickening of the bony vertebral ring would be more apt to manifest itself at this level.[2]

Cauda equina compression resulting from Paget's disease of the lumbar spine is quite rare. The only case I have personally encountered with cauda equina compression involved sarcomatous degeneration of osteitis deformans.[11] It is estimated that 4 percent of all patients with symptomatic Paget's disease have superimposition of a malignant tumor, either osteosarcoma or fibrosarcoma, which occurs in an area previously affected by Paget's disease.[4,12,13,17,21,22,24]

Treatment

While there is no specific treatment for Paget's disease of the lumbar spine, the symptoms may be relieved.

I have treated seven patients with radiculitis secondary to foraminal compression from Paget's disease. Three did reasonably well with bed rest and a low back support. Two improved with intrathecal instillation of methylprednisolone acetate. Two did not derive adequate relief with conservative measures and required foraminotomies.

With regard to surgical technique, greater than usual care is required in performing a subperiosteal paravertebral muscle dissection when the underlying laminae are involved by Paget's disease. Direct downward pressure with the periosteal elevators may fracture a softened lamina and damage the underlying neural elements.

Following the subperiosteal paravertebral muscle dissection, the lumbar laminae and spinous processes may often appear as a single monolithic sheath of bone. Certainly, the anatomy will be sufficiently distorted to make precise localization uncertain. A cross table "marker film" with an instrument at the site of the presumed involved interspace is often most helpful in localization.

There is an increase in vascular attachments between the paraspinal muscles and diseased lamina. The blood flow through bone affected by osteitis deformans has been measured and found to be increased many times over that of normal bone. This observation is well confirmed by the difficulties in achieving adequate hemostasis during the performance of a laminectomy.

REFERENCES

1. Alexander, E., Jr.: Achondroplasia (Significance of the small lumbar spinal canal). J. Neurosurg., *31*:513, 1961.
2. Amyes, E. W., and Vogel, P. N.: Osteitis deformans (Paget's disease) of the spine with compression of the spinal cord: Report of three cases and discussion of the surgical problems. Bull. Los Angeles Neurol. Soc., *19*:18, 1954.
3. Armstrong, J. R.: Lumbar Disc Lesions; Pathogenesis and Treatment of Low Back Pain and Sciatica. Edinburgh, E. and S. Livingstone, Ltd., 1965.
4. Bird, C. E.: Sarcoma complicating Paget's disease of the bone: Report of 9 cases, 5 with pathologic verification. Arch. Surg., *14*:1187, 1927.
5. Caffey, J.: Achondroplasia of pelvis and lumbosacral spine. Some roentgenographic features. Am. J. Roentgenol., *80*:449, 1958.
6. Duvorsin, R. C., and Yahr, M. D.: Compressive spinal cord and root syndromes in achondroplastic dwarfs. Neurology, *12*:202, 1962.
7. Ehni, G., Clark, K., Wilson, C. B., and Alexander, E.: Significance of the small lumbar spinal canal (5 parts), J. Neurosurg., *31*:490, 1969.
8. Elsberg, C. A.: Experiences in spinal surgery. Observations upon 60 laminectomies for spinal disease. Surg. Gynecol. Obstet., *16*:117, 1913.
9. Epstein, J. A.: Diagnosis and treatment of painful neurological disorders caused by spondylosis of the lumbar spine. J. Neurosurg., *17*:991, 1960.
10. Epstein, J. A., Epstein, B. S., and Levine, L.: Nerve root compression associated with narrowing of the lumbar spinal canal. J. Neurol. Neurosurg. Psychiatry, *25*:165, 1962.
11. Finneson, B. E., Goluboff, B., and Shenkin, H. A.: Sarcomatous degeneration of osteitis deformans causing compression of the cauda equina. Neurology, *8*:82, 1958.
12. Geschickter, C. F., and Copeland, M. M.:

13. Gruner, O. C., Scringer, F. A. C., and Foster, L. S.: A clinical and histological study of a case of Paget's disease of the bones with multiple sarcoma formation. Arch. Intern. Med., *9*:641, 1912.
14. Hoelein, B. F.: Canine neurology: Diagnosis and Treatment. Philadelphia and London, W. B. Saunders, 1965.
15. Latimer, F. R., Webster, J. E., and Gurdjian, E. S.: Osteitis deformans with spinal cord compression: Report of three cases. J. Neurosurg., *10*:583, 1953.
16. Paget, J.: On a form of chronic inflammation of bones (osteitis deformans). Med. Chir. Tr., *60*:37, 1877. Also reprinted in Med. Classics *1*:29, 1936.
17. Sachs, B., and Fraenkel, J.: Progressive ankylotic rigidity of the spine. J. Nerve Ment. Dis., *27*:1, 1900.
18. Sarpyener, M. A.: Spina bifida aperta and congenital stricture of the spinal canal. J. Bone Joint Surg., *29*:817, 1947.
19. Schmorl, G.: Ueber Ostitis Deformans Paget. Arch. path. anat., *283*:694, 1932.
20. Schwarz, G. A., and Reback, S.: Compression of the spinal cord in osteitis deformans (Paget's disease) of the vertebrae. Am. J. Roentgenol. *42*:345, 1939.
21. Sear, H. R.: Some notes on diagnosis of bone tumors. Brit. Med. J., *1*:49, 1936.
22. Sear, H. R.: Osteogenic sarcoma as a complication of osteitis deformans. Brit. J. Radiol., *22*:580, 1949.
23. Sherman, R. S., and Soong, K. Y.: A roentgen study of osteogenic sarcoma developing in Paget's disease. Radiology, *63*:48, 1954.
24. Summey, T. J., and Pressly, C. L.: Sarcoma complicating Paget's disease of bone. Am. J. Surg., *123*:135, 1946.
25. Verbiest, H.: Sur certaines formes rares de compression de la queue de cheval. Hommage a Clovis Vincent. Paris: Maloiue, 161, 1949.
26. Verbiest, H.: A radicular syndrome from developmental narrowing of the lumbar vertebral canal. J. Bone Joint Surg., *26B*:230, 1954.
27. Verbiest, H.: Further experiences on the pathological influence of a development narrowness of the bony lumbar vertebral canal. J. Bone Joint Surg., *37B*:576, 1955.
28. Vogl, A.: The fate of the achondroplastic dwarf (Neurologic complications and achondroplasia). Exp. Med. Surg., *20*:108, 1962.
29. Williams, P.C.: The Lumbosacral Spine. New York, McGraw-Hill, 1965.

11
Spondylolysis and Spondylolisthesis

SPONDYLOLYSIS

Etiology
Clinical Features

Treatment

SPONDYLOLISTHESIS

Pseudospondylolisthesis

Isthmic Spondylolisthesis

Classification
Mechanical Factors
Establishing a Skeletal
   Weight-Bearing Line
Causes of Pain Production

Signs and Symptoms
Physical Findings
X-ray Findings
Management

Reverse Spondylolisthesis

Lateral Vertebral Displacement

SPONDYLOLYSIS

Spondylolysis is the term used for a defect, or so-called pseudoarthrosis, involving the lamina or neural arch of the vertebra. This defect occurs in that portion of the lamina midway between the superior and inferior articular facets called the "pars interarticularis."[4]

When the defect in the neural arch of a vertebra is bilateral, separation at the sites of these defects of the vertebral body from the neural arch may occur as a result of mechanical pressure which will allow a forward displacement of the deficient vertebra. This displacement is called spondylolisthesis.

Etiology

There seems to be little question that there is a congenital aspect to this condition.[11,10] Heredity plays a significant role; and in 60 percent of the cases where both father and mother have spondylolysis, the children will have it. Spondylolysis is associated with an increased incidence of other congenital spinal defects. Spina bifida is 13 times as common with pars defects in comparison to the general population; scoliosis is often seen. Stewart has noted wide racial differences in the occurrence of spondylolysis; finding 6.4 percent in white Americans, 2.8 percent in the black American, and 27.4 percent in the Alaskan Eskimo.

This condition is never present in the lumbar region at birth (the youngest case on record is 4 months of age), and it is felt that the pars defects develop as a result of stress in those persons born with structurally inadequate neural arches. As a result of torsional and rotational stress, "microfractures" occur at the site of the inadequacy and eventually progress toward dissolution of the pars interarticularis. Pars interarticularis defects are never seen in four-legged creatures, since it requires the trauma and stress of the upright position to create this pseudoarthrosis. Children who are born with mental and motor dysfunction, preventing assumption of the upright posture, do not seem to develop spondylolysis or spondylolisthesis, despite a

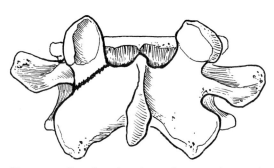

Fig. 11-1. Pseudoarthrosis at the pars interarticularis.

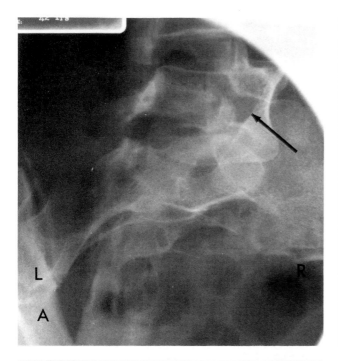

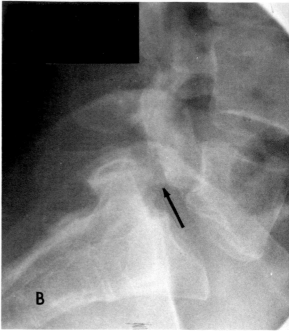

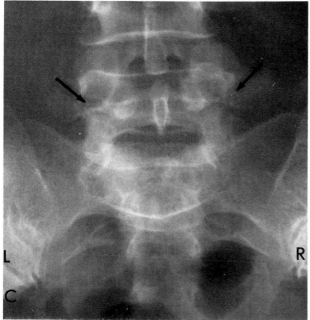

Fig. 11-2. Bilateral spondylolysis L5 in a 42-year-old female. The bony defect (*arrow*) in the pars interarticulares is clearly visualized on the oblique (A) and lateral (B) views. The diagnosis is rarely made on the A-P view (C) but after the lesion is identified, it can often be seen on this view also.

high percentage of other congenital defects, spinal and otherwise, in this group.

On the basis of studies carried out by Ramband and Reanault in 1864 and[7,8] Schwegel in 1859, 2 centers of ossification in each lateral half of the neural arch were found, and they advanced the theory that a pars interarticularis defect occurs because the ossification centers fail to unite. For years, this theory was widely accepted until subsequent investigations revealed that there are 3 primary ossification centers, 1 for each half of the neural arch and 1 for the centrum, thus discounting the original theory.

A study of 90 fetuses was carried out by Hitchcock[5] who demonstrated that the pars interarticularis was an area of potential weakness, being filled with large nutrient vessels. He further indicated that "although ossification begins in juxtaposition to the isthmic region and spreads thence to the pedicles and laminae, the isthmus itself consists very largely of cartilage until after birth, the long connection between remaining somewhat narrowed."

Approximately 4 percent of the population

has either spondylolysis or spondylolisthesis, but a large percentage of these patients have no significant back pain or disability.

Clinical Features

This condition is characterized by a pars interarticularis defect, either unilateral or bilateral with no significant separation at the site of the defect or forward displacement of the affected vertebral body. There is uncertainty as to the mechanism of symptom production with spondylolysis and, in fact, there may be some doubt as to the validity of this condition being an active symptom-producing entity.

The diagnosis is made only by x-ray. A linear defect of the pars interarticularis with some surrounding sclerosis is readily demonstrated by good oblique views of the lumbar spine. These findings will not usually be visualized when A-P and lateral views only are taken but are often seen as incidental x-ray findings.

Physical examination findings are not particularly revealing with minimal muscle spasm and possibly slight restriction of extremes in lumbar mobility. No reflex, motor or sensory changes are elicited.

Occasionally, patients experience mild low back pain of a generalized aching nature. This pain may be referred to the gluteal area and rarely to the posterior thighs.

Treatment

The pain is rarely severe enough to incapacitate and is usually relieved by rest and

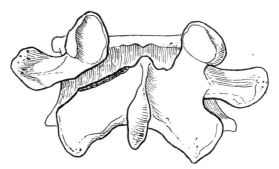

Fig. 11-3. Pseudoarthrectomy.

aggravated by activity including prolonged standing, walking, extensive auto driving and heavy lifting.

Infrequently, pain associated with spondylolysis is not responsive to conservative measures and in such instances surgery involving either excision of the loose vertebral arch or spinal fusion has been advocated.

At the 1971 American Association of Neurological Surgeons' meeting, John Collis presented a paper discussing a new operation performed on 8 patients spanning an 8-year period: excision of only the pseudoarthrosis. This procedure is based on the supposition that the pain associated with spondylolysis is due to motion at the pseudoarthrosis. After excision of this lesion with a small 3 mm. angled laminectomy punch, "every patient has been relieved of his pain and has continued to be pain free." This pseudoarthrectomy is performed only on the symptomatic side; if both sides are symptomatic, then a bilateral pseudoarthrectomy is performed.

SPONDYLOLISTHESIS

The segment of the vertebra between the lamina and superior articular process is identified as the isthmus; and since a bony defect at that site permits anterior luxation of the vertebral body, it is identified as "isthmic" spondylolisthesis. This is in contrast to forward displacement of the vertebra without an actual bony disruption which is identified as pseudospondylolisthesis.

PSEUDOSPONDYLOLISTHESIS

There are 3 types of pseudospondylolisthesis.

1. If there is an abnormally long isthmus between the laminae and the superior articular process, no break in the bony continuity is necessary to allow slight forward displace-

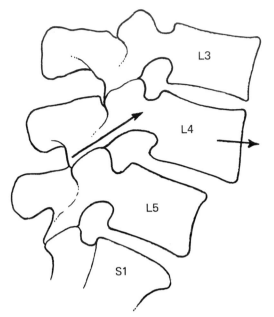

Fig. 11-4. Long isthmus pseudospondylolisthesis.

ment of the affected vertebral body in relationship to the adjacent vertebral bodies.

2. At the lumbosacral articulation, the sacral articular surfaces of the superior facets are positioned in a more sagittal plane than normal. This abnormality, in association with

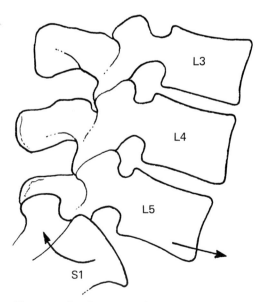

Fig. 11-5. Lordotic pseudospondylolisthesis.

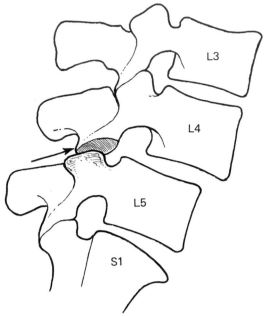

Fig. 11-6. Pseudospondylolisthesis secondary to the flattened apophyseal articular surfaces.

a more acute lumbosacral angle, may permit forward luxation of the fifth lumbar inferior articular process, causing the entire vertebral segment to be anteriorly displaced.

3. When the angle or plane of the apophyseal joints is more sagittal or flatter than those above and below, an anterior displacement of the vertebral body may occur. This condition is seen more often at the L4 vertebra. The oblique position of the articular surfaces may be congenital or more likely may develop gradually as a result of degenerative changes affecting the apophyseal joints.

ISTHMIC SPONDYLOLISTHESIS

Classification

The degree of slippage is classified in increasing increments of severity from 1 to 4.[6] The progressive nature of this slippage varies, and in many patients the forward displacement reaches a certain degree after which further displacement does not occur. In others, the forward slippage continues

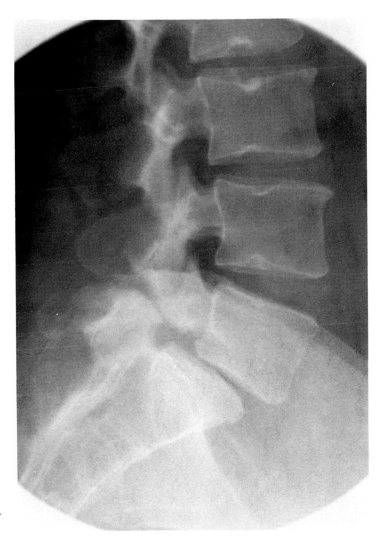

Fig. 11-7. Grade 1 spondylolisthesis L5 on S1.

unabated until the body of the lumbar vertebra slips completely off the sacrum. Although the fifth lumbar vertebra is the most
common site, it is seen in the fourth lumbar
vertebra and occasionally in the third lumbar
segment.

Mechanical Factors

With the normal spine in the upright position, the weight of the trunk transmitted to
the sacrum through the fifth lumbar vertebra
is in a downward and forward direction because of the downward tilt of the sacrum
upon which the fifth lumbar vertebra rests.
This forward shearing force is opposed by

the inferior articular processes of the fifth
lumbar vertebra, which hook down and behind the superior articular processes of the
sacrum. Any break in the continuity of this
opposing lock results in a tendency for the
fifth lumbar vertebral body to slip forward
carrying with it the superimposed vertebral
column.

A normally intact intervertebral disc at the
L5-S1 interspace will prevent forward displacement of the vertebral body. However,
this disc is subjected to increased stress in
the absence of articular bony support and
may develop early degenerative changes.

An altered postural attitude will attempt

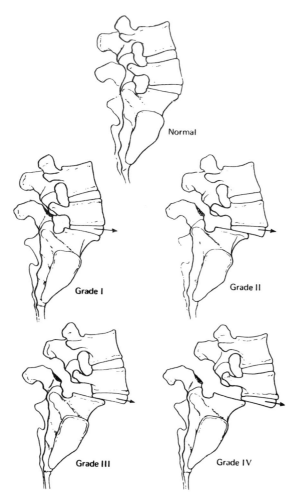

Normal

Grade I

Grade II

Grade III

Grade IV

Fig. 11-8. Classification of spondylolisthesis.

to compensate for the forward shift of the lower trunk which displaces the center of gravity forward. By activating the erector spinal muscles, the upper trunk is thrust farther backward. This increased muscular activity tends to tilt the pelvis forward, increasing the lumbar lordosis and hamstring muscle tension, and further increasing the stress upon the involved interspace.

Establishing a Skeletal Weight-bearing Line

1. The spinous process of the fourth lumbar vertebra may settle into contact with that of the fifth in association with contact between the inferior articular processes of the fourth lumbar vertebra with the superior aspect of the lamina of the fifth lumbar vertebra at the site of the defect. Once such bony contact is established, the major weight of the trunk is transmitted to the sacrum abnormally through these posterior skeletal structures which may serve to prevent further forward luxation of the fifth lumbar vertebra, barring severe trauma.

As the inferior articular processes of the fourth lumbar vertebra settle into the pars articularis defect of the fifth lumbar vertebra, they tend to act as a wedge, forcing the body and the superior articular processes of the fifth lumbar segment forward in relation to the body of the fourth lumbar segment. This results in displacement of the superior articular processes upward and forward into the

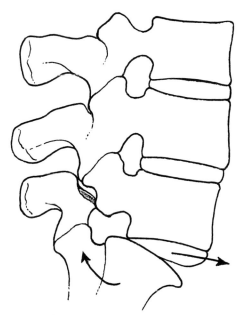

Fig. 11-9. Increased "slippage stress" with increased sacral angle.

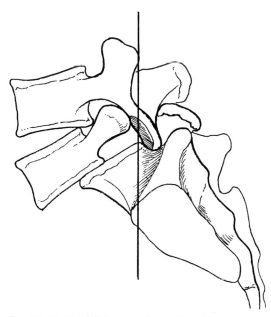

Fig. 11-11. Establishing a skeletal weight-bearing line with L5 spina bifida.

intervertebral foramen between the fourth and fifth lumbar vertebrae subjecting the nerve root to foraminal compression. A further potential source of nerve root compression at the L4-5 level is the frequently noted degeneration of the intervertebral disc from increased stress at that site.

2. As mentioned previously, there is an increased incidence of spina bifida associated with spondylolisthesis. When the posterior structures of the fifth lumbar vertebra are absent or underdeveloped, the parenchyma, in order to establish a skeletal weight-bearing line to the sacrum using the posterior structures, is limited allowing the fifth lumbar vertebral body to slip far forward, in

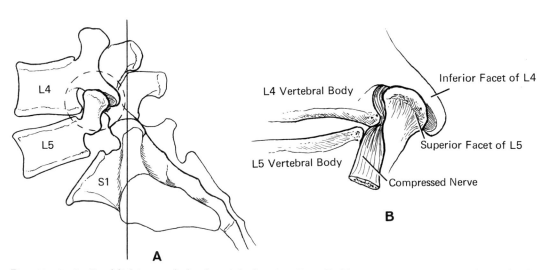

Fig. 11-10. A, Establishing a skeletal weight-bearing line. B, Nerve root compression from the L5 superior facet.

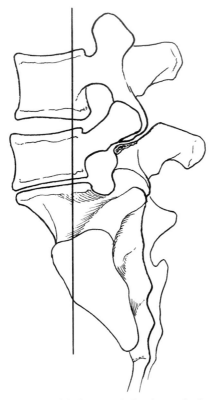

Fig. 11-12. Establishing a skeletal weight-bearing line with a flattened (decreased) sacral angle.

some instances completely off the sacral table.

3. The sheer stress at the lumbosacral joint is related to the lumbosacral angulation. When the plane of the sacral table more nearly approaches the horizontal plane, the tendency for forward luxation of the fifth vertebral body is reduced, despite lack of support by the posterior structures. This allows the body of the fifth lumbar vertebra to seat itself directly upon the sacrum, establishing a skeletal weight-bearing line through the posterior aspect of the vertebral bodies.[9]

Causes of Pain Production

1. The postural adjustments associated with spondylolisthesis may be pain producing. They involve the stretching of the anterior and posterior longitudinal ligaments, the intervertebral discs and the articular joint capsules of the fourth and fifth lumbar vertebrae.

The frequently associated lumbar lordosis converts the lower lumbar articular joints into weight-bearing structures bringing the lower lumbar spinous processes, which also function as weight-bearing structures, into close approximation. This causes compression of the interspinous ligaments and may be pain producing.

2. The above-formed compensatory weight-bearing pseudoarthroses develop hypertrophic osteoarthritic degenerative changes which may be another source of pain.

3. A third source of pain is nerve root irritation and compression. This may occur from impingement of the fifth lumbar superior articulating facet into the L4-5 intervertebral foramen, degeneration and extrusion of the L4-5 disc, or displacement and stretching of nerve roots caused by the step or ledge in the anterior wall of the vertebral canal caused by the vertebral displacement.

Nerve root pressure is less likely to occur from an extruded L5-S1 disc, because, as a result of the forward displacement of the body and superior articular processes of the fifth lumbar vertebra, the spinal canal is enlarged at that level, making root entrapment less likely.

However, despite the extra room afforded by displacement, root irritation at the L5-S1 level can possibly be produced by the ill-defined mass of fibrous tissue in which there are areas of mucoid degeneration surrounding the site of bony disruption and which may also envelop the root.

Signs and Symptoms

I am often surprised at the rather large spondylolisthesis one may occasionally find when viewing lumbar spine radiographs obtained for reasons other than for low back pain, such as for a large bowel or genitourinary study. When these patients are questioned regarding the low back symptoms they have manifested in the past, they com-

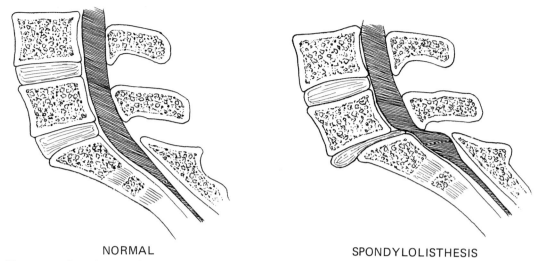

NORMAL   SPONDYLOLISTHESIS

Fig. 11-13. Stretching and compression of nerve roots may be caused by the "step" or ledge of the anterior wall of the vertebral canal which in turn is caused by the vertebral displacement.

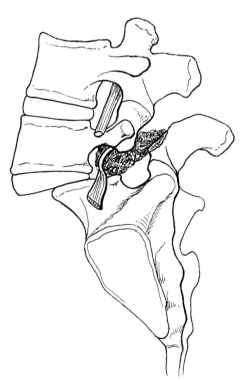

Fig. 11-14. Root irritation at the L5–S1 level may be produced by the fibrous tissue surrounding the pseudoarthrosis enveloping the nerve root.

pletely deny having any symptoms at all in many cases; in other instances a series of leading questions will bring forth an admission of occasional, mild low back discomfort. It is not unusual to find patients with moderately severe spondylolisthesis who have never sought medical attention for low back symptoms. The most frequently encountered symptoms are generalized aching or low back discomfort which is aggravated by activity and eased by rest. Activities such as prolonged stooping, bending, climbing of ladders or lifting tend to aggravate the pain; rest in bed eases it. Sciatica is occasionally present and may be unilateral or bilateral. Occasionally, the cauda equina may be stretched sufficiently to create motor weakness involving both lower extremities and occasionally sphincter disturbances with bladder and rectal symptoms associated with saddle sensory changes.

Physical Findings

The physical findings will vary according to the severity of the spondylolisthesis. A compensatory increased lumbar lordosis is usually apparent, and this is often seen in association with slight flexion of the knees in the erect position. Palpation reveals a step

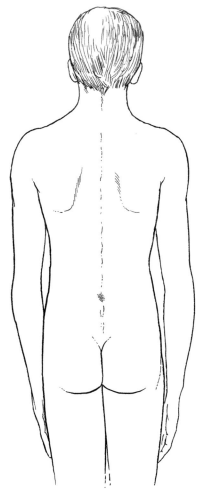

Fig. 11-15. The step or dimple characteristic of spondylolisthesis marks the spinous process of the forward displaced vertebral body which has not moved forward with its body but remains in its proper position and projects more posteriorly than the spinous processes above it.

between the spinous processes of the fourth and fifth lumbar vertebrae, which can be visualized as a "dimple" in the midlumbar crease. This step marks the spinous process of the forward displaced vertebral body which has not moved forward with its body but remains in its proper position and will project more posteriorly than the spinous processes above it. There is often some paraspinal muscle spasm and tenderness in the lumbar region with some limitation of mo-

bility of all lumbar movements and pain at the extremes of all lumbar movements. Sensory, motor and reflex changes are rarely elicited unless cauda equina compression symptoms are present.

X-ray Findings

X-rays of the spine will confirm the diagnosis of spondylolisthesis. The lateral views will indicate the amount of forward slipping and the oblique views reveal the linear bony defect of the pars.

Management

Spondylolisthesis can be managed adequately if the patient avoids strenuous activities, adheres to instructions regarding proper lifting postures and the use of other mechanically efficient methods of daily activities, and with general overall low back care. Mild analgesics and occasionally the use of a low back support, either a brace or a corset, are often helpful during strenuous activities or painful intervals.

The pain of impacted spinous processes may be managed by steroid injection into the interspinous ligament.

If conservative measures do not afford adequate relief of symptoms or the slippage is noted to be progressive on serial x-rays, surgery must be considered.

Any of the following are an indication for surgery:

1. Intractable pain.
2. Progressive anterior luxation.
3. Persisting nerve root pain.
4. Neurological symptoms, including saddle hypesthesia and sphincter dysfunction.

Prior to consideration of surgery, a lumbar myelogram is in order to determine the degree of spinal canal deformity and to help establish radiographic localization of nerve root compression.

The Gill procedure,[1] involving the removal of the neural arch, was introduced in 1955 and for some time thereafter was advocated as the surgical procedure of choice for severe persisting pain with spondylolisthesis. The clinical improvement derived from this decompressive procedure is primarily due to the reduction of nerve root irritation and compression. Some degree of this improvement was probably achieved by removal of the fibrous tissue mass surrounding the pars defect. Many patients appreciated no significant improvement in their pain and occasionally further anterior vertebral slippage occurred, which might be attributed to the surgical reduction of skeletal supporting tissue. Because of the danger of further luxation, this procedure is rarely indicated in children or young adults. It does have a place in the management of the older patient with symptoms of nerve root pressure who is not as apt to enter into strenuous physical activities productive of severe sheer stress upon the weakened joint.

For younger patients the procedure of choice is posterior root decompression followed by either a posterolateral fusion or posterior lumbar interbody fusion of the least number of vertebral bodies that will provide stability. This will usually involve the sacrum and the last 2 lumbar vertebrae for posterolateral fusion and the L5-S1 interspace for the posterior lumbar interbody fusion. When a spina bifida occulta is present with a fibrous shield over the sacrum rather than bone, presenting a poor "bed" for a satisfactory posterior bone graft, the fusion is limited to the facets and the transverse processes. It is most important to include the pars interarticularis defect in the fusion to prevent motion at that site. If pseudoarthrosis develops with posterolateral fusion, an anterior discectomy and fusion of the major interspace involved should be considered as a secondary procedure.[3,2]

REVERSE SPONDYLOLISTHESIS

This condition occurs when for some reason there is marked narrowing of the intervertebral space. It can follow severe degenerative disc involvement, tuberculous spondylitis or a bacterial intervertebral disc infection. Any such destruction of the inter-

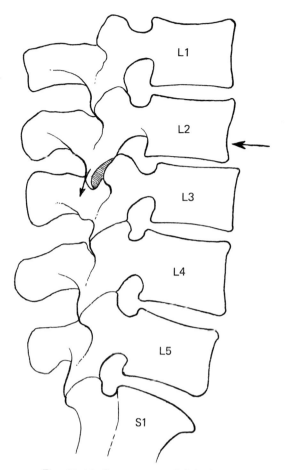

Fig. 11-16. Reverse spondylolisthesis.

space, which leads to a decrease in the height of the disc space, causes the adjacent vertebral bodies to approximate each other. In association with this, the corresponding articulating facets will contract or "accordion" together and due to the oblique inclination of the articular processes will sheer the facet of the superior vertebra into an inferior posterior direction. This tends to pull the affected vertebra posteriorly and is visualized on x-rays as a posterior steplike displacement of the vertebral body. Such a reverse spondylolisthesis is usually seen in the upper lumbar spine most often at L1 or L2.

Clinically, these patients manifest increased pain with movements of the spine that result in stretching of the involved articular facets. They usually have a great deal of compensatory paraspinal muscle spasm which maintains the spine in a fairly stiff, immobile position. Lateral bending may not cause much pain, but forward bending is quite uncomfortable; and attempted hyperextension is often particularly excruciating. There is usually considerable tenderness to pressure over the involved site.

LATERAL VERTEBRAL DISPLACEMENT

Lateral vertebral displacement can occur only when there is extensive destruction of the vertebrae including the facets and the body. This may be seen following severe spinal trauma or malignancy. Lateral vertebral displacement may seem to occur radiographically when there is rotational displacement, but this is invariably associated with a severe scoliosis.

REFERENCES

1. Gill, G. G.; Manning, J. G., and White, H. L.: Surgical treatment of spondylolisthesis without spine fusion. Excision of the loose lamina with decompression of the nerve root. J. Bone Joint Surg., *37A*:493, 1955.
2. Goldner, J. L., McCallum, D. E., and Urbaniak, J. R.: Anterior Disc Excision and Interbody Spine Fusion for Chronic Low Back Pain. American Academy of Orthopedic Surgeons, Symposium on the Spine. St. Louis, C. V. Mosby, 1969.
3. Anterior intervertebral discectomy and arthrodesis for treatment of low back pain with or without radiculopathy. *In* Ojemann, R. G. (ed.): Clinical Neurosurgery. The Congress of Neurological Surgeons, vol. 15, ch. XVI, pp. 352–383, 1968.
4. Hilel, N.: Spondylolysis; its anatomy and mechanism of development. J. Bone Joint Surg., *41A*:303, 1959.
5. Hitchcock, H. H.: Spondylolisthesis, Observations on its Development, Progression, and Genesis, J. Bone Joint Surg., *22*:1, 1940.
6. Meyerding, H. W.: Spondylolisthesis as an etiologic factor in backache. JAMA: 1971, 1938.
7. Ramband, A., and Reanault, C.: Origine et developpement des os, Paris, 1864.
8. Schwegel, A.: Uber Knochenvarietaten, Ztschr. rat. Med. *5*:283, 1859.
9. Williams, Paul C.: The Lumbosacral Spine, New York, McGraw-Hill, 1965.
10. Wiltse, L. L.: Etiology of spondylolisthesis. Clinical Orthop., *11:* Fall, 1959.
11. Wiltse, L. L.: The etiology of spondylolisthesis. J. Bone Joint Surg., *44A*:539, 1962.

12
Vertebral Osteoporosis and Backache

OSTEOPOROSIS

Known Causes of Osteoporosis
Etiology of Postmenopausal
  (senile) Osteoporosis
X-ray Diagnosis

Laboratory Data
Signs and Symptoms
Differential Diagnosis
Treatment

12
Vertebral Osteoporosis and Backache

OSTEOPOROSIS

Bone should be considered not only as a supporting structure for the body but also as an important metabolic mineral deposit which is in constant motion. In the latter regard bone has a regulating function in phosphorus and calcium metabolism which is comparable to that of the liver in carbohydrate metabolism. This guiding and controlling function of bone is influenced by many variables including congenital factors, hormones, vitamin deficiences or overdoses, enzyme disturbances and infectious processes and trauma.

Osteoporosis is the most common of all of the abnormalities involving bone. It can be defined as a reduction in the amount of bone present in any part of the skeleton. Although this commonly found condition may be categorized as resulting from a number of known medical diseases or alterations in body physiology, the largest segment comprises a rather ill-defined entity identified as postmenopausal, senile or idiopathic osteoporosis.

The important change in the physiologic process is decreased osteoblast activity while the osteoclasts are unchanged, and the result is the typical picture of osteoporosis.

Osteoporosis may affect the entire skeletal system but seems to involve the vertebral column in particular and is often radiographically identified only in the spine. A possible explanation for this seeming predisposition toward the spine may be related to the hematopoietic functions of the vertebral marrow in association with an abundant blood supply, which would induce a more rapid metabolic response of the vertebral skeleton to physiologically and pathologically increased calcium demands.

Known Causes of Osteoporosis

1. Genetic abnormalities such as mongolism or hypogonadal states.

2. Nutritional dysfunction associated with severe calcium deficiencies, scurvy and long-standing protein deficiencies.

3. Endocrine diseases including acquired hypogonadism, Cushing's syndrome, thyrotoxicosis and acromegaly.

4. Long-standing administration of corticosteroids in large doses.

5. Prolonged immobilization as is sometimes necessary with severe fractures or in paralyzed extremities.

6. Pregnancy.

7. Prolonged periods of weightlessness. Those active in the space program hope that programmed exercises while on prolonged space voyages will stop or at least reduce this tendency.

All of these known causes of osteoporosis are responsible for a minority of the verified cases with the majority categorized as postmenopausal and senile.[7] This disorder involves the entire population to some degree and starts at the age of 35 to 40 years and results in a loss of bone during the last 4 to 5 decades under "normal" conditions. It is estimated that there are 4.5 to 5 million postmenopausal women with osteoporosis in the United States. In many instances the process is asymptomatic but the disorder is a potentially serious condition because of the high risk of future fractures.

Etiology of Postmenopausal (Senile) Osteoporosis

Despite much study and speculation, the etiology of postmenopausal osteoporosis has not been defined. The role of the menopause in this condition remains uncertain even after many years of study. Deficiencies of estrogen, calcium, protein, phosphate, overproduction of heparin, chronic acidity and deficiency of growth hormone have all been considered.[9] Calcium deficiency results in osteoporosis in certain animal species but is unproved as an etiology in man.

Most investigators agree that there seems to be an increased rate of bone resorption with the rate of bone formation being either normal or decreased, when normally this system is in dynamic equilibrium. Whether this is a physiologic or pathologic process is not at all clear.

Elderly people are osteoporotic in the sense that they have less bone than younger persons. It is difficult to distinguish between the process of normal aging of the skeleton and the condition of senile osteoporosis.

Gross and microscopic examination of osteoporotic bone reveals that the reduction in the amount of cancellous bone is more the result of decrease in number, hence wider spacing of bone trabeculae, than of a reduction in the thickness of these structures.[10] In the vertebral bodies, there is a preferential loss of transverse trabeculae.[3,2]

Histological measurements of the cancellous bone of the iliac crest reveal a normal progressive decrease in the amount of bone with age, with a 40 percent loss occurring

between 20 and 80 years of age in both men and women. When the cortical bone of the iliac crest is similarly measured, the rate of bone loss is more rapid in females.[11]

Senile osteoporosis is more common in females and is found in a much higher incidence in Caucasians. Some attribute this racial difference to less strenuous physical activities of Caucasians in comparison to other races. This may not be valid, since recent studies on Israelis living in Jerusalem demonstrated a higher incidence in Jews of European stock compared to those of Asiatic origin.

Since there is a variable, but steady, loss of skeletal mass after maturity, those patients with a generous skeleton in early adulthood may best be protected against the inroads of skeletal decline which occurs with age.

X-ray Diagnosis

X-rays reveal radiolucency of the skeleton as a whole with the skull usually spared.

X-rays[4] of the spine reveal the radiolucency noted above with decreased bone density and loss of the horizontal striations with the vertical striations usually remaining. The cortical margins are very well defined, being razor sharp and thin. Despite the fact that this condition occurs in elderly patients, there are remarkably few osteophytes in the presence of senile osteoporosis, and the discs are usually in excellent condition with little evidence of degeneration. Occasionally, osteoporosis will sufficiently weaken the vertebral body to allow expansion of the intervertebral disc into the upper and lower cartilaginous plates, producing the characteristic ballooned discs or biconcavity of the vertebral bodies. Any other condition which will weaken the vertebral body, such as multiple myeloma or other malignancies, may cause similar ballooning of the intervertebral disc. Compression fractures are seen with this condition and must be looked for very carefully.

Because of the occasional difficulty in diagnosing and estimating the severity of this condition, a variety of x-ray comparison tests have been devised in which the density of the spine is compared with aluminum or ivory step wedges to establish a measurable index of osteoporosis. However, the varying degree of soft tissues about the spine, particularly in obese patients, leads to a problem in interpretation, so that there is no universally adopted or widespread system which will enable radiologists to readily classify the degree of osteoporosis.

Laboratory Data

Biochemical investigation is not helpful in the definitive diagnosis of osteoporosis. However, serum calcium, inorganic phosphorus and alkaline phosphatase determinations should be obtained to help exclude osteomalacia and osteitis fibrosa. Following osteoporotic fractures, there may be a slight elevation of the alkaline phosphatase, but rarely over 8 Bodansky units. The excretion of calcium in the urine is within normal limits, but there is usually an increased excretion of calcium in the feces.

The cellular and chemical makeup of osteoporotic bone is normal.

Signs and Symptoms

Osteoporosis is associated with a high incidence of low back pain and it is presumed that a reduction in the amount of bone within the vertebral bodies is not likely, by itself, to be a cause of symptoms.

The apparent rarefaction of the spine visualized radiographically does not always correlate with symptomatology. Some hold to the view that symptoms occur mainly when there is a recent progression of the disease, although this impression is admittedly difficult to substantiate. Symptomatic intervals are often interspersed with long pain-free periods. The cause of such pain is probably due to pressure of fractured bone on spinal nerve roots or upon sensory fibers in the periosteum as a result of pathological fractures and vertebral body wedging. In many instances, pain occurs before a fracture can be satisfactorily defined by x-ray and it is

presumed that this represents microfractures which may not be large enough to be adequately visualized radiographically.

Investigation[5] reveals abundant nerve innervation in the articular capsules of the facets, anterior and posterior ligaments, outer zones of the annulus fibrosis and the vertebral periosteum. This nerve supply provides a possible explanation for low back pain when it is difficult to correlate the roentgenographic findings with the clinical signs and symptoms.

Osteoporosis may exist for years without causing any symptoms until trauma causes collapse of one or more vertebral bodies. This trauma may be quite minor—coughing, turning in bed, stepping down from a high curb or bending forward to pick up a relatively light object. In some cases, no specific trauma can be recalled. Generalized low back pain of an aching nature is usually associated with localized tenderness over the collapsed vertebra. Examination may reveal a kyphosis in the area of vertebral body wedging, especially if 2 or more adjacent vertebrae are affected. Measurement may reveal an unexpected loss of height. Paraspinal muscle spasm and limitation of spinal mobility are present. Tenderness over all the long bones, particularly those near the surface of the skin, such as the tibia or the ulna, is noted when the condition is generalized.

Although the back pain may be severe, actual spinal cord compression is a rare occurrence as a result of vertebral compression in osteoporosis.[6]

Differential Diagnosis

Several conditions may be confused with postmenopausal osteoporosis and it is important to rule them out.

Osteoporosis Secondary to Specific Diseases. The several forms of osteoporosis secondary to specific diseases often respond to appropriate therapy. For example, thyrotoxic osteoporosis is curable and should be investigated.

Osteomalacia. Patients with osteomalacia,

which is primarily a vitamin D deficiency, can occasionally be misdiagnosed as having osteoporosis, since they also frequently complain of low back pain and leg pain aggravated by weight bearing. In addition to pain, diffuse primary muscle weakness of the lower extremities is occasionally seen resulting in a peculiar, shuffling, waddling gait utilizing the hips and trunk in ambulating which may be confused with a cauda equina compressive lesion.

Most adults with osteomalacia have some form of intestinal malabsorption or renal tubular acidosis. Some patients have primary or idiopathic osteomalacia in which the specific etiology is difficult to define. There is also a familial form occurring in childhood and persisting into adulthood.[1]

Laboratory studies reveal certain alterations especially the serum alkaline phosphatase which is usually elevated. The serum inorganic phosphate is depressed in the fasting specimen; the serum calcium may be normal but is frequently depressed.

X-rays may be diagnostic if a typical pathognomonic pseudofracture is identified, usually in the ribs, scapulae or pubic bones. These fractures do not necessarily occur at sites of bony pain, so a complete skeletal survey is indicated. If a suspicious area is identified on routine films, laminograms of that region may be necessary to define a pseudofracture.

Biopsy of a pseudofracture is frequently diagnostic and will reveal increased osteoid tissue with many osteoid seams.

Treatment. Osteomalacia is treated with appropriate doses of vitamin D supplemented with oral phosphate and will produce disappearance of bone pain within 2 months. If intestinal malabsorption or renal tubular acidosis is determined to be present, this should be managed by appropriate means.

Hyperparathyroidism. Occasionally hyperparathyroidism due to a parathyroid adenoma will give rise to skeletal involvement with osteitis fibrosa, producing spinal pain and in rare instances spinal cord compression.[8]

Many of these patients give a history of kidney stones, peptic ulcer, pancreatitis, muscle weakness and manifest symptoms of psychiatric disturbance.

Laboratory studies usually reveal elevation of the serum calcium; although if the disease is intermittent, this level may be normal for varying periods of time. If skeletal involvement is extensive, the plasma alkaline phosphatase is usually elevated. Less than half of these patients have lowered serum inorganic phosphorus levels.

X-rays may sometimes reveal only nonspecific demineralization but will occasionally disclose characteristic periosteal resorption in the digital bones or lateral end of the clavicles.

If this disease can be identified and successful parathyroid surgery follows, a most gratifying result can be achieved.

Multiple Myeloma and Metastatic Carcinoma. The conditions most frequently misdiagnosed as senile osteoporosis are multiple myeloma and metastatic carcinoma. These conditions should be considered and ruled out before establishing a diagnosis.

X-rays will usually reveal vertebral destruction and collapse in both conditions. When the pedicle of a collapsed vertebra is "washed out," the diagnosis is almost always metastatic carcinoma. Multiple myeloma primarily involves the cancellous body of the vertebra and will produce vertebral collapse without destroying the cortex of the pedicle; therefore, the pedicle will appear intact on x-ray.

Treatment

There is no treatment for postmenopausal osteoporosis that is clinically satisfactory and we have no specific criteria to measure the effectiveness of the various treatments. The response to therapy may be impossible to measure clinically because postmenopausal osteoporosis develops over a period of 20 to 30 years and effective therapy may require an equal time to manifest clinically satisfactory improvement.

Combinations of estrogens and androgens have been used for years in the hope that production of bone matrix would be stimulated. On the basis of this long experience it is now generally believed that there is no significant long-term advantage to be derived from this method of therapy and that the complications of such treatment, including dangers of stimulating pelvic malignancies, contraindicate its use.

If at all possible, the patient should not be permitted to remain immobilized in bed for prolonged periods of time. Increased activity is of value in producing deposition of calcium in the affected bone by allowing osteoblasts to receive the necessary stimuli. Any means of encouraging early activity in these elderly uncomfortable patients should be utilized including analgesics, physiotherapy, and a low back support to reduce discomfort during ambulation.

A palatable high protein diet is important, since the general nutritional state is often inadequate. At present, I recommend that 1 gram of calcium daily should be given along with sufficient vitamin D to assure calcium absorption. In addition, 45 milligrams of sodium fluoride should be given daily.

Possibly the best management is prophylactic with adequate calcium intake and an active physical existence in early and middle years.

REFERENCES

1. Arnstein, A. R., Frame, B., and Frost, H. M.: Recent progress in osteomalacia and rickets. Ann. Int. Med., *67:*1296, 1967.
2. Atkinson, P.: Variation in trabecular structure of vertebrae with age. Calcif. Tissue Res., *1:*24, 1967.
3. Cassucio, C.: An introduction to the study of osteoporosis (biochemical and biophysical research in home aging). Proc. R. Soc. Med., 55:663, 1962.
4. Frame, B.: Metabolic bone disease as a cause of neckache and backache. Neckache and backache proceedings of a workshop. *In* Gurdjian, E. S., and Thomas, L. M., (eds.): Charles C Thomas.
5. Jackson, H. C., Winkelmann, R. K., and Bickel, W. H.: Nerve endings in the human lumbar spinal column and related structures. J. Bone Joint Surg., *48A:*1272, 1966.
6. Kempinsky, W. H., Morgan, P. P., and Boniface, W. R.: Osteoporotic kyphosis with paraplegia. Neurology, *8:*181, 1958.
7. Rose, G. A.: A critique of modern methods of diagnosis and treatment in osteoporosis. Clin. Orthop., *55:*17, 1967.
8. Shaw, M. T., and Davies, M.: Primary hyperparathyroidism presenting as spinal cord compression. Brit. Med. J., *5625:*230, 1968.
9. Wachman, A., and Bernstein, D. S.: Diet and osteoporosis. Lancet, *1:*958, 1968.
10. Wakamatsu, E., and Sissons, H. A.: Calcif. Tissue Res., *4:*147, 1969.
11. Wolanski, N.: Changes in bone density and cortical thickness of the second metacarpal between the ages of 3 and 74 years. Acta Anat., *67:*74, 1967.

13
Infections of the Lumbar Spine

INFECTIONS SUBSEQUENT TO LUMBAR DISC SURGERY

Soft Tissue Infections

Signs and Symptoms
Management

Intervertebral Disc Space Infections

Signs and Symptoms
Management

Refractory Infections

Meningitis

INFECTIONS WITHOUT ANTECEDENT OPERATIONS ON THE SPINE

Nontuberculous Infections in Children

Clinical Picture
Mode of Infection in Children
X-ray Findings
Management

Nontuberculous Infections in Adults

Clinical Picture
X-ray Findings

Management
Disc Space Abscess

Tuberculosis of the Lumbar Spine

Signs and Symptoms
X-ray Findings
Management

13
Infections of the Lumbar Spine

Because infections of the lumbar spine are not common, they are often overlooked as a cause of back pain; yet they are common enough to deserve consideration in the differential diagnosis of low back dysfunction of uncertain etiology. The infectious process can be bacterial, tuberculous or my-cotic, but in some instances no organism can be demonstrated on smear or culture. Spinal infections occur more commonly in adults than in children and in equal frequency between men and women. The infectious source may be postspinal surgery, a distant focus of infection or idiopathic.

INFECTIONS SUBSEQUENT TO LUMBAR DISC SURGERY

SOFT TISSUE INFECTIONS

In a personal series of 1,000 cases of lumbar disc disease treated surgically, 241 patients developed wound infections (2.41%). The majority of these infections remained localized to the superficial soft tissues and did not involve, in a clinically identifiable way, the intervertebral disc space. When the infection does involve the disc space, the question arises as to whether the interspace infection developed secondarily to the soft tissue infection; or whether the disc space infection developed first and subsequently spread outward to the soft tissues; or whether both sites were simultaneously infected. The sequence of events is of more than academic consideration, since it relates directly to the proper management of the complication. If disc infection is secondary to soft tissue infection, it follows that an incompletely drained soft tissue infection may spread into the intervertebral disc space which otherwise would be spared.

Signs and Symptoms

An elevated temperature on the fourth to eighth postoperative day, in association with more than the anticipated postoperative incisional discomfort, should direct the physician's attention to the possibility of wound infection. Increased incisional tenderness and swelling may make it impossible for the patient to remain in a supine position which causes direct pressure upon the wound. Careful inspection usually reveals evidence of purulence at the edges of the incision, and sometimes drainage of pus is seen.[7]

Management

Purulent drainage is identified as soon as possible by culture and sensitivity tests in addition to microscopic examination.

The generally accepted method of treatment is to open the wound to allow adequate drainage of purulent material and to place the patient on appropriate antibiotics in accordance with the culture and sensitivity tests.

If the infection is confined to the superficial soft tissues, once the purulent collection is allowed to escape and wound abscess pressure is relieved, the incisional pain abates. Persisting fever, signs of general septicemia and increasing back and sciatic pain signal serious extension of the infectious process and require immobilization, massive doses of antibiotic and major medical supportive efforts.

The vast majority of wound infections are confined to the superficial soft tissues, and some difference of opinion exists regarding the extent of wound reopening in such cases.

Some physicians believe that in the presence of signs of wound suppuration limited aspiration, probing or bedside measures of wound evacuation should give way to a much more radical reopening of the wound in the operating room. Utilizing such wide exposure, all recesses of the wound which evidence infection or necrotic tissue or hematoma may then be saucerized and the wound lightly packed open. The wound will heal from the depths outward and, with healing, gradual removal of the packing is carried out from the deepest portion of the wound outward. Soft rubber catheters are usually placed within the packing for daily instillations of topical antibiotics (equal parts of 0.1% polymyxin, 1.0% neomycin, and 500 units per cc. bacitracin). Systematic antibacterial medication is administered in accordance with the organism culture and sensitivity tests.

The treatment of personal preference involves drainage of the wound through a limited and superficial opening of the incision, with no attempt to probe the depths of the wound. Frequent warm, wet soaks are utilized and the patient is permitted to ambulate. In the absence of fever, signs of general septicemia or increasing back and sciatic pain, the patient may be discharged and can continue warm, wet soaks at home without the use of antibiotics. Close outpatient follow-up on a twice weekly basis is continued until complete wound healing occurs.

INTERVERTEBRAL DISC SPACE INFECTIONS

Two intervertebral disc space infections occurred in 241 superficial wound infections (0.8% of 241 superficial wound infections and 0.2% of 1000 cases).

Most intervertebral disc space infections subsequent to lumbar disc surgery are associated with a superficial wound infection, which may develop before or after the interspace infection. Some cases have been reported with no external evidence of purulence.

Signs and Symptoms

Every intervertebral disc space infection is characterized by excruciating back pain which is diffuse, often spreading into the hips and flanks in association with severe lumbar paraspinal muscle spasm. Any movement tends to aggravate the pain, weight bearing is intolerable and even the most minor trauma, such as the inadvertent jarring of the bed by attendants, aggravates the pain. This clinical picture may occur within a week of surgery or may be delayed as long as 6 weeks after surgery. Ileus and abdominal distention may be associated with the clinical picture.

A low-grade temperature elevation may be present but is often normal. The only significant laboratory finding is an elevated erythrocyte sedimentation rate. Leukocytosis may be present.

X-ray findings are unrevealing until at least 4 to 8 weeks, when the first changes are seen. At that time, in addition to slight narrowing of the involved interspace, some erosion of the adjacent articular surfaces can be visualized. Laminography in the lateral views is often helpful in defining these early changes. Progressive rarefaction of the anterior subchondral area with irregular destruction of the end-plate is seen. This is followed by further diminution of the disc space and destruction of the adjacent portion of the neighboring vertebral body. The end stages progress to bony ankylosis laterally and anteriorly over a variable period of time from several weeks to several months. A significant number of cases do not demonstrate radiographic evidence of complete bony fusion.

Management

Maximal immobilization of the lumbar spine is essential to proper treatment of lumbar intervertebral disc space infection. Although absolute bed rest can be considered, persistence of pain may be an indication of inadequate immobilization, which may be augmented by maintaining the patient for 6 weeks in a plaster body spica extending from the midthorax to below the knees. Large doses of an appropriate broad spectrum antibiotic are given for 8 to 10 weeks.

When the spica is removed after 6 weeks, if the interspace infection is arrested, the patient should be reasonably comfortable at bed rest. Low back and mobilization exercises are initiated in bed, but the spine is supported by a low back support during weight bearing for approximately 3 or 4 months.

REFRACTORY INFECTIONS

Despite appropriate treatment, some interspace infections do not respond kindly, and an indolent slowly extending infection will overrun the intervertebral disc space and produce extensive destruction of the vertebral bodies. Such infections are most commonly seen about the hip following hip surgery when the entire head and neck of the femur may progressively erode and eventually disappear. The persistence of pain usually serves as the best clinical guide to the continued activity of the infectious process, since the radiographic findings are invariably "after the fact" and document what has happened 3 to 6 weeks previously.

Occasionally the infectious process will spread anteriorly, producing retroperitoneal abscesses.

In treating these refractory infections, the diseased spine is maintained in immobilization. Antibiotic therapy is continued or reinstituted until the destructive phase of the bone response is complete and new bone proliferation can be radiographically visualized.

If a collection of retroperitoneal pus is present, it is evacuated through a retroperitoneal abdominal approach. This exposure can be utilized for a direct surgical attack upon the involved interspace with evacuation of all purulent material, debris and granulation tissue. Continued instillation of topical antibiotics directly into the disc space can be accomplished by means of a polyethylene tube inserted through the abdominal incision into the involved disc space and secured to the surrounding soft tissues.

MENINGITIS

An uncommon but potentially catastrophic complication, resulting from postlumbar disc surgery infection, is meningitis. The rarity of this problem in the presence of wound infections bears witness to the natural barrier functioning of the dura. The integrity of the dura is probably violated during lumbar disc surgery more often than is realized. When the dura is inadvertently cut with the tip of a #11 blade during yellow ligament dissection or is torn by the careless use of a rongeur, the resultant gush of cerebrospinal fluid makes this mishap apparent to the surgeon. Minor tears of the dura, such as that caused by the edge of the root retractor cutting into the enveloping dural root sleeve, may be unrecognized by the surgeon. However, such small tears may open a potential avenue for spread of infection into the subarachnoid circulation.

The signs of meningeal irritation—headache, nuchal rigidity, photophobia, in association with temperature elevation—should alert the physician to this diagnostic possibility.

A lumbar puncture for spinal fluid examination will reveal an elevated white cell count and decreased sugar content in the cerebrospinal fluid. Culture and sensitivity studies on the spinal fluid will establish the organism.

Major medical therapeutic and supportive measures are in order to avert disaster.

INFECTIONS WITHOUT ANTECEDENT OPERATIONS ON THE SPINE

Infections of the lumbar spine without antecedent spinal surgery may be divided into 2 broad groups: nontuberculous and tuberculous. Root involvement in both groups is usually not a major feature, and in many cases the symptoms produced by this condition are confined to the low back. The nontuberculous infections manifest a number of specific characteristics in children that require a somewhat different diagnostic and therapeutic approach than those seen in adults. Intervertebral disc infection usually runs a more benign course in children, and the lower thoracic and lumbar spines are the common sites of infection; whereas in adults, the disease involves all levels of the spine. The marked vertebral body disruption and wedging of vertebrae seen in the adult form of the disease is not evident in children. Although the disease is more acute initially in children, it tends to be self-limiting, in adults, the infection follows a more insidious course and has a more destructive nature.

NONTUBERCULOUS INFECTIONS IN CHILDREN

In all probability, many children who have had nontuberculous interspace infections were never diagnosed as suffering from this disease. The early manifestations of this condition are back pain and paraspinal lumbar muscle spasm with normal x-ray findings. After 3 or 4 weeks, when evidence of interspace narrowing can be radiographically documented, the symptoms are greatly diminished; and the physician may be content to "let well enough alone" and not obtain follow-up x-ray films. The following case report demonstrates this typical course of events.

The patient (J. D.), a 4-year-old white male, was hospitalized by Dr. James Thomas on December 2, 1970, with a history of a fall producing direct trauma to the back in November of 1970. No immediate significant low back dysfunction resulted from this fall; but 2 weeks later, when stooping down to pick up a box of matches, he was unable to straighten up into an erect position. From that time until admission, he remained in excruciating pain aggravated by motion of the back or legs. A complete evaluation including an orthopaedic, neurosurgical, urologic and pediatric work-up revealed no specific etiology for his complaints. The only significant positive laboratory finding was a persistently elevated sedimentation rate from 90 to 100 mm. per hour initially and then dropping to 54 mm. per hour just prior to discharge. He had no temperature elevation.

During hospitalization on bed rest, his sedimentation rate declined in association with improvement in his pain. He tolerated more activity; however, he continued to stand with marked flattening of his normal lumbar lordosis and paravertebral muscle spasm.

The patient was discharged on December 31, 1970, on no medication with a diagnosis of "spondylitis of unknown etiology." At the time of discharge, he was able to ambulate stiffly and manifested considerable lumbar paraspinal muscle spasm causing him to stand in a position of slight lumbar flexion. He was maintained at bed rest at home with bathroom privileges. On a follow-up visit, repeat x-rays revealed narrowing of the L2-3 intervertebral disc space. A repeat sedimentation rate was in the 25-30 mm. per hour range. With this radiological finding he was treated empirically with antibiotic therapy and was placed in a plaster body spica for 6 weeks. The antibiotics were continued for

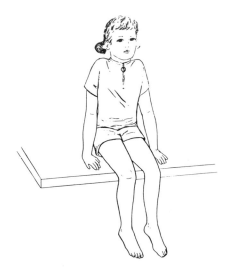

Fig. 13-1. Characteristic sitting position of children with intervertebral disc space infection; placing hands on either side of bed in an attempt to reduce weight bearing of the spine.

6 weeks, after which the spica was removed, and the patient has had an excellent clinical course.

Clinical Picture

A history of abrupt onset of malaise, fever and low back pain in a child should alert the physician to the diagnostic possibility of intervertebral disc infection. A few of these infections arise from known foci, such as superficial wound infections or following an appendectomy; but in most instances the disease develops spontaneously without any recognizable antecedent infection elsewhere. Staphylococcus aureus is the organism usually responsible. In children under 5 years of age, the first symptom may be refusal to walk followed by back pain, stiffness, irritability and fever, most often of less than 3 weeks' duration. Anorexia and weight loss often accompany these symptoms.

On examination the child shows rigid back with extremely restricted mobility. If the examiner attempts to sit the child, he places his hands on either side of the bed behind his back in an attempt to stabilize the spine because of increased pain on weight bearing. Local tenderness of severe degree over the affected part of the spine may be noted. If the child can walk at all, ambulation is stiff, guarded and performed in a gingerly fashion, since any motion or jarring causes an extreme exacerbation of pain. The child will often limp, favoring one or the other hip.[5,2,4]

When the lesion is within the lumbar spine, hamstring tightness is common and a positive iliopsoas sign is present, which may cause the examiner to consider hip disease. The iliopsoas sign is the production of pain when the hip joint is flexed beyond 30 degrees causing the insertion of the iliopsoas into the lesser trochanter to move forward to the extent that its action becomes that of flexion. The Patrick's test involving external rotation of the hip is usually negative.

A low-grade temperature elevation is usually present early in the course of the disease. Laboratory studies usually reveal an elevated white cell count, and an elevated sedementation rate is almost invariably present and may be the only laboratory abnormality.

Mode of Infection in Children

The exact mode of infection of the intervertebral disc in children is not completely clear, but it is thought that the infecting organism is carried through the intervertebral disc space by the blood stream or lymphatics. This can probably best be explained on a developmental basis. The intervertebral disc of the embryo and the young child receives its blood supply from the surfaces of the adjacent vertebral bodies. Blood vessels pass through the disc proper to permit perfusion of nutrients. These vessels gradually disappear with maturation of the vertebral body and the intervertebral disc, and the blood supply to the disc is completely obliterated by the end of the second decade. The vertebral plate of a preadolescent child, which is essentially a growth plate, demonstrates hyaline cartilage with vascular capillary buds penetrating through the cartilage. Organisms lodging in these capillaries may easily involve the disc space.[10]

The vertebral plate of a 16-year-old demonstrates a transverse bony trabecular structure, with blood vessels approaching but not penetrating the vertebral disc cartilage. This closely resembles the adult anatomy with a bony plate and closure or essentially near closure of the growth plate. Intervertebral disc infection in the older child, therefore, closely resembles the process in the adult and may result in destruction along the margins of the vertebral body.

Review section on Embryology for details of intervertebral disc vascularization, pages 2–7.

X-Ray Findings

The roentgenographic findings are meager in the early stages of the disease. At least 2 or 4 weeks elapse after the onset of clinical symptoms before the disc space narrowing appears. There may be, however, a widening of the paravertebral shadows at the site of the involvement and occasional areas of marginal bony destruction in the older child. It is imperative, therefore, that any child with this symptom complex be closely followed at 1- or 2-week intervals for clinical examination and repeated x-rays until the intervertebral disc narrowing at the site of maximum tenderness confirms the diagnosis. Tomograms are helpful in carefully defining the suspected interspace.

The symptomatic course of the disease varies from 2 to 6 weeks after treatment is initiated. However, the roentgenographic changes continue for a considerable period of time. In younger children, the initial reduction of the disc space may be followed in 6 to 12 weeks by a restoration of the original height of the intervertebral disc. In others, it may remain narrow indefinitely. Occasionally, in the older child, a gradual diminution of the disc space with eventual spontaneous fusion is the end result.

Management

Tuberculosis is not, currently, a very common disease while pyogenic infections have not diminished and are much more likely to occur in children than in adults. If there is any doubt regarding the nature of the disease, tuberculin skin tests are most helpful, since they are usually negative in children,

who ordinarily have minimal exposure to tuberculosis.

In addition to tuberculosis, the differential diagnosis must include spinal cord tumors, brucellosis, and salmonella infections. Aspirations and biopsy of the involved interspace with a Turkel needle or surgical exposure for culture and biopsy purposes are frequently indicated in adults, but such aggressive methods to document the organism are not usually necessary in children.

Staphylococcus aureus is the organism usually responsible, and treatment with appropriate antibiotics and bed rest usually leads to a satisfactory outcome. The antibiotics are continued empirically for 6 weeks, and the child is immobilized in a body spica extending from the midthorax to below the knees for 6 to 8 weeks. If the elevated sedimentation rate falls to a normal range and pain subsides, the spica can be removed within 6 to 8 weeks and replaced with a low back support which can be worn during ambulation for an additional 4 months.

NONTUBERCULOUS INFECTIONS IN ADULTS

Clinical Picture

Pyogenic spondylitis in adults may occur spontaneously without any recognizable antecedent infection elsewhere or may follow skin infections, extension from an adjacent infection, or urinary tract infection, either through catheterization or genitourinary surgical procedures. When the urinary tract is the primary focus, the infection probably spreads to the vertebral bodies through the paravertebral veins described by Batson. A significant number of adults who develop this condition have preexisting diabetes mellitus.[8]

In adults it is believed that the infectious organism spreads from a focus within that portion of the vertebral body adjacent to the cartilaginous end-plate. The exact etiology of the infection remains in some question. The literature on this condition reveals that almost one-half of the cases subjected to aspiration or biopsy of a radiologically visualized lesion have sterile or negative cultures. As a result, some investigators are of the opinion that the disc space collapse and subchondral bone opacification are due to an avascular process similar to the avascular necrosis seen in the small bones of the hands and feet and the head of the femur. Since the widespread use of antibiotics, an indolent, slowly developing bone infection is encountered characterized by extensive destruction of bone. This is most commonly seen following hip joint surgery in which the entire head and neck of the femur progressively erodes and disappears over a period of weeks or months. This condition is invariably associated with an elevated white cell count and erythrocyte sedimentation rate. Although positive cultures are not always obtained from the abscess sites, in the final analysis staphylococcus aureus is almost always found to be the causative organism. When these infections occur in the spine, their relative inaccessibility makes accurate establishment of the affecting organism even more difficult than in other areas.

The patient complains of severe pain in the lumbar region which is aggravated by almost any movement or exertion but is not relieved by rest. The onset is usually abrupt but occasionally may be insidious. The exact etiology of the pain is uncertain, since ordinarily "dead bone or cartilage" is not painful.

Examination reveals local tenderness over the affected vertebrae, marked muscle spasm and limitation of all spinal movements. An elevated white cell count and sedimentation rate, in association with a low-grade fever, are usually present.[3]

X-ray Findings

Early in septic spondylitis, roentgenograms are likely to be essentially normal. The bone scan, while not specific as to the nature of the condition, may be useful in localizing the disease process before x-ray changes are evident.

X-ray changes do not develop until 3 or 4 weeks after the onset of pain. After that period of time, x-rays reveal rarefaction of the anterior subchondral area with irregular destruction and erosion of the subchondral bone plate, rapid loss of the disc space and destruction of the adjacent portion of the neighboring vertebral body. The process may advance to bony ankylosis laterally and anteriorly over the course of a few weeks or months.

Some cases do not go on to fusion but undergo progressive destruction of vertebrae, with possible extension of the infection anteriorly into the retroperitoneal space or pass through the natural barrier of the dura into the subarachnoid pathway developing meningitis.

Management

Because of the potentially progressive nature of this disease in the adult, attempt at documentation of the infecting organism is advocated by many.

Aspiration and biopsy of the involved interspace with a Turkel needle may be necessary to establish a bacteriologic diagnosis and to exclude neoplasm or granulomatous disease, such as brucellosis and tuberculosis. The main difficulty with needle biopsy of the intervertebral disc is not obtaining sufficient material with this method for either culture or pathologic diagnosis. Complications such as bleeding or irreversible damage to neurological structures are not particularly common.[1]

When efforts to obtain such materials are unsuccessful or, as in the thoracic region, unsafe, it might be necessary to consider open surgery. If tissue diagnosis and culture is needed in the thoracic region, a costotransversectomy is usually done.

Because of the significant number of patients in whom such diagnostic efforts result in negative or sterile cultures, some authorities defer such attempts and will treat with bed rest, antibiotics and a body spica. They will rely on the clinical course as manifested by relief of pain, improvement in leukocytosis, sedimentation rate and temperature, plus serial x-rays of the spine to determine success or failure of therapy. Some are not convinced of the effectiveness of antibiotics in the absence of temperature or white cell count elevations.

My personal preference in adults is to utilize an attempt at documentation of organisms by needle biopsy and to use antibiotics in addition to immobilization with a body spica.[9,6]

Occasionally myelography is necessary from a diagnostic point of view.

Disc Space Abscess

Very rarely a disc space abscess is encountered which will simulate a disc herniation. My personal experience is limited to one case of this nature. The patient (T.D.), a 58-year-old man, was admitted to the hospital on March 8, 1957, with low back pain and radiation into the left lower extremity. Examination revealed a diminished but present left Achilles reflex and an inconstant zone of hypersthesia extending into the lateral aspect of the foot. The temperature was normal, blood count and laboratory studies unremarkable. The back pain was excruciating and aggravated by any movement; the sciatica was less painful. Pelvic traction was instituted but discontinued because of increased discomfort. A myelogram revealed a filling defect at the L5-S1 interspace on the left which was thought to be compatible with a disc herniation. Because of the severity of his pain, surgery was performed March 12, 1957, the day following myelography. An interlaminar exploration of the L5-S1 interspace on the left was performed; and upon retracting the nerve root, 5 cc. of creamy white purulent material escaped from the interspace which, upon being cultured, grew staphylococcus aureus coagulase-positive organisms. Inspection of the area revealed no free fragments of disc material; and after aspiration of the pus, no attempt was made to enter the intervertebral space. The wound was irrigated with bacitracin solution and closed with stainless steel wire technique. Three drains were allowed to exit through the skin incision. The patient's postoperative course was remarkably benign and unevent-

ful. He was maintained on antibiotics for 6 weeks. The patient was followed for 6 months after surgery and had a good clinical course and returned to work in 3 months. Preoperative x-rays of the lumbar spine had revealed a somewhat narrowed L5-S1 interspace but no evidence of bone destruction was noted. Postoperative x-rays of the lumbar spine were not obtained; the patient left the geographical area and has not since been seen.

TUBERCULOSIS OF THE LUMBAR SPINE

Tuberculous disc space infections are usually secondary to tuberculous infection of the adjacent vertebral body. The negative tuberculin skin test will usually, but not always, preclude the diagnosis of tuberculosis spondylitis. In occasional cases, the disc space will be the primary site of the infection. If this is the case, vascularity must be present in the disc, and thus it will occur in the younger age group.

Signs and Symptoms

A tuberculous infection of the lumbar spine is more insidious in its onset and course than a pyogenic infection. The patient complains of dull, aching pain in the low back that is aggravated by exertion but not relieved by rest. On examination there is localized tenderness over the affected vertebra, marked rigidity of the lumbar muscles and an almost complete loss of all lumbar movements. There are usually some general signs of infection even in the early stages, the most reliable being a slight evening rise of temperature and a raised sedimentation rate.

X-ray Findings

Roetgenographically, narrowing of the disc space will occur before bony destruction when the disc is primarily involved. The characteristic osseous changes of osteolysis and sclerosis will be present before disc thinning if the infection is primarily in the bone. The presence of a paraspinal mass is

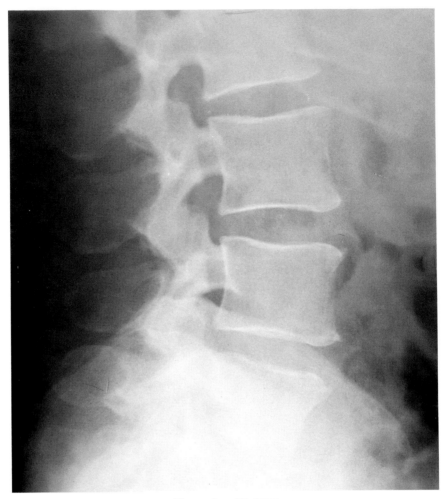

November 17, 1954

Fig. 13-2. The insidious course of tuberculosis of the spine is demonstrated by these films. This 56-year-old man with pulmonary tuberculosis first developed a dull aching low back pain in October 1954 and spine films obtained November 17, 1954 were nonrevealing. Early vertebral body destruction of the L5 vertebra was visualized four months later. The film taken December 14, 1956 reveals extensive destruction of L5 with significant destructive changes involving L4. The interspace is spared, indicating that the infection is primarily in the bone.

strongly suggestive to tuberculosis. Usually the loss of disc space occurs much later in tuberculosis than in pyogenic infections.

Management

Management of tuberculosis of the spine, as any other form of tuberculosis, requires the general treatment of the patient.

The treatment directed toward the spine initially consists of immobilization with a body spica for a period of at least 3 months and the use of antitubercular drugs for 4 to 6 months.

Operative procedures which are rarely necessary, involve excision of diseased tissue and placement of drains for instillation of specific chemotherapeutic agents directly into the focus. The approach for the exposure

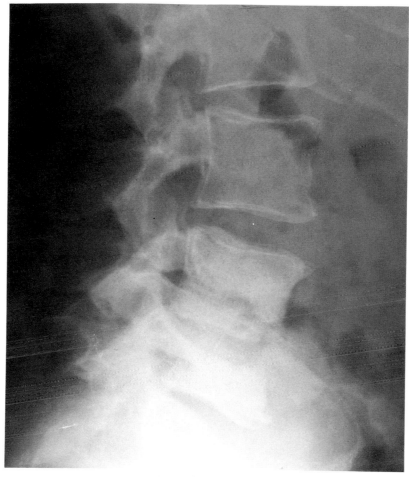

December 14, 1956

Fig. 13-2. (*Cont'd*)

of the spinal focus may be posterolateral with partial removal of the transverse process, or abdominal, either lateroretroperitoneally or transperitoneally.

REFERENCES

1. Craig, F. S.: Vertebral-body biopsy. J. Bone Joint Surg., *38A:93*, 1956.
2. Keiser, R. P., and Grimes, H. A.: Intervertebral disk space infections in children. Clin. Orthop., *30:163*, 1963.
3. Mella, B.: Inflammatory spondylitis. J. Neurosurg., *22:393*, 1965.
4. Smith, R. F., and Taylor T. K. F.: Inflammatory lesions of intervertebral discs in children. J. Bone Joint Surg., *49A:1508*, 1967.
5. Spiegal, P. G., Kengla, K. W., Isaacson, A. S., and Wilson, J. C.: Intervertebral disc-space inflammation in children. J. Bone Joint Surg., *54A:284*, 1972.
6. Stern, E. W., and Balch, R. E.: Surgical aspects of nonspecific inflammatory and suppurative disease of the vertebral column. Am. J. Surg., *112:314*, 1966.
7. Stern, W. E., and Crandell, P. H.: Inflammatory intervertebral, disc disease as a complication of the operative treatment of lumbar herniations. J. Neurosurg., *16:261*, 1959.
8. Sullivan, C. R.: Diagnosis and treatment of pyogenic infections of intervertebral disk. Surg. Clin. N. Am., *41:1077*, 1961.
9. Sullivan, C. R., and Symmonds, R. E.: Disk infections and abdominal pain. JAMA, *188:655*, 1964.

14
Tumors of
the Spine

BENIGN TUMORS

Hemangiomas

Pathology
X-ray Findings

Signs and Symptoms
Treatment

Osteomas

MALIGNANT TUMORS

Sarcomas

Multiple Myeloma

METASTATIC TUMORS

Symptoms
Physical Findings

X-ray Diagnosis
Management

INTRADURAL TUMORS

Neurilemmomas (Schwannoma Neuro-fibroma)

Meningiomas

SURGERY OF SPINAL CORD TUMORS

Tumors of the spine present the physician with a considerable challenge both in evaluation and in management. Sometimes a problem of this nature is, at first glance, unpromising, and yet, with a planned approach, the results of proper management may be quite gratifying. Both primary and metastatic tumors involve the bony spine, with the ligaments and discs rarely affected. Intraspinal tumors originating from neural or meningeal cells may produce pressure erosion of the adjacent bony spine.

BENIGN TUMORS

HEMANGIOMAS

Hemangiomas are the most commonly occurring tumors of the vertebrae, found in approximately 10 percent of all spines when subjected to careful anatomical serial examination. They occur with greatest frequency between the twelfth thoracic and fourth lumbar vertebrae and with least frequency at the upper cervical spine and the lowermost part of the sacrum. Women are more often affected than men by two-thirds. The incidence of hemangiomas increases with age, indicating that if these lesions are all truly congenital, they become progressively larger and more apparent with the passage of years. Most hemangiomas are revealed as incidental autopsy findings without clinically apparent symptoms.[14]

Pathology

Vertebral hemangiomas cause diminution in the number of bony trabeculae, with coarsening of the remaining trabeculae and transformation of some trabeculae into vertically extending strands which lend support to the diseased vertebral body. In addition to these characteristic vertical reticular stripes, one occasionally sees a coarse honeycombed bony configuration. Large hemangiomas involving an entire vertebral body cause a "ballooning" of the body with the normally concave or indented sides of the vertebrae assuming a straight or even convex configuration. Large hemangiomas occupying the entire vertebral body occasionally extend into the laminae and spinous processes; and with involvement of a thoracic vertebra, hemangiomas occasionally extend into an adjoining rib, causing these structures to become thickened and honeycombed.[4,3,10]

X-ray Findings

The characteristic radiographic signs are the coarse vertical supportive strands, honeycombing and the ballooned configuration of the vertebral body.[13]

Signs and Symptoms

Most vertebral hemangiomas are noted as incidental findings, with clinical symptoms not commonly associated with the condition. The occasional symptoms that develop usually arise from nerve root pressure due to

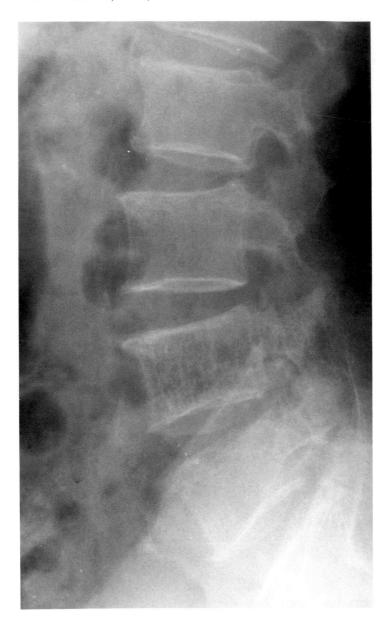

Fig. 14-1. Hemangioma of the fourth vertebral body. This lesion was noted as an incidental (symptom free) finding in a 71-year-old man who was involved in a vehicular accident.

thickening of the vertebral body and arches or perforation of hemangiomatous tissue into the neural canal.[1,6]

Despite extensive vertebral involvement, compression fractures or wedging are rather uncommon because of the support provided by the vertical reinforcing lamellae. Interestingly enough, even in the face of trauma sufficient to fracture neighboring vertebral bodies, the diseased vertebra often remains intact.

Treatment

No treatment is required if the lesion is symptom free. When the condition is associated with nerve root pressure, radiation therapy may be effective.

OSTEOMAS

Osteomas may occur within any portion of the vertebra but are more apt to produce clinical symptoms when located within the

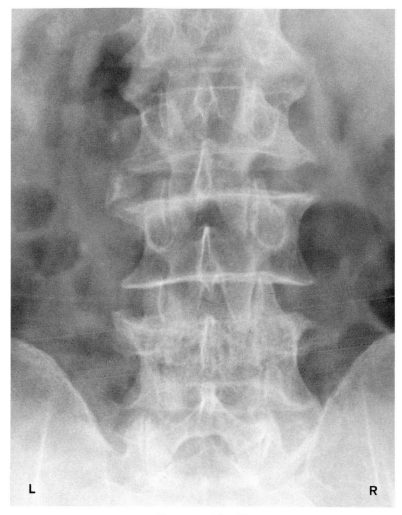

Fig. 14-1. (*Cont'd*)

laminae or spinous processes. These exostosis-like lesions in the laminae will produce direct impingement upon the cauda equina or individual roots and in the spinous processes may produce spinal malalignment and deformity.

Osteoid osteomas, also called benign oste- oblastomas, destroy the bony parenchyma. Although they do not metastisize, they do extend locally and may be associated with compression of the nervous structures within the neural canal.[9,12] Treatment is directed at a radical excision of the lesion and spinal fusion, followed by radiation therapy.

MALIGNANT TUMORS

SARCOMAS

Sarcomas of the spine are extremely rare, with less than 1 percent of all bone sarcomas originating in the spine. These lesions cause extensive bony destruction within the verte- brae, which is associated with vertebral body collapse. Occasionally, sarcomas produce osteosclerosis producing the so-called "ivory vertebra," a radiographic term used to imply a pathologic bony condensing process of the vertebra. As a result of the proliferation of tumor tissue and malformation and malalignment of the spine, compression of the neural elements is almost invariably associated with this lesion. An increased paravertebral shadow is seen on x-ray which differs from the rather elongated spindle shape of the paravertebral shadow seen in tuberculosis, with a more ovoid mass surrounding only the vertebra or vertebrae which are involved with tumor.

Roentgenologic evaluation of this lesion is generally nonspecific, so that a needle biopsy or possibly a surgical biopsy is necessary to obtain a satisfactory diagnosis. Because of the rapidly growing nature of this neoplasm, surgery is best confined to biopsy, with minimal benefits to be achieved by palliative decompression. The treatment of choice both to alleviate pain and to arrest the rapid progression of the disease is x-ray therapy.

MULTIPLE MYELOMA

A large percentage of patients with multiple myeloma present with low back pain, resulting from involvement of this disease with the lower lumbar vertebrae. As the vertebral bodies are penetrated and destroyed by the myeloma, all possible forms of vertebral body collapse with associated spinal deformities can be seen—wedging, marked flattening, compression of the vertebral bodies, sometimes so flat that they are less than the height of the adjacent intervertebral discs. Osteosclerosis and periosteal proliferation, or reactive bony proliferation, surrounding the site of metastasis are not seen in multiple myeloma; thus, differentiating it from other osseous metastatic lesions where they are common. This condition occurs most commonly between the ages of 35 and 65 and is rarely found in children.

The characteristic symptoms of multiple myeloma begin with somewhat vague and poorly localized low back pain, which is often worse when lying in bed at night. This diagnosis is not often made in its early stages because the x-rays may be unrevealing or, if they are abnormal, resemble diffuse osteoporosis. With the passage of time, sufficient destruction of the vertebra occurs to produce vertebral collapse, often associated with nerve root compression symptoms. At this stage of the disease, the character of the pain undergoes a change, both with regard to radiation from radicular compression and to its becoming more related to activity, so that any movement, particularly jarring or percussion over the lumbar region, produces an acute aggravation of the pain. If the patient is followed by serial x-rays of the spine, the fairly rapid development of multiple lytic lesions can be identified, in addition to diffuse osteoporosis.[8]

In differentiating this condition from metastatic carcinoma, the radiologists use, as a general rule of thumb, the criterion that when a pedicle is destroyed, in association with a collapsed vertebral body, the cause is metastatic carcinoma rather than multiple myeloma. The latter usually causes vertebral body collapse without destroying the cortex of the pedicle; therefore, the pedicles appear intact on the x-ray.

The diagnosis can be aided through the use of laboratory studies which demonstrate a markedly elevated sedimentation rate, a normocytic anemia and a strikingly elevated gamma globulin concentration, with a characteristic configuration on the paper electrophoretic pattern. The urine may reveal Bence Jones protein. Bone marrow aspiration yields characteristic myeloma cells and is necessary to confirm the diagnosis. Occasionally, some cases of multiple myeloma present themselves as localized lesions, and the diagnosis may require a needle biopsy or even an open biopsy of the involved area.[7]

Operative intervention is generally contraindicated; but treatment with cytostatic drugs and x-ray therapy may produce long-lasting improvement.

METASTATIC TUMORS

Metastatic disease of the spine is one of the most common abnormalities involving the bony elements of the spine. Almost 70 percent of all spinal tumors are metastatic, with the remaining 30 percent divided between primary spinal tumors and direct tumor invasion from adjacent structures or from neoplasm arising from dural tissues within the spinal canal. The magnitude of metastatic carcinoma to the bone becomes evident when one reviews the literature and finds that metastatic disease to the skeleton ranges from about 20 percent in one series to about 70 percent in autopsy cases reviewed by Jaffe.[11] The vertebrae are the most common site for metastatic disease, followed by the pelvis, proximal long bones and ribs. It is quite rare to find metastatic disease distal to the elbow or knee joints. Certain cancers have distinct predilections for bone, with breast and prostate being the most frequent, followed by lung, kidney and thyroid. In the Institute for Spinal Column Research in Frankfurt, Germany, established by Dr. Georg Schmorl, it is the practice to routinely remove the entire spinal column in every autopsy. Each spinal specimen is then subjected to a planned and most meticulous examination. Using this method, 1,000 patients with cancer were investigated (500 women and 500 men) in order to establish the incidence of spinal involvement. This method revealed that 17.6 percent of patients with cancer had metastasis to the spine, representing a 19.6 percent incidence in men, and a 15.6 percent in women. Most other series are considerably lower, but no other clinic follows the painstaking method utilized by the Schmorl Institute.

At one time considerable confusion and speculation existed regarding the route by which carcinomas metastasized to the vertebrae. The hematogenous route was thought to be the principal pathway for metastatic disease, but no adequate explanation was offered at the time for the frequent absence of lung lesions in the face of widespread bony metastasis. It was considered by some that lymphatics were the root of most metastatic diseases, but advocates of this mechanism had difficulty explaining the frequency of bony metastasis, in view of the fact that bone is largely alymphatic. Batson, an anatomist, was responsible for rediscovering the vertebral vein complex. Through his specialized latex injection studies, he demonstrated that this venous system is quite complex, involving extensive anastomoses with the portal system, the upper thorax by way of the intercostals and the superior vena caval system.[5] This is known to be a valvular system; and with any increase in intra-abdominal pressure, such as through coughing or straining, the flow of blood can be reversed through this system carrying tumor emboli with it. When tumor cells are experimentally injected into the femoral veins of rabbits, there is a marked increase in the number of vertebral bodies involved by tumor when the intra-abdominal pressure has been increased. We still are unable to fully explain why certain tumors, such as bladder carcinomas or carcinomas of the cervix, do not frequently metastasize to the spine as do prostatic tumors.

Symptoms

A patient with a history of previous surgery for malignant disease who has the insidious onset of low back pain must be suspected of having possible metastatic disease to the spine. A prolonged lapse of time from the primary surgical procedure would not allay one's suspicions concerning metastatic disease, since it is well known that carcinomas of the breast frequently metastasize quite late following a radical mastectomy. It is not rare to see patients 5, 7, 10, and even more years following breast surgery who develop low back pain, which turns out to be a metastatic tumor from the original breast lesion.

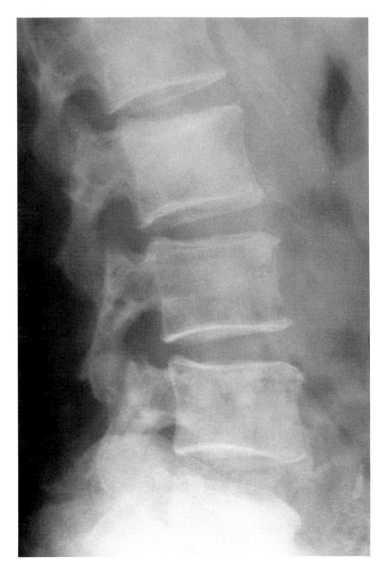

Fig. 14-2. Osteoblastic and osteoclastic metastasis simultaneously involving the vertebral bodies. Patient is a 59-year-old man with carcinoma of the prostate.

The pain produced by metastatic and primary tumors is characteristically of insidious onset, more frequently worse at night, and gradually increasing in severity with the passage of time. However, sudden onset of pain, or an acute exacerbation of pain in the back following little or no trauma, may represent a pathologic fracture and occasionally may be the presenting complaint with metastatic disease to the spine.

Physical Findings

Physical examination is of considerable importance, although initially the examination may not be rewarding aside from noting some local tenderness over the area of pain and some paraspinal muscle spasm with limited spinal mobility. Occasionally, with advanced metastatic disease associated with wedging and collapse of a vertebra, one can detect the presence of a gibbous formation, resulting from the malalignment of the spine. When a gibbous formation can be palpated and visualized, there is usually considerable point tenderness over the site. When malignant disease is suspected, a most comprehensive inspection and examination of the entire body is important to determine either the primary site or an accessible area of biopsy. This examination should, of course, include examination of the breasts, and if any suspicious areas of resistance or possible nodules are present, special techniques such as mammography may be helpful. The vaginal and rectal examination is important, and the examiner must always keep in his mind that many unnecessary biopsies of the spine have been done because the physician failed to slip on a rectal glove and missed a very obvious hard prostatic nodule or some other rectal mass.

X-ray Diagnosis

Tumor metastasis to the spine may occur in two different forms: osteoclastic, or bone-destructive metastases, and osteoblastic, or bone-forming metastases. Both of these forms may occur simultaneously and, in fact, sometimes the same vertebral body will display both forms of metastasis in apposition. The osteoblastic metastases are characteristically seen when the primary tumor is prostate or breast. They are seen on x-ray as areas of increased density and are often described by the radiologist as "ivory-like" tumor foci. The osteoclastic tumor metastases are more frequently associated with vertebral body collapse. Metastatic lesions may involve any portion of the vertebrae and sometimes extend beyond the boundaries of the vertebrae and proliferate externally.

The x-ray appearance of tumor metastasis to the spine is quite variable, due to the frequent simultaneous existence of osteoclastic and osteoblastic metastases, which may present difficulties in differential diagnosis. It must be recognized that at least 35 percent of the vertebrae must be involved by neoplasm before these changes are readily appreciated by x-ray. Often, the axis of the defect in relationship to the axis of the x-ray beam is a factor in how readily the lesion can be seen radiographically. If there is an equivocal lesion, tomography will be most helpful in more specifically determining the nature and true extent of a metastatic lesion. Because of these difficulties in making a

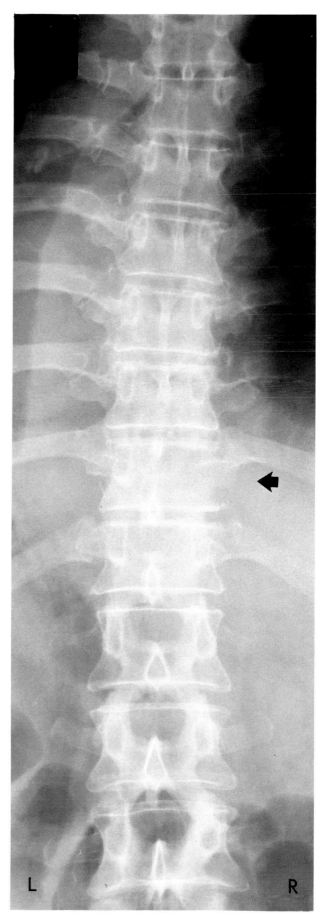

Fig. 14-3. Destruction of Pedicle T11 on right from metastatic bronchogenic carcinoma.

radiographic diagnosis and, since symptoms often precede roentgenographic changes, we must not stop in our diagnostic efforts with a presumably normal spine x-ray, if there is a suspicious history indicative of possible metastatic disease. When neoplasm is suspected, spine films must be carefully examined—each pedicle, each transverse process, each spinous process, the laminae, to eliminate lesions arising in these sites. There must also be a careful inspection of the vertebral bodies in which tumor pathology is more readily recognized when a metastatic lytic lesion produces some vertebral wedging or collapse.[2]

Management

Histological verification of these lesions is a necessity for proper management. If no other more accessible lesions are apparent, a biopsy of the affected vertebral body should be carried out. In some cases, a closed biopsy of the spine can be performed using several types of needles specifically designed for this purpose, such as the Craig needle with a 2 millimeter diameter bore. The advantage of this technique, which can usually be carried out under local anesthesia with biplane x-ray control, is its relative simplicity, which does not interfere with the patient's activities or with any treatment being carried out simultaneously. The greatest disadvantage of all needle biopsies is the relatively small fragment of tissue obtained, resulting in an indecisive diagnosis. When

using a needle biopsy technique, the pathologist should have some understanding of the problem, be aware of the inherent difficulties and be prepared to give additional attention to the small fragments of tissue obtained. In addition, there are some potential dangers involving damage to surrounding structures and nerves. Occasionally, the lesion itself may be vascular so that a biopsy may result in considerable bleeding at that site. When needle biopsy is either not feasible or not successful, an open biopsy may be in order which may usually be accompanied with an attempt at operative decompression. When gross neurological deficit is caused by tumor compression from an absolute block, such decompression is often helpful. However, when the aim of decompression is to relieve pain, in many cases relief obtained by decompression of the nerves from the enveloping tumor is often temporary. Then cytostatic drugs and x-ray therapy, which remains the mainstay of treatment in most lesions, should be employed. Even when tumors are considered to be somewhat x-ray resistant, there is often significant alleviation of some pain, and such therapy tends to slow down the rapidity of growth. The fact that breast and prostatic tumors are hormonal dependent should be kept in mind, and occasionally relief is achieved by pituitary ablation or hormonal therapy. In some cases, steroids are effective in relieving pain for limited durations, their action being primarily a reduction of edema resulting from tumor compression.

INTRADURAL TUMORS

NEURILEMMOMAS (SCHWANNOMA NEUROFIBROMA)

Neurilemmomas are usually intradural and arise from the sheaths of the spinal nerve roots, usually as oval or rounded tumors causing intradural compression of the neurological elements at the level of the tumor. These circumscribed, encapsulated growths, into which a portion of the nerve root can

usually be traced, are usually single and may grow to enormous size, particularly in the cauda equina, before they produce symptoms which are easily recognized. By contrast, in von Recklinghausen's disease, there may be multiple tumors involving the cauda equina and conus medullaris, which are associated with cutaneous evidence of neurofibromatosis. It is felt by most authorities that the solitary neurilemmoma or schwannoma is indistinguishable from the multiple neurofibroma of von Recklinghausen's disease. Often neurilemmomas grow along the spinal nerve root through the dura mater and the vertebral foramen into the surrounding tissues, extending either into the abdomen in the lumbar region and into the thoracic cavity if involving the thoracic spine. As the tumor passes through the intervertebral foramen, it becomes constricted, taking an hourglass or dumbbell shape. Microscopically, the spinal cord neurilemmoma shows palisading of nuclei in association with degenerative changes, such as interstitial masses of lipoid deposits, hyaline substances and cellular debris.

These tumors are usually separated from either the cord or nerve roots and can be totally removed, along with any root fibers incorporated within the body of the tumor. In carrying out the surgery, magnification technique using a dissecting microscope, or sometimes high-powered löups, may be helpful. When a dumbbell tumor is found to extend into the abdomen or in the higher spinal regions (the thorax), it should be pursued extradually and removed during the same procedure, if possible. In extremely large tumors, where the extradural extension is so great that total excision through a laminectomy incision might be hazardous, it is helpful to use silver clip markers on the portion of the tumor that is visible through the laminectomy incision. The markers will help the general surgeon when he plans subsequent removal of this lesion as a secondary procedure. I have used this technique on several occasions, and have been surprised,

on taking postoperative x-rays, to realize how far anterior or lateral to the spine my dissection had carried me. Following removal of a neurofibroma, a watertight dural closure is always performed.

MENINGIOMAS

Meningiomas are occasionally seen in the cauda equina, arising in most instances from the inner surface of the dura mater or from the arachnoid membrane. These are usually a bit softer and occasionally more vascular than neurofibromas and are more likely to fit over the surface of the cauda equina and conform to its irregularities. They may vary from a round or oval shape to a large irregular mass, resembling the contour of that portion of the canal in which they are located. Histologically, the spinal meningiomas closely resemble the intracranial meningiomas and are composed of masses of cells which do not form an intercellular substance. Just as is the case in the intracranial meningioma, though this tumor is benign, if it is adherent to the dura, it may be necessary to completely excise the dura around the site of tumor origin to prevent recurrence. It will then be necessary to patch the dural defect in watertight fashion; and a sheet of fascia, which can be obtained from the paraspinal muscles, is usually suitable. After the patch has been sutured in place, the original dural incision should, of course, be closed. As in excision of neurofibromas, magnification is most helpful in completely excising such lesions.

SURGERY OF SPINAL CORD TUMORS

The surgery of intraspinal tumors requires careful attention to certain details of technique. For instance, prior to surgery, one must consider the character and extent of the lesion and plan the location of the incision in relation to the lesion. The time-honored method of establishing the desired vertebral

level in the lumbar region is to start from the sacrum and to count the interspaces from the solid sacral bone. For the upper lumbar level, the twelfth rib may serve as a useful guide; and the spinous process of L1 is broader and larger than the thoracic spine. Further accuracy can be obtained in planning

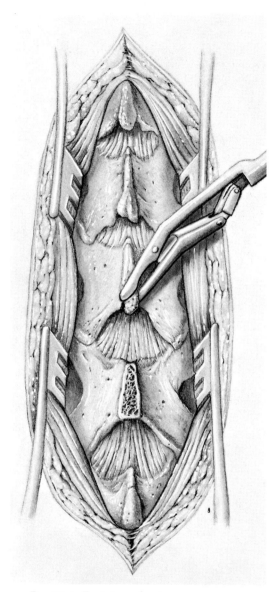

Fig. 14-4. Excision of spinous processes.

is flexed on the operating table. The position of the patient for surgery is usually prone with maximal flexion of the spine at the level of the lesion.

During the performance of the laminectomy, a few factors should be considered. Blood loss is kept at a minimum by performing a strictly midline incision of the fascial attachments. Over the spinous processes and laminae great efforts should be made to peel the fascia cleanly without penetrating muscle, which is often the principal source of bleeding. While carrying out a subperiosteal muscle dissection, care should be used with the periosteal elevators to avoid direct downward pressure. Such care is necessary because with both benign and malignant tumors, erosion and thinning of the laminal arches can occur, allowing a carelessly used instrument to plunge through this abnormal bone and produce damage to the underlying neural structures. Not long ago I carried out surgery on a neurofibroma in which the overlying lamina on the side of the tumor was paper thin.

Following complete exposure of the spinous processes and laminae, the spinous processes are removed with rongeurs; and any bleeding from their base can be controlled with the use of bone wax. Controlling bleeding as it occurs allows a far more orderly procedure and, of course, avoids the excessive loss of blood throughout the procedure. As an aid in identifying the upper and lower edges of each lamina the edges may be curetted clear of ligamentum flavum. As much of the laminal removal is done "en face," to avoid introducing a rongeur blade beneath the lamina, by holding the rongeur vertically so that the bone is actually rongeured away from above downwards. When the surgeon cannot avoid introducing a rongeur blade beneath the lamina, he should use a thin underblade, such as a thin-bladed laminectomy punch with an angled tip. Adherence to this technique will prevent added cauda equina compression that may result in permanent neurological dysfunction. After carrying out the medial portion of the lami-

a laminectomy incision by placing a metal marker on the skin at the exact location of the tumor during myelography. An x-ray which is taken with the marker in place is followed by marking that site with indelible ink or in some cases, subcutaneously injecting a dot of methylene blue. It is most important to take the marking film while the patient is flexed in the prone position, which is the position planned for laminectomy, to avoid shift of the cutaneous mark when he

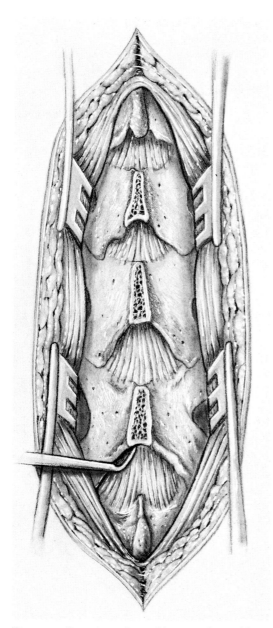

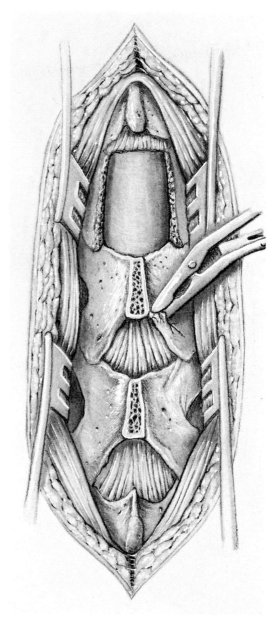

Fig. 14-5. Curetting edges of lamina clear of ligamentum flavum.

Fig. 14-6. Removing lamina "en face" to avoid excessive pressure upon dural contents.

nectomy, it is then helpful to go to either side and carry out a more lateral decompression; and again the angled thin-bladed laminectomy punch is most helpful in performing this procedure without producing dural compression. Following this portion of the procedure, complete hemostasis of all bleeding structures should be achieved. Bleeding from muscles may be controlled with cautery; venous oozing from the rongeured bony edges with bone wax; epidural venous bleeding, in most cases, with a small pledget of Gelfoam.* If epidural bleeding persists,

*Trademark Upjohn.

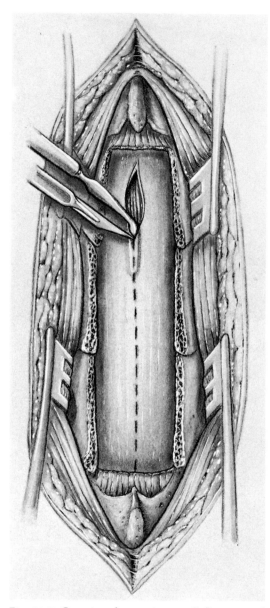

Fig. 14-7. Opening dura using small flat grooved director.

cauterization with the use of a Mallis bipolar cautery may be necessary.

At this point a search for an extradural tumor, disc or bony spur can be carried out. Most extradural spinal tumors are malignant with metastatic tumors being the most frequent. Usually both meningiomas and neurofibromas are intradural; however, an occasional neurofibroma or meningioma may be extradural and frequently referred to as a "dumbbell tumor" with extension through the intervertebral foramen into tissues adjacent to the spine. This type of lesion extends along either side of the dura, and the extradural extension can project through the intervertebral foramen into the peritoneal space or, if it is in the thoracic or cervical region, into the lung and sometimes into the soft tissue of the neck. Lipomas, congenital cysts and osteomas are rarely found as benign extradural tumors.

The dura should almost always be opened in the midline, beginning the incision at the safest point above the area of obstruction, and extending it past the lesion, so that the tumor can be completely exposed. The dura is opened with a No. 11 blade, attempting to keep the arachnoid intact. A small flat grooved director can be introduced between the dura and the arachnoid and may be used to guide the No. 11 blade over the lesion. After opening the dura, if it is found that the tumor had not been completely exposed, the laminectomy should, of course, be extended further until an adequate exposure can be obtained.

Surgery of an extradural malignancy should be done without undue delay. A decompressive laminectomy is carried out as widely and as thoroughly as possible using all means, including rongeurs and curettage, to achieve as extensive a tumor removal as can be done. On completing the laminectomy and tumor removal, particularly when the vertebral bodies are grossly involved, the spinal column may be so weakened that a spinal fusion should be considered at time of operation. A method which has been utilized by Dr. William Scoville, with patients who had advanced malignant involvement of one or more contiguous vertebrae, is to fill the bony defect with a plastic substance, methyl methacrylate. In his technique, he inserts a metal screw partially into the center of each healthy vertebral body, above and below the defect; these screws provide an

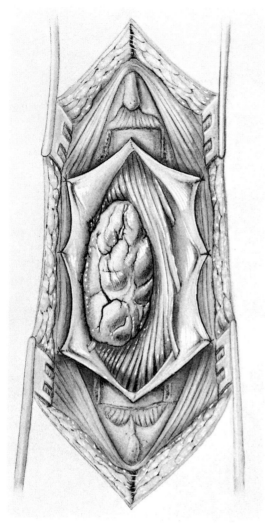

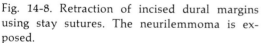

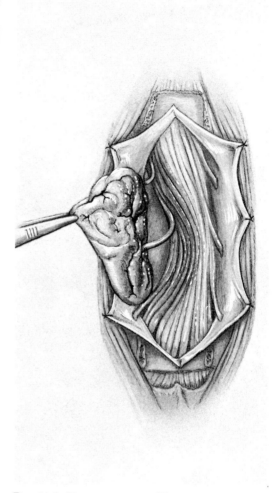

Fig. 14-8. Retraction of incised dural margins using stay sutures. The neurilemmoma is exposed.

Fig. 14-9. Tumor excision. The L4 nerve root is incorporated within the body of the tumor and will be sectioned.

anchor for the methyl methacrylate that is poured in to fill the defect. In using this technique, to prevent the heat of polymerization of this plastic from damaging the cord, he uses a protective layer of Gelfoam over the dura and continues to irrigate the wound during polymerization with cool saline solution. Following surgery, x-ray therapy or chemotherapy may be considered if indicated by the nature of the pathology.

REFERENCES

1. Askenasy, H., Behmoaram, A.: Neurological manifestations in haemangioma of the vertebrae. J. Neurol.; *20*:276, 1957.
2. Austin, G. M.: The Spinal Cord. Charles C Thomas, Springfield, (Ill.), 1961.
3. Baily, P., Bucy, P.: Cavernous hemangioma of the vertebrae JAMA, *92*:27, 1929.
4. Barnard, N.: Primary haemangioma of the spine. Am. Surg., *97*:19, 1933.

5. Batson, O. V.: The vertebral vein system. Am. J. Roentgenol. *78:*195, 1957.

6. Bell, R: Hemangioma of a dorsal vertebra with collapse and compression myelopathy. J. Neurosurg., *12:*570, 1955.

7. Cohen, D. M., Dahlin, D. C., and MacCarty, C. S.: Apparently solitary tumors of the vertebral column. Mayo Clin. Proc., *39:*509 July, 1964.

8. Davison, B.: Myeloma and its neurological complications. Arch. Surg. *35:*913, 1937.

9. Freiberger, R. E.: Osteoid osteoma of the spine. A cause of backache and scoliosis in children and young adults. Radiology, *75:*232, 1960.

10. Ireland, J.: Haemangioma of the vertebrae. Am. J. Roentgenol *28:*372, 1932.

11. Jaffe, H. L.: Tumors and Tumorous Conditions of the Bonesand Joints. Philadelphia, Lea & Febiger, 1958.

12. Lichtenstein, L., and Sawyer, W. R.: Benign osteoblastoma. J. Bone Joint Surg., *46A:755,* 1964.

13. Lindqvist, I.: Vertebral haemangioma with compression of the spinal cord. Acta. radiol. (Stockh.), *35:*400, 1951.

14. Schmorl, G., Junghanns, H., and Besemann, E. F.: The human spine in health and disease. Grune and Stratton, 1971.

15
Uncommon Causes of Low Back Pain and Sciatica

PELVIC DISEASE

LOW BACK PAIN AND PREGNANCY

INTRA-ABDOMINAL VASCULAR DISEASE

SCIATIC NEURITIS

Entrapment Neuropathy   Primary Sciatica
Trauma   Tumors Involving the Sciatic Nerve

ENTRAPMENT NEUROPATHIES

Obturator Neuropathy   Technique of Obturator Nerve Block

ILLIOHYPOGASTRIC AND ILIOINGUINAL NEURITIS (INGUINAL NEURITIS)

Anatomy   Technique of Block
Mechanism of Injury   Management

MERALGIA PARESTHETICA

Pathophysiology   Diagnosis
Signs and Symptoms   Treatment

ADHESIVE ARACHNOIDITIS

ARTHRITIS OF THE HIPS

ILIUM-TRANSVERSE PROCESS PSEUDOARTHROSIS

Treatment

ANKYLOSING SPONDYLITIS

Symptoms	X-ray
Examination	Treatment
Laboratory	Confusion with Lumbar Disc Disease

CHARCOT'S DISEASE OF THE SPINE (VERTEBRAL OSTEOARTHROPATHY)

SACRAL CYSTS

15

Uncommon Causes of Low Back Pain and Sciatica

The diseases included in this section are either rarely encountered or not commonly considered in connection with low back pain and sciatica. However, an awareness of their existence may be helpful in considering the occasional clinical problem that does not lend itself to ready classification.

PELVIC DISEASE

Low back pain of variable severity is manifested during menstrual periods by approximately 10 to 20 percent of females. These pains often described as "bearing down," a sensation of heaviness, a tired feeling, are not particularly severe and are usually adequately managed with mild analgesics, so that the patient is able to carry on with routine activities of daily living. In rare cases, the pain, often referred to by gynecologists as "pelvic backache," is of such severity that the patient may be confined to bed for 1 or 2 days each month. Examination usually reveals nothing, even during the painful intervals.

Pelvic tumors, particularly those within the retroperitoneal space, may cause irritation and compression of the lumbosacral plexus and be productive of low back pain and sciatica. Occasionally, endometriosis may actually invade the lumbar or sciatic plexus or the sciatic nerve itself producing severe hip and sciatic pain. In such cases, reflex, motor and sensory changes may be elicited on physical examination.

LOW BACK PAIN AND PREGNANCY

During the end of pregnancy a moderate degree of low back pain is common in part because of the increased mechanical demands on the low back imposed by the burden of carrying the fetus. During the latter half of pregnancy also there is a generalized softening of the fibrous structures in the lumbosacral spine and pelvis, attributed to hormonal effect, which produce some tissue laxity, allowing increased stretching of the involved ligaments. Several months may elapse before these fibrous structures regain their original tensile strength.

The vast majority of pregnant women who complain of low back pain are easily managed with a program of reduced physical

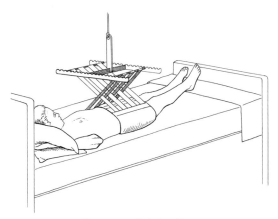

Fig. 15-1. Pelvic sling.

activities, mild analgesics and a supporting corset. In some instances, the low back symptoms are so severe that prolonged periods of bed rest are necessary. Occasionally, joint diastasis is seen on x-rays, with some separation of the symphysis pubis and a slight widening of the sacroiliac joints.[2]

The most severe problems are usually in multiparas who have had a diastasis during a previous pregnancy. The pain is often quite severe in the low back and both hips and may also be present in the lower abdomen and over the symphysis pubis. Sometimes, the pain is not adequately relieved by resting in a non-weight-bearing position and will require the use of a canvas pelvic sling suspended from an overhead bar. The sling is attached to traction weights and is most effective if it crosses in front of the body, reducing the sacroiliac and symphysis pubis separations.

Postpartum improvement in low back dysfunction is generally seen and is attributed to passage of the mechanical burden imposed by the fetus and recovery of the

fibrous structures to normal tensile strength. Infrequently, the sacroiliac and pubic pain persists and, with increased physical activity, may even worsen. The typical sacroiliac waddling gait is associated with increased lumbar lordosis and protrusion of the abdomen resulting from relaxation of the lower abdominal muscles, which are painful at the site of pubic attachment. The "reverse" Patrick's test, using internal rotation rather than external rotation, is painful, since it tends to distract the sacroiliac joint.

Treatment of this condition requires approximately 2 weeks in a pelvic sling, after which a pelvic support is worn for 3 or 4 months.

In addition to softening of the ligaments at the symphysis pubis and sacroiliac joint, similar changes occur in the ligamentous supporting structures of the lower lumbar spine, including the annulus fibrosis of the lower intervertebral discs. Preexisting annular weakness may be aggravated during pregnancy, leading to severe protrusion of the nucleus pulposus, and all of the signs and symptoms of lumbar disc disease will follow. Some low back and sciatic pains, attributed by the obstetrician to pressure of the fetal head, are caused by lumbar disc disease.

This type of problem is best managed prophylactically, when dealing with a patient who has a past history compatible with lumbar disc disease. Restriction of all activities likely to cause undue stress on the low back structures is helpful.

Severe pain is best treated with prolonged bed rest and mild analgesics. The only indication for disc surgery during pregnancy is severe neurologic dysfunction, such as a cauda equina syndrome.

INTRA-ABDOMINAL VASCULAR DISEASE

Thrombosis of the terminal aorta may be the cause of lumbar pain, while occlusion of the common iliac or internal iliac may produce low back and hip pain. Occasionally, this pain is quite severe and may be the

predominant symptom. It is described as a constant, deep, severe, aching pain and is poorly localized. Other symptoms of arterial obstruction, including intermittent claudication with numbness and tingling of the legs and temperature changes in the feet, are seen on examination. The femoral and dorsalis pedis pulses are diminished or absent.[1]

Compression of the lumbosacral plexus by an aneurysm of the common iliac artery is a rare cause of sciatica.

A dissection aneurysm of the aorta may produce as its initial symptom excruciating low back pain which spreads into the buttocks and legs. The pain is usually associated with pallor, sweating and with the patient close to shock. The femoral pulses may be absent, and bruits may be heard along the course of the aorta or its branches. Occasionally, paraplegia may develop suddenly as a result of ischemia to the spinal cord.

All of these vascular lesions are delineated by aortography.

SCIATIC NEURITIS

Entrapment Neuropathy

An entrapment neuropathy of the sciatic nerve is extremely rare. The piriformis syndrome may occur when the nerve is tightened against the greater sciatic notch by a hip flexion posture with a compensatory lordosis. The pressure against this nerve by the rotator group of muscles is increased when, because of inadequate low back stabilization, the pelvic and femoral muscles are in a state of compensatory spasm. If this condition is sufficiently severe, operative neurolysis of the sciatic nerve is necessary, exposing the ring of the sciatic notch and carrying the incision down to the thigh where the nerve passes under the hamstring muscles to visualize the distal portion of the sciatic trunk.

Trauma

Probably the most frequent cause of sciatic trauma is an inadvertently placed intramuscular injection in the buttock, with the needle situated too low and medial. At the time of the injection, the patient may experience a painful radiation down the leg. Depending on the severity of damage to the nerve from the injection, the symptoms can vary from mild discomfort and "tingling" paresthesii along the course of the sciatic nerve to severe motor changes, with a complete foot drop and anesthesia along the lateral aspect of the calf and dorsum of the foot.

Sciatic trauma may occur from a posterior dislocation of the femur. Occasionally, a fall in the sitting position on a hard projecting object will traumatize the nerve where it is quite superficial, just below the edge of the gluteus maximus. This sudden trauma may not only cause direct injury to the nerve but also may impinge the nerve against the sharp edge of the sciatic notch, which may be a significant factor in the prolongation of persisting symptoms. Contusions of the sciatic nerve, in addition to causing pain, may produce motor and sensory dysfunction. Given a history of injury either from blunt trauma or injection, the diagnosis is generally obvious.

Primary Sciatica

This is an extremely rare condition involving pain along the distribution of the sciatic nerve, which will vary in intensity from a dull ache to severe episodic lancinating pain.

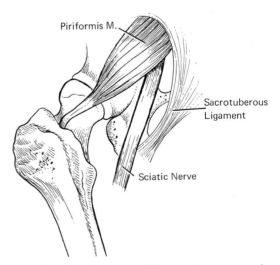

Fig. 15-2. Relationship of the piriformis muscle and the sciatic nerve.

The exact nature of this condition remains unknown. I have treated two patients who complained of extremely severe lancinating pains, which were similar in intensity and character to the pain of tic douloureux. Improvement occurred with bed rest, sedation and Dilantin, often helpful in controlling the pain of tic douloureux, (100 milligrams every 6 hours) within several days. This condition seems to be self-limiting in nature, and symptomatic measures seem to suffice.

Tumors Involving the Sciatic Nerve

Tumors involving the sciatic nerve are quite painful and often difficult to diagnose, particularly if the lesion is hidden by the mass of the buttock. Tumors of the nerve sheath, such as a neurofibroma, may occur and should be suspected if the patient has von Recklinghausen's disease. Occasionally, the sciatic nerve is invaded by metastatic tumor. I have seen one such patient who complained of hip and sciatic pain as the only manifestation of this condition. He continued to complain of this pain for 6 months and was considered by his physician to be a neurotic. Unfortunately, I did not diagnose the cause of his pain, and he was later seen by a medical neurologist, who palpated along the course of the sciatic nerve and located a tender area of swelling. The patient was subsequently explored, and biopsy revealed evidence of a neoplasm which was eventually determined to be a renal carcinoma.

ENTRAPMENT NEUROPATHIES

Obturator Neuropathy

Obturator neuritis may occur from either an obturator hernia or from osteitis pubis. The pain characteristically radiates from the groin along the inner aspect of the thigh; in the case of an obturator hernia, coughing or sneezing, which increases the abdominal pressure, will be productive of pain.[3]

Why obturator neuritis is so often seen in association with osteitis pubis is not completely clear to me; but it is attributed to the surrounding tissue edema associated with this condition. Osteitis pubis, as intervertebral disc space infection, must be diagnosed on the basis of history and physical findings, since in both conditions the characteristic x-ray changes are not apparent for 3 to 6 weeks after onset of pain. By the time radiographic evidence is discernable, the clinical syndrome is usually improving and is another example of an "after the fact" x-ray diagnosis.

In addition to pain, obturator neuritis is associated with weakness of thigh adduction. However, thigh adductor atrophy is not seen, even in patients with long-standing obturator neuritis, because the adductor magnus is supplied, in addition, by the sciatic nerve, and the adductor longus frequently has supplementary innervation by the femoral nerve.

In association with the pain radiating along the inner aspect of the thigh, a dysesthesia or paresthesia may be appreciated. Sensory examination may reveal some loss of sensation but, more frequently there is none, despite painstaking examination.

A characteristic "obturator neuritis gait" abnormality, with an increased outward swing of the involved leg, is helpful in diagnosing this condition, because of the partially unopposed action of the thigh abductors.

If rest and medication do not relieve the symptoms, an obturator nerve block may be helpful on two counts—relief of pain following the block provides further verification of the diagnosis, and it can be utilized as a therapeutic trial for intrapelvic section of the obturator nerve, if intractable pain makes this procedure necessary.

TECHNIQUE OF OBTURATOR NERVE BLOCK

With the patient lying in the supine position, both thighs are abducted. The pubic tubercle on the side to be blocked is palpated and a local anesthetic wheal made one-half

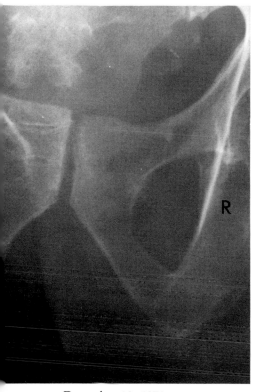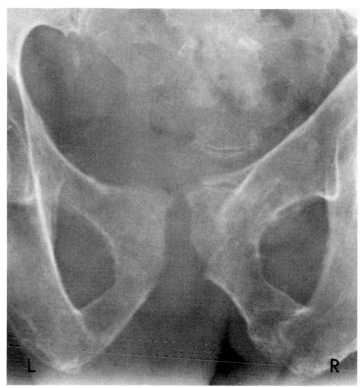

December 20, 1971   March 22, 1972

Fig. 15-3. This 69-year-old man developed severe pain characteristic of obturator neuritis, December 1971. Films of the symphysis pubis (12/20/71) were nonrevealing. Clinical improvement began two months after the onset of the symptoms and the radiologic changes were most evident in March 1972 (3/22/72) at which time the patient was quite comfortable and almost symptom free.

inch lateral and inferior to it. A 22-gauge, three-and-a-half inch spinal needle is introduced through this wheal perpendicular to the skin, until the upper portion of the inferior ramus of the pubis is contacted. The depth gauge is placed one inch above the skin. The needle is withdrawn to permit an altered lateral and slightly superior needle direction, allowing the needle bevel to glide along the inferior border of the superior ramus of the pubis. When the depth gauge is flush with the skin, the stylet is removed and aspiration attempted, in order to rule out blood vessel penetration. If aspiration is negative, 10 cc. of 1 percent Xylocaine are injected, and the obturator nerve will be blocked by diffusion of the anesthetic agent. In addition to the increased thigh adductor weakness, a zone of hypesthesia on the medial aspect of the thigh may develop.

ILIOHYPOGASTRIC AND ILIOINGUINAL NEURITIS (INGUINAL NEURITIS)

The most frequent cause of iliohypogastric and ilioinguinal neuritis is nerve damage following a surgical procedure. Because of the long course of these nerves within the abdominal muscle layers, incisions at several sites may tear or sever one of these nerves. Much less frequently, "inguinal neuritis" occurs without preceding surgery. Trauma,

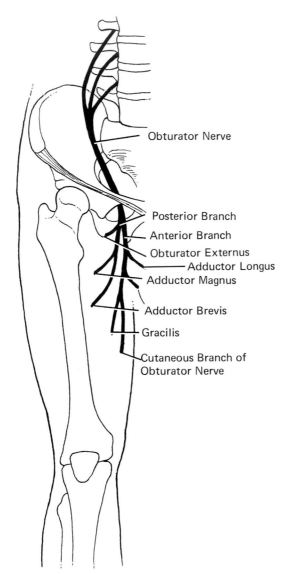

Fig. 15-4. Obturator nerve.

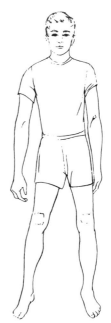

Fig. 15-5. Characteristic gait of obturator neuritis with increased lateral swing of the involved leg.

either direct, in the form of a blunt impact over the course of the nerve, or indirect, in association with a sudden violent spasm of the abdominal musculature, may be implicated.

Anatomy

Both nerves arise from the upper branches of the anterior primary divisions of the first and second lumbar nerve roots. The course parallels the twelfth thoracic nerve and both nerves follow the basic pattern of an intercostal nerve. Leaving the anterior rami of the lumbar roots, these nerves course laterally and inferiorly through the psoas muscle and then between the quadriceps lumborum muscle and the parietal peritoneum until reaching the region medial to the iliac crest, where they pierce the transversus abdominis and course between the transversus and the internal oblique muscles. Both nerves anastomose at this point, to some degree, but retain individual integrity. The iliohypogastric provides sensation to the suprapubic region, minimally innervating the abdominal muscles. The ilioinguinal nerve pierces the internal oblique, enters the inguinal canal, joining the spermatic cord and exits the inguinal canal through the external inguinal ring. It partially innervates the lowermost abdominal muscles and provides sensation to a strip of skin over the inguinal ligament and the base of the scrotum or labia.

Mechanism of Injury

Because of the oblique downward course of the nerves, injury may result from a variety of incisions. A high flank incision as for kidney surgery, a low McBurney muscle-

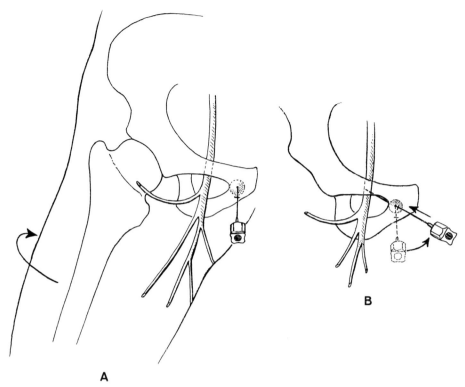

A

B

Fig. 15-6. Technique of obturator nerve block.

splitting incision, or the incision of an inguinal herniorrhaphy may be associated with "inguinal neuritis." Complaints range from a mild aching dysesthesia to severe lancinating pain within the cutaneous innervation of these nerves but inguinal pain rarely extends into the medial aspect of the thigh. Relief is often obtained in the supine position and sometimes hip flexion on the painful side is helpful. Standing tends to worsen the pain and occasionally any maneuver causing a sudden tightening of the abdominal muscles, such as coughing or sneezing, will aggravate the pain.

The infrequent cases of "inguinal neuritis" not postoperative in etiology are not clearly explainable. Some physicians identify these problems as "entrapment neuropathies" with the presumption that the shifting course of the nerves from one abdominal muscle interface to another makes them vulnerable for abdominal muscle spasm. I have difficulty completely accepting this theory but have

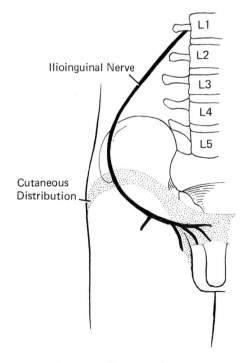

Fig. 15-7. Ilioinguinal nerve.

nothing better to offer in way of explanation. Whatever the cause, the spontaneous onset of this condition occasionally occurs and can be mistaken for various forms of renal disease, because of its pain distribution, or the patient is sometimes labeled a psychoneurotic.

If "inguinal neuritis" is a diagnostic possibility, a nerve block at the anterior iliac spine may be helpful.

Technique of Block

A line drawn from the umbilicus to the anterior superior iliac spine is divided into thirds. An anesthetic wheal is formed at the lateral third of this line through which 3 cc. of local anesthetic are deposited in 5 closely approximated sites as the needle is progressively moved perpendicular to the original line.

Management

If relief is obtained with a local block, a series of blocks may be utilized with hydrocortisone. Rest and oral anti-inflammatory medication may also be helpful. If conservative measures are ineffective, a neurolysis may be in order.

MERALGIA PARESTHETICA

Neuralgia of the lateral femoral cutaneous nerve causes burning pain and numbness in the anterolateral aspect of the thigh, and may be confused with sciatica.

Pathophysiology

Pressure on the lateral femoral cutaneous nerve at any point along its long course may produce the syndrome. The nerve arises from the second and third lumbar nerve roots, and hypertrophic arthritis of the upper lumbar spine may cause nerve root compression; and it emerges at the lateral border of the psoas major muscle, and can be involved at this site by a psoas abscess. The nerve then runs across the iliacus muscle in the pelvis just beneath the iliac fascia. Because of the superficial position in its long course within the pelvis, it is quite vulnerable to pressure produced by intrapelvic lesions, including pregnancy, tumors and infections. A traction neuritis of the nerve may occur as it passes over the brim of the iliac crest and emerges from the fascia under Poupart's ligaments, just medial to its attachment to the anterior superior spine of the ilium. At this site, the nerve may be angulated and stretched as the patient stands or walks. Patients who have gained weight and have developed pendulous abdomens are particularly susceptible to involvement at this site. Braces, corsets and trusses may cause compression in this region. We once treated a dentist for this problem who was accustomed to standing for long periods with his right anterior iliac spine compressed against the arm of the dental chair, producing compression neuritis of the lateral femoral cutaneous nerve.

Signs and Symptoms

The pain of meralgia paresthetica, frequently described as burning, glowing, tingling and pins and needles, involves the anterolateral thigh. The onset is usually spontaneous, but occasionally the patient may relate the development of pain to an unusually long walk or a prolonged period of standing. Symptoms are usually unilateral, although rarely both thighs may be involved. The pain is usually decreased by lying down or sitting and is aggravated by walking about or prolonged standing. Although firm pressure upon the affected area may not be uncomfortable, light stroking of the skin may provoke an unpleasant tingling sensation. Men often complain that the fabric of their trousers brushes their thighs when they walk and causes this unpleasant dysesthesia.

Diagnosis

Although little difficulty is encountered in diagnosing this rather distinct clinical entity,

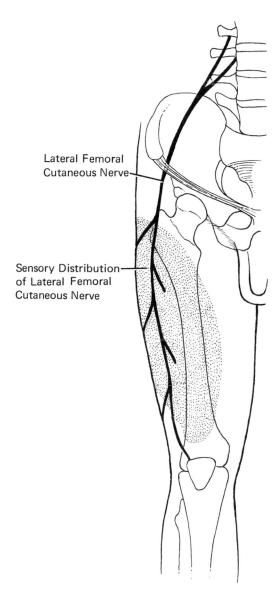

Fig. 15-8. Lateral femoral cutaneous nerve.

Lateral Femoral Cutaneous Nerve

Sensory Distribution of Lateral Femoral Cutaneous Nerve

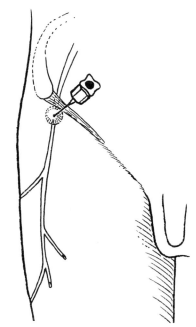

Fig. 15-9. Lateral femoral cutaneous nerve block.

determining the nature and site of the causative factor may be a problem. If the nerve is involved as it passes over the brim of the iliac crest, an analgesic block of the lateral femoral cutaneous nerve will relieve the pain. This block will be ineffective if the lesion is located proximally. In such instances, a complete neurologic survey, including x-rays of the lumbar spine, should be carried out. When the lesion is within the spine and is due to compression of the nerve roots by

osteoarthritis or a herniated disc in the upper lumbar region, diminution of the patellar reflex and weakness and atrophy of the quadriceps muscle may be evident. Rectal and vaginal examination should be done, and in some cases, myelography may be necessary.

Treatment

If the lesion is located at the anterior-superior iliac spine and is confirmed by subsidence of pain after analgesic block, repeated injections may create progressively longer pain-free intervals. If after 3 blocks no significant improvement beyond the pharmacologic action of the local anesthetic is noted, they are not likely to be of therapeutic value.

Lateral Femoral Cutaneous Nerve Block. The technique of blocking the lateral femoral cutaneous nerve in the thigh is simple. A 25-gauge, one inch hypodermic needle is inserted at a site one-half inch medial and one inch below the anterior superior iliac spine. This is carefully advanced through the skin until paresthesii occur from contact with the nerve, at which point 10 ml. of Xylocaine

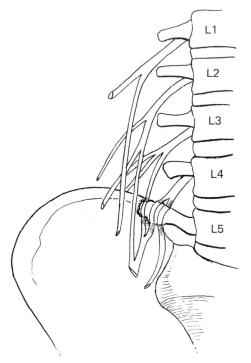

Fig. 15-10. The relationship of the ilium-transverse process pseudoarthrosis and lower lumbar roots.

is infiltrated. There is a tendency to insert the needle too deeply, thus causing the anesthetic to be injected into the sartorius muscle and resulting in an ineffective block.

The patient should be placed on a reducing diet directed at elimination of the pendulous abdomen. Constricting straps around the abdomen must be eliminated—women must discard tight corsets or girdles; men must substitute suspenders for belts.

At one time, section of the lateral femoral cutaneous nerve or neurolysis and transposition into a slot in the ilium was the treatment of choice. These procedures have not withstood the tests of time particularly well. When the nerve is sectioned, the pain may return because of the formation of a painful neuroma, which may also occur with transposition of the nerve. Spontaneous subsidence of the pain is likely to occur if a conservative regimen as previously outlined is carried out. When the syndrome is caused by a proximal lesion of the nerve or its spinal roots, proper therapy is directed appropriately.

ADHESIVE ARACHNOIDITIS

A number of patients with low back and sciatic pain have had their symptoms attributed to adhesive arachnoiditis which was demonstrated by myelography. In many instances spinal anesthesia, which had been carried out years previously, was attributed as the etiology of this condition; in some cases, no history of spinal anesthesia was obtained.[4,5]

A number of physicians advocated performing a laminectomy, opening the dura and separating the roots from their adhesive constrictions. This is no longer a widely accepted or commonly performed procedure. It is now believed that some of those patients who improved following this procedure, did so as a result of the decompressive laminectomy, since some of them may have had an unrecognized stenotic lumbar spinal canal, with a misinterpreted myelogram.

ARTHRITIS OF THE HIPS

Pain of arthritis of the hips is usually quite characteristic and readily identified. It is usually confined to the hip and is aggravated by all hip movements.

Occasionally, this pain radiates not only down into the posterior thigh to the knee but also up into the buttock and lumbar region. In such infrequent instances, the physician may confuse hip pain with sciatica. Sometimes, the associated muscle spasm of hip disease may cause diminution of deep tendon reflexes.

Hip pain is almost invariably aggravated by external hip rotation, and the Patrick's test is probably the single most reliable sign to aid in the diagnosis. X-ray evidence of hip disease is sometimes equivocal in the early stages of the condition.

ILIUM-TRANSVERSE PROCESS PSEUDOARTHROSIS

A rare cause of low back pain occurs when an elongated transverse process of the fifth lumbar vertebra comes into contact with, but is not fused to, the ilium. As a result of normal fifth lumbar vertebra movement, the site of such bony impaction is subject to trauma, and hypertrophic osteoarthritic changes at the site of contact occur.

The primary symptom resulting from such a pseudoarthrosis is low back pain with rather specific referral to the site of pseudoarthrosis. Examination reveals tenderness to pressure over the site, with paraspinal muscle spasm particularly on the involved side. The pain is aggravated by specific movements of the lumbar spine, particularly lateral flexion and rotation, which in most other causes of low back dysfunction are not hampered or productive of increased discomfort.

Occasionally, either the fourth or fifth lumbar nerve root in its extrathecal course may become involved with the mass of degenerated fibrocartilaginous tissue formed in reaction to the pseudoarthrosis. This may produce a radiculitis of the affected nerve root, with lower extremity pain and a positive straight leg raising test on the affected side. The root affected depends upon the relative position of the sacrum with regard to the pelvis.

Treatment

This condition is improved with bed rest, anti-inflammatory and analgesic medication and the wearing of a low back support.

If pain persists, injection of hydrocortisone into the site of the pseudoarthrosis may be in order.

If pain persists despite adequate conservative management, surgery may be necessary. At surgery, the site of the pseudoarthrosis is exposed and the elongated transverse process rongeured away.

ANKYLOSING SPONDYLITIS

This condition, also called Marie-Strumpell disease, is a form of rheumatoid arthritis with certain features identifying it as a specific entity. The disease is often familial, is predominant in males at a 5 to 1 ratio and presents with an absence of rheumatoid factor or rheumatoid nodules. In common with rheumatoid arthritis, typical rheumatoid peripheral joint disease occurs sporadically in more than half of these patients and a significant proportion suffer from chronic peripheral joint disease.

Symptoms

The onset usually occurs between 25 and 35 years of age and is manifested by low back discomfort, involving one or both buttocks, and usually described as an aching or stiffness, which is often more apparent after remaining in the same position for prolonged periods and particularly so upon awakening in the morning. This onset is rather insidious, tends to be episodic, is not likely to require medical attention initially and is usually vaguely recalled by the patient during the history in retrospect. With the passage of time, the episodes of discomfort become progressively more severe and may awaken the patient from a sound sleep during the night. Unlike most pains associated with low back dysfunction, it is not particularly aggravated by physical activity.

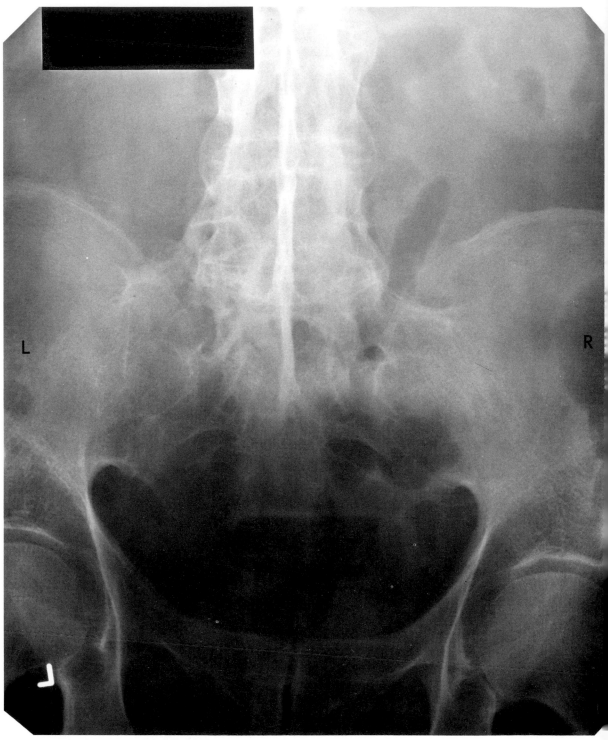

Fig. 15-11. Ankylosing spondylitis. Note the almost obliterated sacroiliac joint margins, fusion of the apophyseal joints, and interspinous ligamentus ossification. This 62-year-old patient was hospitalized subsequent to relatively moderate trauma which produced a compression fracture of L1. The rigidity of the spine makes this structure vulnerable to mechanical stresses which are easily tolerated by a normally mobile skeleton.

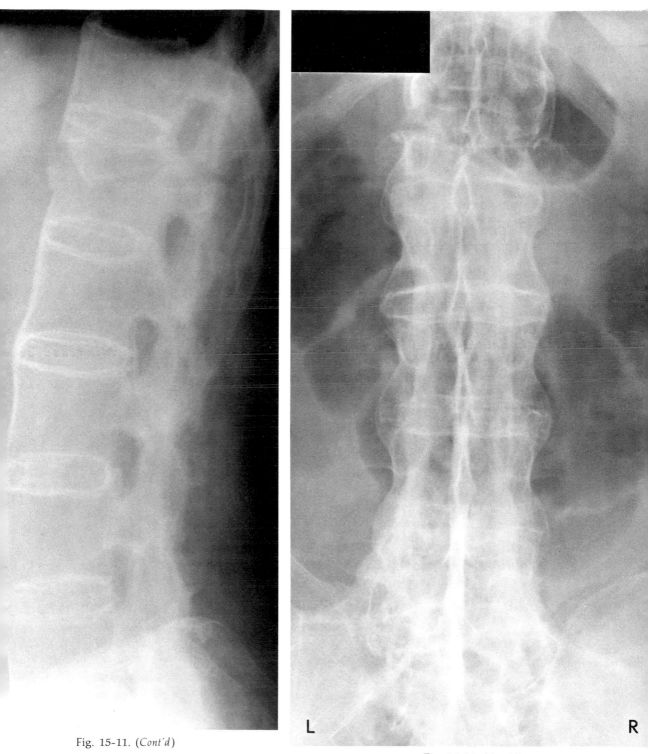

Fig. 15-11. (*Cont'd*)

Fig. 15-11. (*Cont'd*)

Approximately 75 percent of the patients with this condition have some form of sciatica—unilateral, alternating, or bilateral—usually occurring during the early phases of the disease. Eventually, these radicular pains are superceded by increased aching and stiffness, aggravated by inactivity.

The increasingly severe episodes of pain over a period of years will be associated with increasing rigidity of the spine.

Occasionally, an episode of iritis occurs as one of the early symptoms.

Examination

In the early stages of this disease, physical examination may reveal nothing, but later findings include paraspinal muscle spasm, with flattening of the lumbar lordosis. Tenderness over the sacroiliac joints may be quite striking and can be elicited not only by pressure or percussion posteriorly but also by digital pressure applied per rectum. Eventually, a flattening of the lower thoracic curvature and restriction of cervical mobility are noted, with restriction of chest expansion a relatively late sign.

Despite a history of radicular signs, sensory, motor or reflex changes are rare.

Eventually, the entire vertebral column becomes fixed.

Intermittent low-grade fevers may occur.

Laboratory

An elevated sedimentation rate may be most helpful, but this may remain normal even during active exacerbations in 10 to 20 percent of patients.

X-ray

Convincing roentgen diagnosis of ankylosing spondylitis is usually apparent only after several years. The earliest x-ray abnormalities are usually seen in the sacroiliac

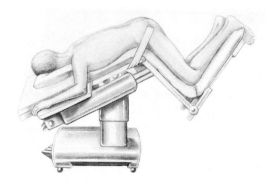

Fig. 15-12. Positioning of the patient for unroofing of the sacrum. If the patient is obese, it may be necessary to use adhesive strapping to laterally retract the gluteii.

joints, the joint space at first being somewhat wider than usual, with irregular margins due to bony erosion and a slight increase in density at the margins of the joints. In almost every case this condition ultimately progresses to destructive sacro-iliitis. The spine eventually progresses to ligamentous ossification with narrowing and fusion of the apophyseal joints.

Treatment

In the early stages of the disease, symptomatic relief is obtained with local heat, salicylates and mild exercise. X-ray therapy is of value in relieving acute symptoms.

Confusion with Lumbar Disc Disease

Each year I encounter a patient or two with ankylosing spondylitis who was subjected to lumbar disc surgery in the early stages of disease. A positive familial history for spondylitis, a past history of peripheral joint disease or iritis, the typical morning stiffness and absence of positive neurological signs should warn off the surgeon. In the late stages of this diseases, the diagnosis is apparent.

CHARCOT'S DISEASE OF THE SPINE (VERTEBRAL OSTEOARTHROPATHY)

One of the rare causes of low back pain is tertiary syphilis which produces bony changes in the vertebral bodies. The bone and joint changes involving the lumbar spine basically resemble those of osteoarthritis in the earlier stages of this disease. However, with progression in the tabetic arthropathy, the eburnation of bone and the proliferative changes at the margins of the vertebral bodies are more extensive than those seen in ordinary osteoarthritis.

The appreciation of pain, which normally protects the joints from injury or from excessive use after injury, lessens as a result of tabes dorsalis. It is thought to be responsible for fragmentation of the hypertrophied margins of the vertebrae and extensive degeneration of the intervertebral discs at multiple levels. There are those who feel that this neurotrophic disease affects the vertebrae directly through disturbance of bone metabolism and point to the fact that the bones of patients with tabes are not exposed to extraordinarily excessive trauma.

As a result of considerable new bone formation with posterior and posterolateral bony ridges, cauda equina compression may occur, thus further complicating the neurological dysfunction caused by tabes dorsalis. Myelography in these instances reveals marked generalized narrowing of the subarachnoid space as a result of bony proliferation and thickening of the ligaments of the vertebral canal. Bilateral constriction resulting from this narrowing is seen at multiple layers both in the A-P and lateral views. Frequently, the bony encroachment is severe enough to cause a partial or complete myelographic block. When this occurs, surgical decompression for relief of cauda equina compression is indicated.

SACRAL CYSTS

Uncommonly, patients with low back and sciatic pain will be found to have sacral cysts on myelography. The etiology and pathogenesis of these lesions are obscure, as is the mechanism of symptom production. These cysts usually occur at the junction of the posterior root and the dorsal ganglion and can be found on the dorsal ganglia of any of the spinal nerve roots. They are most commonly seen on the second and third sacral roots. They may either be asymptomatic or associated with low back and sciatic pain and may be single or multiple.

Beginning in 1938, Dr. I. M. Tarlov has written extensively on cysts of the posterior sacral roots. He believes that these lesions are caused by hydrostatic pressure dissecting the nerve root sheath at a site where the arachnoid investing the nerve roots is relatively weak. This results in a splitting of the nerve root sheath with formation of a space between the pia-derived endoneurium and the arachnoid-derived perineurium. Others attribute the formation of these cysts to trauma and some consider them purely congenital in etiology.

Plain x-rays are usually negative but occasionally, with extremely large cysts, localized thinning and erosion of the sacrum occurs, best seen in the lateral view.

Myelography is essential to establishing the diagnosis and may demonstrate a free and readily patent communication between the subarachnoid space and the cyst or there may be a partial communication; and in some instances no communication between the subarachnoid space and the cyst can be demonstrated. When the communication is partial, the Pantopaque may be forced into the cyst either by bilateral jugular compression or a Valsalva type maneuver with the patient straining. If the partial communication between the subarachnoid space and the cyst is minimal, Pantopaque will not enter the cyst until 24 or 48 hours after the initial subarachnoid injection of the radiocontrast material. Some authorities advocate intentionally leaving 1 cc. of dye within the subarachnoid space and obtaining a follow-up film 48 hours later in order to determine the possible existence of such lesions. A number of these cysts were discovered when a complete withdrawal of Pantopaque was technically unsuccessful and follow-up x-rays unexpectedly revealed their presence. When no communication exists between the

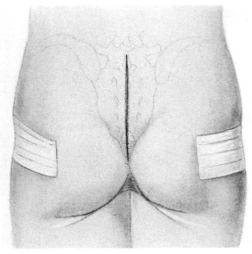

Fig. 15-13. Incision.

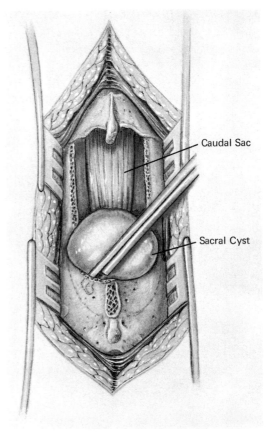

Fig. 15-15. Unroofing of sacrum.

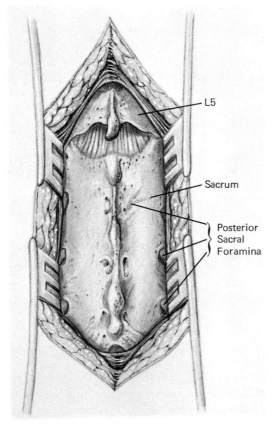

Fig. 15-14. In retracting and carrying out a sub-periosteal muscle dissection, avoid carrying out the dissection beyond the posterior sacral foramina to prevent damage to the dorsal division of the sacral nerves emerging through the foramina under cover of the multifidus.

subarachnoid space and the cyst, the presence of such a lesion can only be inferred by displacement of the caudal sac in association with bony erosion.

One should be relatively cautious in the surgical removal of these lesions for two reasons. First, in many instances they are asymptomatic; and after obliteration of the cyst, the patient notes no abatement of the pain. Second, excision of a sacral nerve root cyst may result in some sensory dysfunction within the sacral distribution. If this numbness extends over the shaft of the penis in males, it may be associated with alteration and impairment of sexual functions. Before considering surgery on a sacral cyst, particularly in a male, this potential complication should be discussed at some length with the patient. Failure to alert the patient to this potential problem has led to a number of lawsuits.

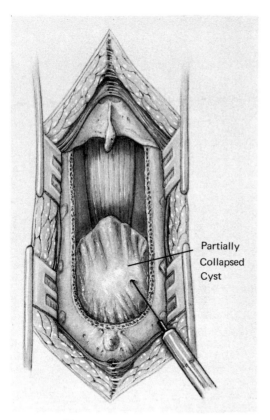

Fig. 15-16. Tapping the cyst to reduce the pressure, permitting cyst wall mobilization in all directions for visualization of the exiting sacral nerves.

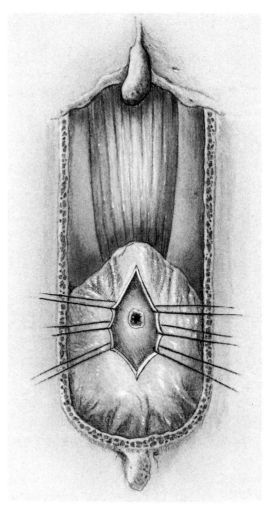

Fig. 15-17. Incision into cyst and visualization of connection between neck of cyst and the terminal position of the caudal sac.

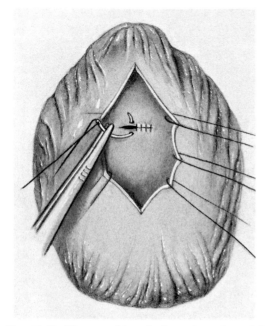

Fig. 15-18. Closure of terminal portion of caudal sac.

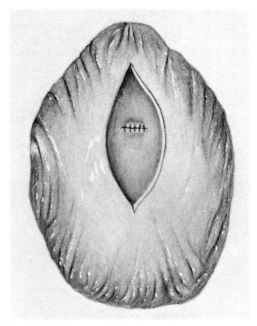

Fig. 15-19. Cyst wall is allowed to remain open so that it will not reform.

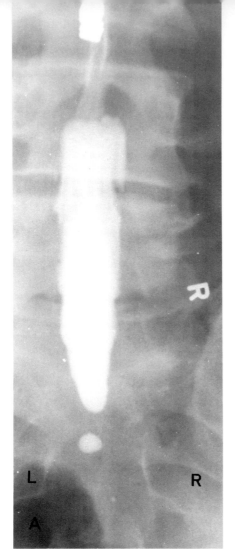

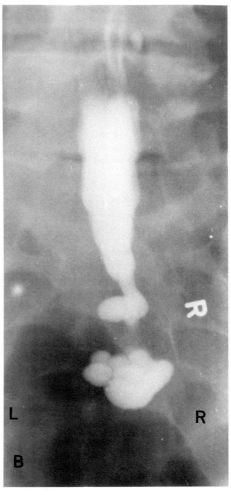

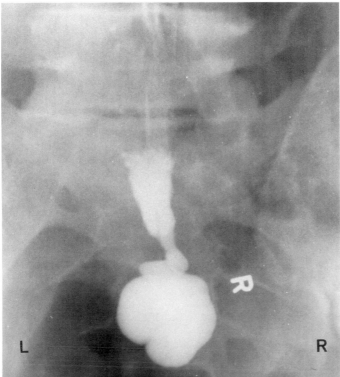

Fig. 15-20. Myelography of sacral cyst.

A, Normal lumbar myelogram with droplet of Pantopaque indicative of possible sacral cyst.

B, Sacral cyst gradually filling by placing patient in upright (standing) position and having him strain ("bear down").

C, Sacral cyst filled with Pantopaque.

The following case history will indicate my caution with regard to this lesion.

G. L. (49542), a 34-year-old policeman, was hospitalized on July 19, 1970, because of long-standing low back pain and right sciatica which did not respond to conservative management. A myelogram revealed a large sacral cyst measuring approximately $1\frac{1}{2}$ inches in diameter. After Pantopaque removal (some remained within the cyst and could not be removed), 80 milligrams of methyl prednisolone acetate were injected through the lumbar puncture needle used for myelography, prior to needle withdrawal.

The patient noted some improvement with this medication and was discharged from the hospital on July 24, 1970. He was followed at intervals on an outpatient basis for 2 years,

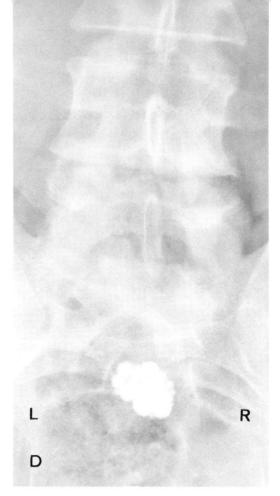

Fig. 15-20. D, After Pantopaque withdrawal some remained trapped within the sacral cyst.

E, Lateral view of the "trapped" Pantopaque within the sacral cyst. Note the bony erosion of the sacrum at the site of the cyst.

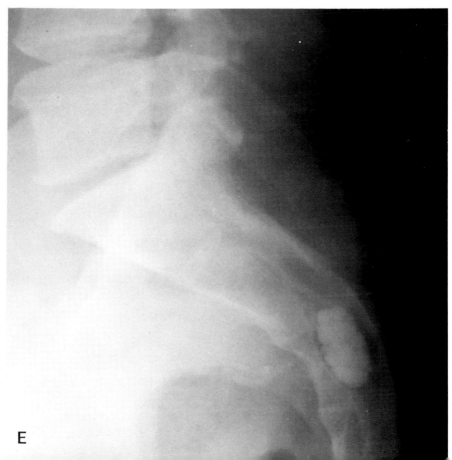

and during this interval he continued to complain of severe and intense low back pain and right sciatica. Because of the persistence of his symptoms, he was rehospitalized and the sacral cyst was excised June 7, 1972. The postoperative course was benign and uneventful, and the patient has had no recurrence of pain. During the 2-year interval between discovery of the sacral cyst and its excision, the patient was followed regularly and was fully aware of the potential sexual complications of surgery. After patient and surgeon were satisfied that he would not appreciate any significant improvement, we mutually agreed that surgery was in order.

REFERENCES

1. Filtzer, D. L., and Bhanson, H. H.: Low back pain due to arterial obstruction. J. Bone Joint Surg., *41B*:244, 1959.
2. Finneson, B. E.: Diagnosis and Management of Pain Syndromes, ed. 2, W. B. Saunders, 1969.
3. Kopell, H. P., and Thompson, W. A. L.: Peripheral Entrapment Neuropathies. Baltimore, William and Wilkins, 1963.
4. Schwarz, G. A., and Bevilacqua, J. E.: Paraplegia following spinal anesthesia. Clinicopathologic report and review of literature. Arch. Neurol., *10*:308, 1964.
5. Thorsen, G.: Neurological complications after spinal anesthesia and results from 2,493 follow-up cases. Acta. Chir. Scand., Suppl. 121, *95*:1–272, 1947.

16
Lumbar Spinal Fusion

Surgical Techniques

Posterior Fusion
Vertebral Body Fusion

Complications of Anterior Interabdominal Lumbar Fusion

Indications for Lumbar Spinal Fusion

16
Lumbar Spinal Fusion

Lumbar spinal fusion has been utilized as a treatment for low back pain for many years. Even prior to the development of lumbar disc surgery, spinal fusion was occasionally resorted to for the management of severe intractable low back pain. With the increased acceptance and utilization of lumbar disc surgery, a parallel increase occurred in the use of spinal fusion. The majority of these were carried out with the disc excision and spinal fusion performed as a combined procedure. However, the objective of each half of the combined procedure is separate and distinct, with disc excision performed for decompression of a nerve root and fusion to eliminate mobility between the vertebrae. In the face of such differing objectives, one might presume that the indications for each procedure would differ and invite speculation regarding the necessity or the advisability of performing the two procedures simultaneously. In the past thirty years, significant modifications and innovations have evolved in both the surgical techniques and clinical indications for lumbar spinal fusion.

SURGICAL TECHNIQUES

Individual surgeons have developed so many variations of surgical technique in performing lumbar fusion procedures, and these enbody such vast differences in surgical philosophy and diagnostic criteria, that review of various reported series of lumbar fusion procedures do not lend themselves to valid statistical analyses.

Posterior Fusion

The so-called posterior fusion is the traditional method of fusing the spine and involves the positioning of osseous tissue or bone chips upon some or all portions of the posterior bony elements of the spine.

Nonosseous materials including wire, metallic plates and screws have all been employed for immobilization of the lumbar spine but have few advocates at present. The combined stress of weight bearing and mobility tend to loosen these foreign substances, causing them to loose their initial effectiveness in immobilizing the vertebral segments. Failure of the nonosseous material is usually not due to weakness of the appliance and subsequent breakdown but is more often related to bony pressure erosion at the site of fixation between the vertebral arch and the foreign substance. The use of "living bony callus" to produce fixation of the vertebral arches achieves a greater degree of success. However, even with a solid bony posterior fusion, less than the desired vertebral immobility is achieved. Experimental investigation, by Rolander,[14] of lumbar stability following posterior fusions, including the spinous processes, laminae and the transverse processes, demonstrate surprising residual mobility between the vertebral bodies. An additional disadvantage of "posterior fusion" is that the relative spinal fixation is achieved in association with narrowing of the intervertebral disc space and relative constriction of the intervertebral foramina.

Despite these presumed shortcomings, the type of lumbar spinal fusion in most common use remains some form of posterior spinal fusion. The general acceptance of this method of treatment is based on a number of factors, the most important of which is the large body of documented long-standing clinical successes associated with this technique. Possibly complete immobilization of the lumbar spine is not mandatory and may even be undesirable, with merely reduced intervertebral mobility required in many cases. A significant factor in the predominant use of this technique is that the traditional posterior approach is part of the standard training of all specialists involved in spinal surgery, both orthopedic and neurological surgeons, and they are generally more comfortable in utilizing this approach.

Vertebral Body Fusion

Theoretically, the optimal lumbar spine fusion should immobilize the vertebral bodies, which are the portions of the vertebrae most involved with weight bearing. In addition, the fixation is best performed with restoration of the normal width of the intervertebral disc space and associated widening of the intervertebral foramina. This has given rise to the lumbar interbody fusion either by the anterior interabdominal approach or by the posterior lumbar interbody fusion technique developed by Dr. Ralph B. Cloward (see chapter 7).

The anterior interabdominal (either transperitoneal or retroperitoneal) approach[7,8,16,17] is used primarily as a method of managing the patient who has had several posterior operative procedures that have failed. In addition to the above-noted theoretical advantages of intervertebral body fusion, it has the major practical advantage of avoiding an area of previous spinal surgery. This eliminates dissection and retraction of a scar-encased caudal sac and adherent nerve roots, which so often is associated with an increased inci-

dence of surgical root trauma, and leads to persisting radicular motor and sensory dysfunction and exacerbation of the originally intolerable presurgical status.

The preferred interabdominal approach is retroperitoneal, with the transperitoneal approach usually reserved for those patients who have had prior multiple abdominal surgical procedures, making a retroperitoneal dissection technically unfeasible. Following surgery, a nonreinforced lumbosacral support is usually necessary, not so much for the bony spine but to support the abdominal musculature in the maintenance of the erect posture.

COMPLICATIONS OF ANTERIOR INTERABDOMINAL LUMBAR FUSION

In addition to a fairly high percentage of pseudoarthrosis (15–25%), a number of complications unique to the abdominal approach may occur. Anticipated thrombophlebitis of the lower extremities, probably related to retraction of the iliac vessels, is treated with the routine postoperative use of anticoagulants. Despite this prophylaxis, the incidence of thrombophlebitis varies between 5 and 8 percent. Urinary tract disturbances including atonic bladder, hydronephrosis and infections are reported. As a result of trauma to the sympathetic chains over the sacral promontory and on either side of the lumbar vertebrae, most males report a significant degree of sexual impotence and failure to ejaculate.

INDICATIONS FOR LUMBAR SPINAL FUSION

There are almost as many opinions regarding the role of spinal fusion in lumbar disc surgery as there are spinal surgeons. The subtle shades of differences elude categorization, but the following 6 criteria list the chief positions of advocacy.

1. *Every lumbar disc excision should be combined with spinal fusion.*

The statistics of simple disc excision without fusion vary in published series from 75 to 90% satisfactory results. These statistics appear to depend primarily on the diagnostic criteria leading to the original surgery. Those series in which surgery is reserved for patients with clearly identifiable nerve root compression syndromes and satisfactory myelographic correlation of the clinical picture have the highest incidence of success with less than a 10 percent failure rate. A considerable difference exists between the hazards of simple disc excision compared to the more prolonged and extensive "combined procedure" involving lumbar fusion. The postoperative convalescence following the combined procedure is much more prolonged and associated with more pain and an increased incidence of complications in comparison to simple disc excision. It is generally accepted that pseudoarthrosis following lumbar spinal fusion occurs at the rate of somewhat less than 10 percent for each interspace fused and is associated with symptoms that are usually severe enough to require surgical correction. It must be further realized that a significant number of patients with solid fusions continue to have low back pain of a mechanical nature, which is relieved by bed rest and aggravated by activity. In the face of these generally accepted statistics, it is difficult to understand the advocacy of lumbar fusion at the time of every lumbar disc excision.

2. *Repeat lumbar disc surgery performed for recurrence or persistence of lumbar disc symptoms following an unsuccessful "simple disc excision" should be combined with lumbar fusion.*

Those who advocate a lumbar fusion at the time of a repeat operative procedure for disc excision presume that if the first operative procedure was properly done, some factor, in addition to simple nerve root pressure, must be causing persisting symptoms; therefore, immobilization of those spinal segments requiring secondary surgery is in order. This point of view does have some validity, since it is based on the fact that the initial surgery was a failure and a persuasion that "more of the same" may again be inadequate to

provide relief of symptoms. Issue may be taken with blanket approval of this criteria, on the basis that if a patient continues to manifest symptoms typical of nerve root pain, this is most likely due to continued nerve root irritation either in the form of inadequately relieved pressure, or root dysfunction secondary to irritation from the original compression, or nerve root trauma from the original surgery. If a second myelogram reveals a filling defect indicative of continued pressure at the site of the original nerve root decompressive procedure, little is to be gained by fusing that interspace, but a second effort at decompressing the nerve root may be advisable. If, however, in addition to persisting nerve root symptoms, the patient has low back pain of clearly mechanical nature, with aggravation by weight bearing and relief by rest, fusion at the time of the second exploration may, indeed, be in order.

3. *Lumbar disc surgery with radiological evidence of hypertrophic osteoarthritic degenerative changes at the involved interspace requires a lumbar fusion.*

Degenerative changes involving the interspace of a protruding lumbar disc is a controvertible indication for fusion at that site. Simple disc excision and foraminotomy compared with combined disc excision and lumbar fusion, in the presence of hypertrophic osteoarthritic degenerative changes at the site of disc protrusion, indicate no significant end result advantage with fusion. Since degenerative changes are more likely to be found in patients of advanced years, the additional rigors and potential hazards of the combined operation would weigh against its use.

4. *Lumbar spinal instability with or without myelographic evidence of disc protrusion requires lumbar spinal fusion.*

The diagnosis of lumbar spinal instability is frequently submitted as an indication for fusion. Undoubtedly, some intervertebral joints are more mobile and seem less "stable" than usual, but clinically consistent signs and symptoms of this entity are not established. Some surgeons believe this diagnosis can be made at the operating table when the lumbar spine is exposed, by placing heavy Kocher clamps upon the spinous processes and rocking the vertebrae, one on the other. The maneuver is of interest but in practice is generally an "after the commitment" diagnosis. Rarely does the surgeon who has planned a spinal fusion stop at this point because the vertebral mobility was less than expected.

5. *Lumbar disc excision upon a patient who performs heavy physical work requires a spinal fusion.*

Considerations of the heavy physical work done prior to lumbar disc surgery as an indication of fusion may be theoretically valid but in practice do not hold up particularly well. Many patients who have had either simple lumbar disc excision or lumbar disc excision followed by fusion are not able to return to heavy physical work. Efforts made to place this patient in an occupation that does not involve excessive stress on the low back structures would seem to be statistically more helpful than the illusory hope that with a fusion he might become strong enough to return to heavy labor.

6. *Lumbar spinal fusion is never indicated under any circumstances.*

This type of "blanket rule" is as unsound as the first criteria, which advocates fusions on all patients undergoing lumbar disc surgery. There are specific indications for fusion, but these are significantly different from those involving excision of the intervertebral disc.

Lumbar spinal fusion is indicated in patients who manifest intractable mechanical low back pain. These are patients who will improve with bed rest and will worsen following weight bearing and activities that incur stress upon the lumbar spine. A further diagnostic criteria would be derivation of at least some relief with the use of external support of the low back. The indications for fusion are occasionally clear enough so that it can be performed as a separate procedure without the need for a second intervertebral disc excision or nerve root exploration.

17
Experimental and Unorthodox Treatments for Low Back and Sciatic Pain

EVALUATING TREATMENT

INTERVERTEBRAL DISCOLYSIS

Chymopapain Injection

Collagenase Injection

INTRADISCAL HYDROCORTISONE INJECTION

PROLOTHERAPY

Proliferating Solutions
Injection Technique
Site of Injection

Complications
Present Status of Prolotherapy

FACET RHIZOTOMY

Principle of Facet Rhizotomy

Technique of Facet Rhizotomy

DORSAL COLUMN STIMULATION

Indications

Surgical Technique

EVALUATING TREATMENT

The ever-present problem of low back pain illustrates how very thin and unsubstantial are theories, with only experience being tangible. The physician must be constantly mindful that no one disease or condition is responsible for low back dysfunction, nor can one single form of treatment be considered as universally effective for the variety of causal entities. The goal of proper management is individualization of the treatment of the patient's specific needs. When deciding upon treatment for such a relatively benign condition, the potential hazards of the contemplated treatment, the residual dysfunction produced by the treatment and the convalescent interval following the treatment must be considered.

In 1949, as an assistant neurology resident, I was exposed to my first clinical research experience. This effort involved the use of a drug which some investigators claimed would arrest the progressive worsening of patients with multiple sclerosis. The natural history of this disease, characterized by occasionally prolonged periods of remission is well known to create short-term, overoptimistic results. However, after two years my enthusiasm for what turned out to be a valueless treatment was realistically cooled. Similarly, the prolonged remissions characteristic of low back dysfunction can easily lead to overoptimistic misinterpretation of the benefits resulting from treatment for this condition.

Some years ago, in an effort to document the "natural history" of lumbar disc disease, a number of my patients with verified lumbar disc protrusions, who were not treated surgically but who received conservative management, were contacted by mail. Slightly more than 50 percent of these patients indicated that they were physically active and reasonably pain free. Three years later a second mailed questionnaire was sent to a somewhat larger group but including most of the previously polled patients. The second mailing again indicated that approximately 50 percent of the patients were satisfied with their status but these were different patients. Careful scrutiny revealed that a sizable shift had occurred, with formerly pain-free patients now being incapacitated and many of the previously incapacitated patients now being comfortable.

At any given time approximately half of all untreated patients with low back dysfunction will be in remission. For a method of treatment to be considered effective, it must improve on the natural history of the disease; that is, achieve a "cure rate" of significantly better than 50 percent.

INTERVERTEBRAL DISCOLYSIS

The concept of nonsurgically diminishing the overall bulk of protruding intervertebral disc, with the presumption that such a contraction of tissue mass would reduce nerve root pressure, has been considered for more than twenty years. A variety of methods to convert the intervertebral disc to scar tissue were considered, including damaging the disc with heavy needles or trocars, injecting bacteria into the disc space and injecting sclerosing solutions into the disc.

Chymopapain Injection

In 1959 Dr. Carl Hirsch discussed the feasibility of injecting a discolytic enzyme into the intervertebral space and this was further discussed by Dr. Mitchell, Dr. Hendry, and Dr. Billewicz in 1961. Dr. Lyman Smith injected chymopapain, the major proteolytic component of *Carica papaya* latex, into the intervertebral discs of rabbits and dogs. On the basis of this animal experimentation, the first humans were so treated by him in July of 1963. Since that time, a number of investigators have conducted similar clinical investigative experiments in man. This substance attacks chondromucoprotein-producing keratosulfate, chondroitin sulfate and protein. There are at present more than forty investigators most of them orthopedic surgeons and six neurosurgeons, carrying out active clinical research on humans with chymopapain. These men are working in conjunction with the drug company that is manufacturing this material and the experiments are being conducted along guidelines established by the Food and Drug Administration.

Technique of Intervertebral Chymopapain Injection. Because of the rather severe pain associated with injection of chymopapain, the procedure is usually performed under general anesthesia. Since intrachecal injection of chymopapain is associated with potentially catastrophic complications, the preferred method of needle placement into the disc is by means of the lateral approach which completely skirts the dura. Occasionally this approach cannot be used at the L5–S1 interspace because of the iliac crest; and when this problem occurs, either the posterior lateral or the posterior approach is utilized. Using the lateral approach, the patient is positioned in the lateral position, and most of the injectors position the patient lying on the left side with the right side up, with no particular consideration given to the side of sciatic symptoms. Six inch, 18-gauge spinal needles are directed from a point 8 centimeters lateral to the spinous process of the disc to be injected, with the needle maintained at an angle of 45° toward the disc. Needle placement of the L5–S1 disc requires a 35° caudal angulation. Sometimes it is impossible to satisfactorily place the needle within the L5–S1 interspace using the lateral approach and the posterior approach will be required. After the needle bevels are positioned as close to the middle of the interspace as possible, 1 cc. of water soluble x-ray contrast material (Hypaque, Conray, Renografin) is injected and lateral discogram films are obtained after each injection.

On the basis of the clinical symptoms, the previously performed myelogram (some of the physicians carrying out this study do not routinely perform myelography), and the discogram, a decision is made regarding the appropriate disc or discs to be injected with chymopapain. The average dosage of this material is 4 mg. with variations from 2 to 12 mg. being given.

Following the chymopapain injection, most patients experience considerable low back pain and require narcotics and general supportive measures. The degree of pain is comparable to the discomfort appreciated by the postoperative laminectomy patient and in some cases even somewhat more severe. Progressive mobilization and physiotherapy are instituted over the next week to ten days, and the patient is usually comfortable enough to be discharged from the hospital a week or ten days postinjection.

Indications for Intervertebral Discolysis. Selection of patients is based primarily on the degree and persistence of pain and the lack of an adequate response to conservative management. Most of the patients selected are those who would in the ordinary course of events be considered for surgery. This procedure is presently utilized as a possible alternative to lumbar disc surgery. Many of the patients who have been selected for chymopapain injection have had previous lumbar disc surgery which was unsuccessful or may have been successful for a time and subsequently developed recurrent symptoms. A few of the patients selected were not considered suitable candidates for surgery for medical reasons, either because of advanced years or because of cardiac or other medical problems.

The number of interspaces injected is somewhat larger than the number of interspaces that would have been subjected to surgery. Since the needles were already in place for carrying out the discogram prior to the contemplated chymopapain injection when there was some uncertainty regarding a possible interspace, this was usually given the benefit of the doubt and injected with this discolytic substance.

Results of Chymopapain Injection. The results of this series varied depending on the individual reporting on the series and the criteria used to report the results. Approximately 50 percent of the patients injected

had been reported as appreciating "good" clinical improvement. The other 50 percent is almost equally divided among those who noted "fair" improvement but continued to manifest significant pain and outright failures with no improvement. Most of the patients who showed no improvement were eventually brought to surgery and a significant percentage of those who reported "fair" improvement eventually came to surgery.

It was felt by most of the injectors that this technique resulted in reducing by 50 to 75 percent the number of laminectomies which would have otherwise been performed.

Following discolysis there is often a significant narrowing of the intervertebral space noted radiographically. This narrowing is seen shortly after the injection of chymopapain into the disc and does not seem to change years later.

If a myelographic defect was seen prior to chymopapain injection, this does not seem to change on a postinjection myelogram even if the sciatic symptoms improve.

Complications of Chymopapain Injection. The most frequent complication is anaphylactic reaction to the chymopapain and several patients had been reported as going into anaphylactic shock. One such patient was reported by Dr. Lee T. Ford who discovered after the injection was given that this patient had previously known that she was allergic to Adolph's meat tenderizer, a product consisting of lytic enzymes. Following this episode he now asks all patients whether they are aware of any sensitivity to this tenderizer. One patient suffered an irreversible paraplegia 10 days following injection; another developed a Brown-Séquard syndrome 6 weeks after injection into the sixth cervical interspace. Other complications include a reported pulmonary embolus and a fractured rib caused either by lying in the lateral position under anesthesia or as a result of moving the patient while under anesthesia. Several disc space infections had been reported following intervertebral discolysis with chymopapain. This method remains experimental and is not in general use.

Collagenase Injection

Collagenase, extracted from culture of *C. histolyticum* and *C. welchii*, is an enzyme which attacks the collagen molecule. It has been utilized in the debridement of dermal ulcers, necrotic tissues and burns. It has been implicated as a possible etiological factor in the early stages of degenerative joint disease. This material has been used to date in vitro studies and in the operative intradiscal injection of dogs.

Dr. Bernard Sussman who advocates the use of collagenase as opposed to chymopapain states that the chemical changes undergone by degenerating discs, both from aging or herniation, increases the collagen content both in the nucleus pulposus and the annulus fibrosus. He further states that since chymopapain has no solubilizing effect upon collagen, collagenase would seem the logical discolytic agent of choice. He states too that chymopapain exerts its principal enzymatic action upon the nucleus pulposus, but many symptom-producing discs are actually a protrusion of the annulus fibrosus over the underlying nucleus pulposus, strengthening his thesis that collagenase is more suitable as a discolytic agent in the degenerated disc.

With regard to the relative toxicity of the two substances, experimental animal intrathecal injection of collagenase did not lead to complications; whereas, a similar placement of chymopapain produced death.

At this time, chymopapain is undergoing extensive clinical investigation in man and collagenase is still in the stage of laboratory studies on effectiveness and toxicity in animals.

INTRADISCAL HYDROCORTISONE INJECTION

Dr. Henry L. Feffer first injected hydrocortisone into an intervertebral disc in 1954. He stated that degeneration of this structure inevitably leads to radial tears and fissures, which cause an inflammatory reaction in the surrounding longitudinal ligaments of the spine to produce a syndrome of low back pain. Progression of this lesion will cause increased widening of the angular fissures and eventually sufficient weakness of the annulus fibrosus so that herniation of nuclear material will occur through this tear. It is assumed by Dr. Feffer that the polymerizing effect of hydrocortisone would reverse or block the degenerative changes within the intervertebral disc and would help recreate the normal physiological role of the nucleus pulposus in supporting the vertical load. He further assumed that the fissures and tears of the annulus fibrosus associated with the clinical syndrome of low back pain would have an opportunity to heal and this treatment, in association with routine low back rehabilitative measures, would be of value to prevent recurrence of low back pain.

His technique involved discograms which were performed by means of a posterior lateral approach using a 23-gauge spinal needle. The injected mixture consists of 25 mg. of hydrocortisone with 1.5 cc. of radiopaque, water-soluble contrast material (Diodrast, and more recently Hypaque). The selection of patients was primarily from those who did not improve with conservative management and in whom the question of low back surgery was considered.

He reported a series of 244 patients who were followed for a minimum of 4 years and a maximum of 10 years. A fraction less than half of these patients (46.7%) obtained permanent remission from this injection or at most a minor backache on occasion; a fraction more than half (53.3%) either showed no initial response or suffered recurrence of symptoms from 1 week to 6 years later. The patients whose pain was primarily in the back rather than radicular, those mainly within the older age groups, seemed to do better. One intervertebral disc space infection was reported as a complication.

On the basis of these reports it seems that the patients with primarily low back pain without sciatic radiation do better with the intradiscal injection of hydrocortisone, while those with radicular symptoms are best served by intervertebral discolysis.

Some authorities object to the use of hydrocortisone in degenerative disc disease, since hydrocortisone, which is widely used in the treatment of soft tissue injuries of all kinds, by its action inhibits fibrous tissue formation and as a result in certain circumstances may help to prevent the formation of painful scarring. If one presumes that the eventual desired result in a degenerative disc lesion is to establish formation of a stable fibrous tissue reaction, locally injecting hydrocortisone into the disc would appear to run counter to this desired end result.

PROLOTHERAPY

In 1956, a monograph was published indicating that the cause of low back pain in many patients was relaxation of the ligaments about the joints of the spine and pelvis.[1] Dr. George S. Hackett, the author of this text, proposed that as a result of "strain, sprain, tearing or degeneration" a weakening of the fibrous tissue at the fibro-osseous junction occurs, causing relaxation of the affected ligaments, impairing the stability of the joints supported by these "incompetent" ligaments and resulting in a painful disability. He defined ligament relaxation as a "condition in which the strength of the ligament fibers has become impaired so that a stretching of the fibrous strands occurs when the ligament is submitted to normal or less than normal tension." The treatment advocated by Dr. Hackett was the intraligamentous injection of a sclerosing solution to develop a maximum amount of fibrous tissue and bone, thereby affording joint stabilization. He called his method "prolotherapy" based on the Latin *proli* meaning offspring, from which the word proliferate derives. He implied by this term "the rehabilitation of an incompetent structure by the generation of new cellular tissue."

Proliferating Solutions

Several proliferating solutions can be used. Sylnasol (G. D. Searle & Co.) is a solution of the sodium salt of a psyllium oil fatty acid. For office treatment, this is combined with an equal amount of local anesthetic solution, usually 1 percent Xylocaine. For hospitalized patients, the Sylnasol is combined with normal saline, which apparently is productive of a greater amount of reactive fibrous tissue and bone. The increased pain appreciated in the absence of a local anesthetic is controlled by the administration of analgesics in the hospital.

Zinc sulfate may be used in combination with either phenol or Pontocaine, or a combination of all three (zinc sulfate, phenol, and Pontocaine).

A dextrose proliferating solution, which is said to give adequate fibro-osseous proliferation with a minimum of discomfort, can be made up by a pharmacist as follows:

Dextrose BP	25.0%
Phenol BP	2.5%
Glycerine BP	25.0%
Distilled water to	100.0%

This solution, which is "self-sterilizing," may be placed in 100 cc. rubber-stoppered bottles. Prior to injection 1 part of this solution is mixed with 3 parts of 1 percent Xylocaine.

Injection Technique

The injection technique utilizes a 22-gauge Luerlock needle of sufficient length to contact bone at the site of the fibro-osseous attachment. The needle is attached to a 10 cc. syringe containing the sclerosing solution combined with a local anesthetic solution. After inserting the needle to contact bone within the fibro-osseous attachment, 0.25 cc. to 1.0 cc. of solution is injected, the needle is withdrawn sufficiently to redirect without bending and recontact bone at approximately one-half inch distance from the original injection. Usually, 3 to 8 injections are made through one cutaneous needle insertion, depending on the size of the area and the amount of solution injected at each needle placement. Forced aspiration prior to injection is stressed, as is the dictum "always touch bone" during the injection.[4] These precautions are taken to avoid inadvertent injection into a blood vessel, nerve root or the subarachnoid space.

Site of Injection

Selection of injection site is based on rather unique guidelines and diagnostic criteria formulated by Dr. Hackett. Confirmation of this diagnosis is obtained during the intraligamentous needling by the precipitation of intense trigger point pain, which disappears within 2 minutes from the effect of the local anesthetic solution.

Posterior sacroiliac "relaxation" is identified by local tenderness over the sacroiliac joint in association with referred pain to the "outer anterior thigh and the outer side of the leg."[2] The treatment for posterior sacroiliac "relaxation" is injection of sclerosing solution into the fibro-osseous attachment of the posterior sacroiliac, sacrospinous and sacrotuberous ligaments.

Other ligaments which are presumably prone to "relaxation" and require treatment with injection are the interspinous ligaments, the lumbosacral ligaments and the lumbar articular capsular ligaments.

Some advocates of this method are less selective in their approach and, rather than injecting one specific ligament, will treat "the entire low back area." This involves injecting the intraspinous ligaments from the third lumbar to the first sacral vertebra, the lumbar articular capsular ligaments, the sacroiliac, sacrosciatic and sacrotuberous ligaments. Injections are made at weekly intervals until all of the ligaments are injected, doing as "many as the patient permits or the operator feels the patient can tolerate." After a series of from 3 to 6 weekly injections is completed, a "rest period" of 6 to 8 weeks is suggested, after which the patient may return for monthly "follow-up" injections for recurrent pain.

Postinjection pain is treated with substantial doses of Demerol.

The advocates of this method consider all patients with low back pain suitable candidates, including those who have previously undergone surgery.

Complications

After publication of Dr. Hackett's monograph in 1956, a number of physicians involved in the management of low back problems explored this method of treatment. Generally, the results were disappointing, much below the 82 percent improvement rate reported by Dr. Hackett. On the heels of indifferent results, two reports of serious complications arising from this method were published in *Journal of the American Medical Association;* the first in August, 1959, and the second a year later.[3,4]

The first case involved a 50-year-old woman with a long history of lumbar and sciatic pain who improved on two occasions on a regimen of pelvic traction, bed boards, bed rest, a back brace and sedation. Following each remission of pain, she developed intermittent recurrence of her symptoms. In June of 1957 she underwent interligamentous injection of sclerosing agent. The patient was placed in a prone position and the sclerosing agent (zinc sulfate in 2.5% phenol solution) was injected in the midline into the ligaments about the lumbosacral joint. She developed immediate severe pain in the legs, became paralyzed from the waist downward and had loss of bladder control. On attempting to arise from the table she fell to the floor. She gradually regained almost complete use of her legs over the next few days but required an indwelling catheter for bladder function and cleansing enemas for bowel care. On October 27 of 1957, she was readmitted to the hospital complaining of nausea, vomiting, paresthesias over the buttocks and legs, perioral numbness, blurred vision, headaches and generalized malaise. She had developed diplopia due to a right sixth nerve palsy. On examining the fundi, two diopters of papilledema were found, with retinal hemorrhages and engorged retinal veins bilaterally. She had a mild peripheral facial paresis on the right, progressive weakness of the right leg, nuchal rigidity and slurred speech. A diagnosis of basilar adhesive arachnoiditis was made. On November 1, 1957, ventriculograms demonstrated a widely dilated ventricular system, and a ventriculostomy was performed to gradually reduce the markedly increased intracranial pressure. On November 4, 1957, exploration of the posterior fossa was performed, which revealed a markedly adhesive arachnoiditis about the rim of the cisterna magna. Technical difficulties were encountered during surgery, and the patient died several hours after surgery. The immediate cause of death was an extradural hematoma in the occipital area, which was a complication of the suboccipital craniectomy. In addition to the changes secondary to surgery, chronic changes involving the spine and brain were attributed to the introduction of sclerosing solution into the subarachnoid space. Adhesive arachnoiditis and chronic scarification were found in the cauda equina, spinal cord, medulla, cerebellopontine angle and the base of the brain.

The second case report of a serious complication of this method involved a 53-year-old woman suffering from low back pain. In March, 1957, she received an injection of "vegetable oil and anesthetic" into each sacroiliac region. After the injection, she developed severe pain which radiated from the site of injection around to the anterior and medial aspect of both thighs and down the medial aspect of the lower extremities to the ankles. The pain in the sacroiliac region persisted for three weeks, but the radiating pain into the lower extremities subsided by the next morning. In May, 1957, she received two more injections into each sacroiliac area

and a third injection into "one side of the spine." She immediately experienced severe pain in the low back, which radiated down both legs, and a numbness over her body below the umbilicus. When she tried to walk, her legs would not support her; and she was unable to urinate for several hours. These symptoms subsided by the next morning. One week later she awakened with a severe headache which recurred daily for two weeks. During this period she had a stiff neck and pain in the right shoulder. In July 1957, she began to drag both feet as she walked, and within three or four weeks she required a cane and had to hold onto furniture or walls. Numbness returned to her lower extremities and grew more severe. In August, 1957, a lumbar myelogram was normal except for an elevated spinal fluid protein of 68 mg. percent. In September, 1957, she was unable to walk. Urinary frequency and occasional incontinence developed; finally, she could not urinate and became severely constipated. By October, 1957, the patient had complete spastic paraplegia with the usual reflex changes. There was analgesia below the fifth rib on the left side and the sixth on the right, complete anesthesia from the eighth thoracic through the third lumbar dermatomes on the left side, and hypesthesia in the remainder of the analgesic area. Vibratory sensibility, sense of position and the perception of numbers written on the skin were all absent bilaterally below the costal margins. Roentgenographic examination revealed a small residue of radiopaque material in the spinal canal at the level of the sixth thoracic vertebra. This did not move as the patient was tipped on the fluoroscopic table.

On October 7, 1957, a laminectomy of the fifth, sixth, and seventh thoracic vertebrae was performed. The dura was closely adherent to the underlying structures throughout the area exposed by the laminectomy, and a subarachnoid cyst was evacuated at the level of the sixth thoracic vertebra and considerable thickened arachnoidal tissue was cut away, including the walls of the cyst.

Following surgery the patient's condition

improved slightly, but soon the spastic paraplegia returned to its original intensity and ultimately grew more severe.

The microscopic examination of the surgical specimens revealed adhesive arachnoiditis.

Present Status of "Prolotherapy"

The authors of the two case reports were critical of this method both as regard to the authenticity of its value and to the potential dangers. It was emphasized that "there are areas in the lower part of the back where a needle can accidentally and easily enter the subarachnoid space. This can occur directly at the lumbosacral joint or laterally at the dural sleeve of the spinal nerve root."

After the second case report was published in 1960, the number of physicians utilizing this method declined sharply; but in the past few years it has enjoyed a mild revival. Most of the patients referred to me who had previously received this treatment did not seem to demonstrate any beneficial deviation from the expected natural course of their dysfunction. Such unevenly weighted material may lead to a biased conclusion, but my overall personal opinion of the technique is not favorable.

FACET RHIZOTOMY

In 1971 Dr. W. E. Shyrme Rees, an Australian physician, reported on a large series of cases with low back and sciatic pain which he treated with an original and unique technique of cutting the nerve rootlets to the spinal facets.[5,6] Dr. C. Norman Shealy of LaCrosse, Wisconsin, impressed by the excellent results, invited Dr. Rees to the United States to demonstrate his procedure. Encouraged by the results of the technique, he performed the Rees procedure on 29 patients. Dr. Shealy subsequently modified this procedure, using a radio frequency lesion rather than a scalpel to perform the rhizotomy.

Principle of Facet Rhizotomy

Many patients with low back pain, who have extension of this pain into a lower extremity, present with sciatic symptoms which are often more diffuse and vague than the characteristic "single root syndrome" associated with nerve root compression. Such nonspecific leg pain does not remain within the distribution of a single root and is usually not associated with reflex changes or valid motor weakness. It is speculated that "facet dysfunction" may be a factor in these problems. A clinical finding associated with facet dysfunction is acute tenderness to pressure over the affected facet. Sometimes this pressure will reproduce not only pain within the back but aggravate extension of the pain into a lower extremity. It is further speculated that the facet dysfunction may occur from derangement and instability of the facet joint, resulting from overriding secondary to a collapsed degenerated intervertebral disc.

The clinical success of this procedure in selected cases causes one to speculate upon the entire symptom complex of many patients with low back and leg pain. It reemphasizes the importance of strict correlation of myelographic findings with the clinical findings before a determination is made that the patient's symptoms are primarily due to a protruding lumbar disc causing the root pressure. Further speculation is invited regarding the clinical improvement occasionally derived from prolotherapy (injection of sclerosing solution). It is possible that sclerosing solution injected in the vicinity of the articular facet is associated with clinical improvement, not because of a beneficial effect on the stability of the facet joint, but is due to destruction of the nerve rootlet innervating the facet.

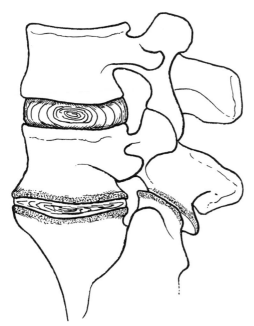

Fig. 17-1. Facet joint "over-riding" secondary to the collapsed degenerated intervertebral disc.

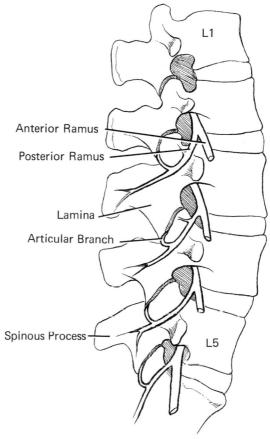

Fig 17-2. Diagrammatic representation of the articular rootlets entering the capsule of the intervertebral joints. (*After* Pedersen, Blunck, Gardener.)[9]

Technique of Facet Rhizotomy

The technique advocated by Dr. Rees involves making a deep stab incision 2 cc. lateral to the spinous process. This incision is extended just lateral to the articular facet to the level of the transverse process, at which level a sweep of the tip of the knife blade is made to assure sectioning of the facet innervation. A determination as to the site of the stab incision is made primarily by the sites of tenderness to deep pressure over the facets. Following this type of stab incision, a considerable hematoma often developed in the paraspinal muscles of the lumbar region, particularly if this procedure was carried out at multiple levels.

Because of the excessive subcutaneous bleeding that occurred in two patients, Dr. Shealy modified the procedure. Using fluoroscopic and x-ray control, a radio frequency electrode is inserted down to the intertransverse ligament slightly lateral to the facets. Local anesthesia is used only to make a skin wheal with no anesthetic injected into the

deeper tissues. Avoidance of deep local anesthetic will allow a further clinical correlation of the facet syndrome, since when the electrode reaches the intertransverse ligament it invariably elicits pain similar to that which the patient originally complained of.

Electrical stimulation with a pulse of 1 millisecond duration, 25 to 50 cycles, evokes tingling at 1 to 2 volts, pain at 2 to 4 volts. If the electrode is inserted too deeply and is impinging upon the nerve root, pain will occur with less than 1 volt and muscle contractions will occur at 1 or 2 volts. This test is done to avoid damaging the root with a radio frequency lesion. A further safety

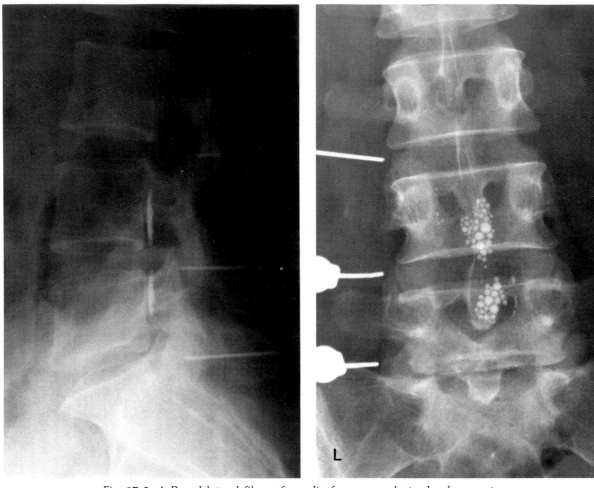

Fig. 17-3. A-P and lateral films of a radio frequency electrode placement.

check is a lateral Polaroid x-ray film to confirm that the depth of electrode penetration is short of the intervertebral foramen and the exiting nerve root.

After the electrode is positioned to satisfaction, a radio frequency generator is activated with the power raised slowly to produce a temperature of 70° centigrade at the electrode tip for 90 seconds. If the elevation of the temperature to 70° is excessively painful, the temperature is reduced to 50°; and after a minute at this temperature, it can then usually be raised to 70° with little or no discomfort.

This procedure using x-ray guidance and radio frequency technique has been utilized for less than a year. My personal experience with this procedure involves 18 patients who had low back and sciatic pain; 10 of these patients were surgical failures; 8 had never previously been subjected to surgery but had normal myelograms; 4 appreciated significant relief of their symptoms; 3 were somewhat improved but continued to have some degree of low back dysfunction; 11 were unimproved. There have been no complications with this procedure to date.

The newness of the procedure and lack of long-term follow-up leaves many questions unanswered. However, in view of what appears to be initially significant results, it can be hoped that this procedure will be useful and play a helpful role in the management of certain forms of low back dysfunction.

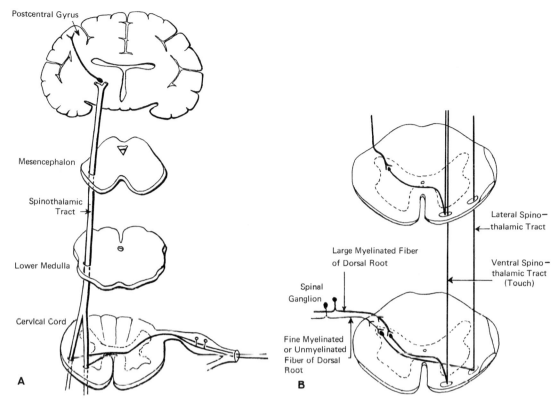

Fig. 17-4. Diagrammatic illustration of the traditional concept of pain conduction. (Courtesy of W. B. Saunders.)

DORSAL COLUMN STIMULATION

This technique is based on a theory of pain mechanism advanced in 1965 by Dr. Ronald Melzack, Professor of Psychology, McGill University, Montreal, Canada, and Dr. Patrick D. Wall, Professor of Psychology, M.I.T., Cambridge, Massachusetts. This theory has been popularly referred to as the "gate theory of pain transmission," and it introduced a number of new concepts regarding pathways of pain. The traditional concept of pain conduction implied that the pain impulses were transmitted into the spinal cord through the dorsal roots and once reaching the cord crossed within several spinal segments to the opposite anterolateral quadrant of the cord. Fibers within the anterolateral quadrant of the cord gathered into a specific bundle identified as the spinothalamic tract, which conducted pain sensa-

tion upward to the thalamus. The anatomical basis of this concept of pain transmission was developed by tracing neural pathways, using the traditional method of following the course of myelin sheath and nerve degeneration with a variety of silver tissue stains and other histologic techniques. These traditional anatomical degenerative studies presented a rather simplistic pain pathway schema and did not allow for consideration of the multiple synaptic connections within the cord and the fact that most of the pain input fibers were of the smaller, unmyelinated type.

It has been demonstrated that pain impulses are transmitted to the spinal cord by way of the smaller gamma-delta or C-fibers, and that stimulation of the larger A-beta fibers is never painful. Physiologically, the painful response consists of prolonged firing

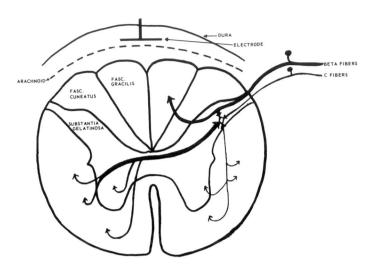

Fig. 17-5. Diagrammatic illustration of the synapse between the large beta fibers and the small C-fibers. Note the position of the stimulating electrode over the dorsal columns. (Shealy, Long, Kahn Pan-Pacific Surgical Association, 1972.)

of many units activating the C-fibers throughout the entire spinal axis, through the medulla into the medial reticular formation of the midbrain, with projections into the cerebellum. It is theorized that activity in the larger beta fibers inhibits at the first spinal synapse immediate subsequent activity from the smaller C-fibers considered essential to pain production. Melzack and Wall suggested that this mechanism normally acts as a gate to balance the input of pain and non-pain sensations. Wall and Sweet tested this theory by employing low-voltage electrical stimulation to the large fibers within a peripheral nerve and reported inhibition of the response to C-fiber input. Painful stimuli to a site within the sensory distribution of the nerve were not appreciated as pain so long as electrical stimulation to the large fibers continued. Conversely, it can be demonstrated that if one blocks the large and intermediate beta-gamma and delta peripheral nerve fibers there is an increase in the amount of the prolonged after-discharge with stimulation of the isolated C-fiber in a peripheral nerve.

Because most pain arises from diffusely injured tissues, and it is impractical to use peripheral nerve stimulation for control of such pain, it was logical to extend experimental work to a more central transmission site of pain; namely, the spinal cord. Since the dorsal columns within the spinal cord contain an almost pure and concentrated grouping of beta fibers, Dr. Shealy hypothesized that the dorsal columns offered the best site for selective stimulation of pain fibers. Experimentally, he applied a stimulating current to the dorsal column of cats; and during such dorsal column stimulation, noxious stimuli did not provoke any apparent pain response in conscious animals. However, if the noxious stimulus was continued and the dorsal column stimulation removed, the experimental animals would react with the normal violent reaction within 5 seconds of cessation of dorsal stimulation. This technique was subsequently applied to human patients with chronic intractable pain.

Prior to the technical implementation of the Melzack-Wall theory, the treatment of chronic intractable pain relied mainly on procedures involving destruction of some portion of the pain transmitting pathway (thalamotomy, cordotomy, rhizotomy, neurectomy) or the use of narcotics in progressively increasing dosage. The goal of dorsal column stimulation is to interfere with pain impulses without destroying any portion of the pain conduction system.

Indications

The prime indication for the application of a dorsal column stimulator is the long-

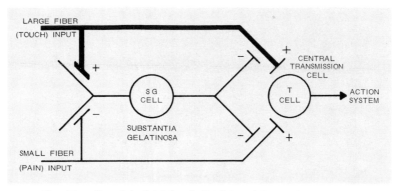

Fig. 17-6. Simplified Melzack-Wall Model. (Medtronic, Inc.)

standing and intractable nature of the pain. The pain should not be amenable to the more traditional methods of managment. For example, in the management of a patient with low back pain secondary to malignancy, if the neoplasm is x-ray sensitive, a trial of radiation is in order prior to consideration of this method. When this device is considered for patients with low back and sciatic pain, who have been failures following disc surgery, a most exhaustive and prying study is required. It must be well established that further low back surgery, or other treatment locally to the involved root or nerve roots, would be fruitless.

Psychoneurosis of severe degree is a significant contraindication to use of a dorsal column stimulator. Narcotic addiction of long-standing duration is a contraindication; however, the severity of the pain should be such that it is refractory to non-narcotic drug therapy. The physician should be particularly hesitant to use this device in those patients whose pain is unusual, suspected of being nonorganic and without any definite explainable etiology.

Routine preoperative screening of the patient involves both psychological and psychiatric evaluation, including the Minnesota Multiphasic Personality Inventory (MMPI). Patients with MMPI's showing elevations or depressions of 2 or more standard deviations in 4 or more personality scales are generally considered poor candidates for dorsal column stimulation. It must be realized, how-

ever, that some patients often have changes in the MMPI related to their long-standing suffering, so that absolute values and rigid standards relating to emotional factors are difficult to establish.

An essential preoperative screening factor is the patient's response to some form of trial electrical stimulation. In most instances, this is easily done by applying skin electrodes at sites which will induce a tingling sensation in some portion of the painfully involved area. Often, a patient who will derive significant improvement from dorsal column stimulation will also appreciate some degree of improvement within the limited anatomical area affected by transcutaneous stimulation. Of even greater importance are those patients who will find the transcutaneous stimulation unpleasant, since they will almost invariably have a poor result from the dorsal column stimulator.

Surgical Technique

Clinical evaluation results indicate that the stimulating electrode is best placed 4 to 6 spinal segments above the highest pain input, and the site of preference for low back and sciatic pain is the third to fourth thoracic level.

With the patient in the sitting position, a laminectomy of T3, 4 and 5 is performed. The bony removal is carried out to the facets to assure adequate exposure of the dura mater to position the electrode. After this portion of the procedure has been completed,

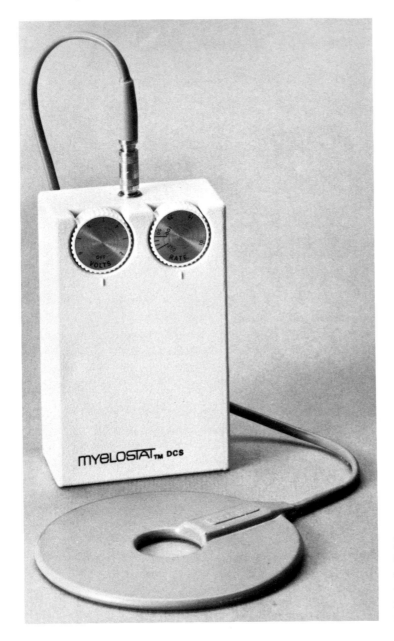

Fig. 17-7. Radiofrequency transmitter and antenna. The antenna is taped onto the skin directly over the subcutaneously implanted receiver. (Medtronic, Inc.)

with all bleeding controlled, a sponge is lightly packed within the laminectomy wound and the subclavicular receiver site is prepared.

A 3-inch transverse incision is made over the right clavical and a small subcutaneous pocket, just large enough to accommodate the receiver, is developed beneath the lower flap of the clavicular incision. With blunt dissection, using a long double-curved uterine packing forceps, a subcutaneous tunnel is extended from the clavicular incision, over the right shoulder to the laminectomy site. Through this tunnel, a one-quarter-inch Penrose drain is passed, and using the drain as a guide, the electrode is pulled back through the tunnel into the laminectomy incision.

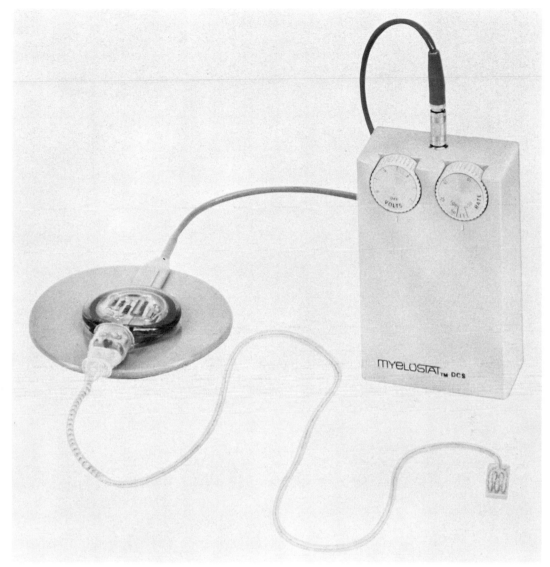

Fig. 17-8. The radio frequency transmitter-antenna, together with the receiver and electrode. (Medtronic, Inc.)

The dura is then opened in the midline, and the electrode is positioned over the dorsal columns between the dura and the arachnoid. The electrode is secured in place using 4 sutures at each corner, and closure of the wound is carried out in the usual fashion.

Postoperatively, the transmitting antenna is placed on the skin overlying the receiver and dorsal column stimulation is instituted with a radio frequency transmitter. When the transmitter is activated, the patient appreciates a tingling sensation below the level of electrode implantation and simultaneous reduction of pain. Patients have individually varying needs regarding duration and frequency of stimulation from several times daily to almost constant stimulation.

In addition to the use of this mechanical appliance, the patient requires considerable

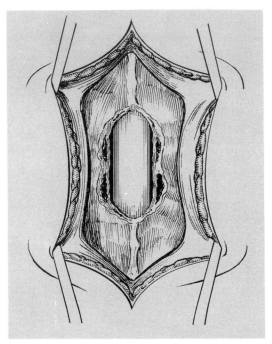

Fig. 17-9. Thoracic laminectomy. (Medtronic, Inc.)

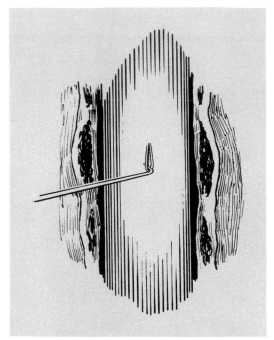

Fig. 17-11. Opening dura in midline. (Medtronic, Inc.)

support to be helped to withdraw from narcotics as rapidly as possible; and in addition, a total program of physical and emotional rehabilitation is generally necessary.

After five years of clinical experience, this device, though still experimental, seems to hold promise for certain selected chronic low back pain problems.

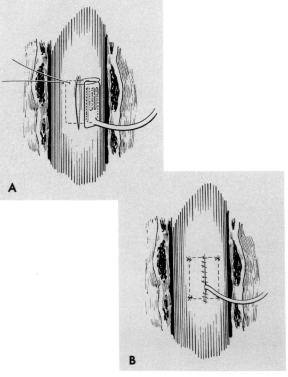

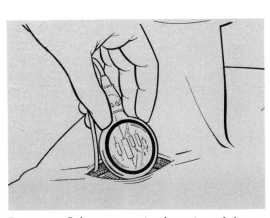

Fig. 17-10. Subcutaneous implantation of the receiver below the right clavicle. (Medtronic, Inc.)

Fig. 17-12. Electrode placement. (Medtronic, Inc.)

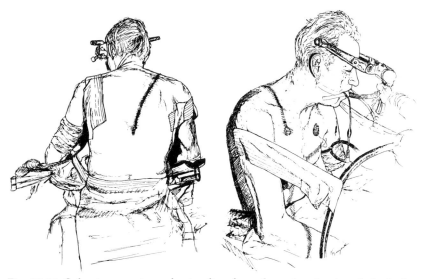

Fig. 17-13. Subcutaneous tunnel extending from thoracic spine to subclavicular region.

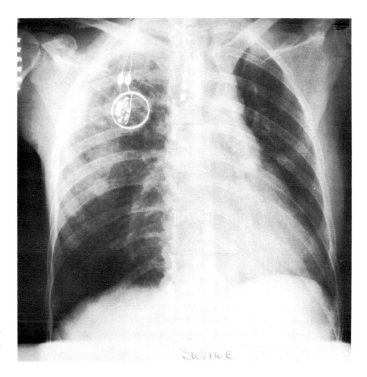

Fig. 17-14. X-ray of implanted spinal cord electrode and sub-cutaneous receiver.

REFERENCES

1. Feffer, H. L.: Thapeutic Intradiscal hydrocortisone Symposium Chemonuclolysis, Clin. Orthop., No. 67, 1969.
2. Ford, L. T.: Clinical use of Chymopapain in lumbar and dorsal disk lesions, Symposium Chemonucleolysis, Clinical Orthop., No. 67, 1969.
3. Garvin, P. J., Jennings, R. B., Smith, L., and Gesler, R. M.: Chymopapain: A pharmacologic and toxicologic evaluation in experimental animals, Clin. Orthop., 41:204, 1965.
4. Hackett, G. S.: Joint Ligament Relaxation Treated by Fibro-osseous Proliferation with Special Reference to Low Back Disability—Trigger Point Pain and Referred Pain, Springfield, Ill., Charles C Thomas, 1956.
5. Hackett, G. S., and Huang, T. C.: Prolotherapy of sciatica from weak pelvic ligaments and bone dystrophy. Clinical Medicine, Vol. 8, No. 12, Dec., 1961.
6. Jansen, E. F., and Balls, A. K.: Chymopapain: A new crystalline protease from Papayalatex, J. Biol. Chem., 137:459, 1941.
7. Keplinger, J. E., and Bucy, P. C. Paraplegia from treatment with sclerosing agents. JAMA, 173:1333, 1960.
8. Myers, A.: Prolotherapy treatment of low back pain and sciatica. Bulletin of the Hospital for Joint Disease. 22:48, 1961.
9. Pedersen, H. E., Blunck, S. F. J., and Gardner, E.: The anatomy of lumbosacral posterior rami and meningeal branches of the spinal nerves (Sinu-vertebral nerves). J. Bone Joint Surg. 38A:377, 1956.
10. Rees, W. E. Shyrme: Multiple bilateral subcutaneous rhizolysis of segmental nerves in the treatment of the intervertebral disc syndrome. Ann. Gen. Tract 16:126, 1971.
11. Schneider, R. C., Williams, J. J., and Liss, L.: Fatality after injection of sclerosing agent to precipitate fibro-osseous proliferation. JAMA, 170:1768, 1959.
12. Shealy, C. N.: Tissue reaction to chymopapain in cats, J. Neurosurg., 26:327, 1967.
13. Smith, L.: Enzyme dissolution of the nucleus pulposus in humans, JAMA, 187:137, 1964.
14. Smith, L., and Brown, J. E.: Treatment of lumbar intervertebral disc lesions by direct injection of chymopapain, Bone Joint Surg., 49B:502, 1967.
15. Smith, L., Garvin, P. J., Jennings, R. B., and Gesler, R. M.: Enzyme dissolution of the nucleus pulpous, Nature, 198:1311, 1963.
16. Stern, I. J., and Smith, L.: Dissolution by chymopapain in vitro of tissue from normal or prolapsed intervertebral disks, Clin. Orthop., 50:269, 1966.

Index

Page numbers printed in *italic* type refer to illustrations.

Abdominal cavity, as spinal support, 31–33, *32*
Abdominal strength, evaluation of, 118–119, *119*
Abductors, of lumbar spine, 23
Acetophenetidin, 108
Acetylsalicylic acid, 107–108
Achilles reflexes, examination of, 44, *43*
Achilles tendon, shortened, exercise for, 136, *136*
Achondroplasia, in dogs, 271
  spinal abnormalities in, 270–271
  spinal degenerative changes in, 271
  stenotic lumbar spinal canal in, myelography in, 271
    signs and symptoms of, 271
    treatment of, 272
Adaptation, definition of, 80
  reactions to pain and, 80
Adhesive arachnoiditis. *See* Arachnoiditis, adhesive
Alcohol, as analgesic, 111
Alphaprodine hydrochloride, 107
Amnion, in embryonic development, 3, *3*
Analgesic blocks, 238–248
Analgesic drugs, non-narcotic, 107–109
  synthetic addicting, 106–107
Anesthesia, in Cloward technique of disc removal, 219
  levels of, amount of anesthetic for, *246*
  for lumbar disc surgery, 177, *180*
  spinal, adhesive arachnoiditis and, 332
Anesthetic, surface, as physiotherapy, 99, *99*
Anileridine, 107
Ankle, plantar flexion strength of, testing of, 46, *46*
Annulus fibrosus, anterior portion of, calcification of, 158–159
  composition and function of, 11–12, *11, 12*
  development of, 6, *5*
  incision of, in lumbar disc surgery, 196, *196*
  in intervertebral disc biomechanics, 26–28, *27*
  in lumbar spondylosis, 264–265, *264, 265*
  and spinal compression, 30, *30*
Anti-inflammatory drugs, 109–111
Aorta, lesions of, low back pain in, 324–325
  relationship of, to anterior lumbar spine, *198*
Arachnoiditis, adhesive, 332
  basilar, following myelography, 59
  following myelography, 59
  following prolotherapy, 355, *356*
Artery(ies), intersegmental, in embryo, 3, *4*
  lesions of, low back pain in, 324–325
  pulses of, assessment of, in physical examination, 48

Arthritis, of hips, 332–333
  hypertrophic. *See* Spondylosis, lumbar
Articulation(s). *See* Joint(s)
Aspirin, 107–108
Athletics, reactions to pain and, 81–82

Back, lower. *See* Low back
Backache, nonorganic, 88–92
  apocryphal diagnosis in, 88–89
  suspected, management of, 89, 92
  preexisting, as symptom in lumbar disc disease, 141–144
Bed rest, mobilization following, 96–97
  positions in, 95–96, *96*
  ineffective, 95, *95*
  prolonged, adverse effects of, 96
  rules for, 96
Biopsy of spine, closed, 314
Bleeding, from epidural veins, following lumbar disc surgery, control of, 202–203, *199*
  skin, in lumbar disc surgery, control of, 187–189
  in surgery of spinal cord tumors, control of, 316, 317–318
Block(s), analgesic, 238–248
  caudal, 240–246, *244, 245*
  lateral femoral cutaneous nerve, 331–332, *331*
  lumbar epidural, 238–240, *239*
  obturator nerve, 326–327, *329*
  paravertebral, 246–248, *247, 248*
Blood, supply, of lumbar spine, 17–18, *17*
Bone, functions of, 290
Bone grafting in posterior lumbar interbody fusion, 231–233, *232, 233, 234*
Bone grafts for posterior lumbar interbody fusion, 230–231, *231*
Brace(s), "chair back," 124–125, 129, *128*
  Knight spinal, 124–125, 129, *128*
  low back, advantages of, 126
  history of, 124–125
  "three-point pressure" principle of, 127–129, *127*
  Taylor spinal, 124, 129–130, *129*
  Williams lordosis, 127–129, *127, 128*
Butazolidin, 109–110

Carcinoma, metastatic. *See* Metastatic disease of spine
Carisoprodol, 111
Cartilaginous end-plates, and spinal compression, 30, *30*

367

Cauda equina syndrome, 205–207, *201, 202–203*
  in lumbar spondylosis with stenotic lumbar spinal
    canal, 268
  surgical technique for, 207–208, *207*
Caudal block, 240–246
  complications of, 245–246
  technique in, 243–245, *244, 245*
Caudal sac, 241
  gradients, spinal manometer recording, 62, *62*
Cervical spine, bone-disc ratio of, *10*
  and root compression lesions, 11, *11*
Charcot's disease of spine, 336–337
Chlormezamone, 111
Chlorzoxazone, 111
Chymopain injection in intervertebral discolysis,
    350–352
  complications of, 351
  experiments in, 350
  indications for, 351
  results of, 351
  technique of, 350
Claudication, cauda equina, and vascular, compared,
    268, *268*
Cloward technique, of disc removal. *See* Intervertebral
    disc(s), lumbar, ruptured, Cloward technique in
  of lumbar fusion. *See* Lumbar spinal fusion,
      posterior interbody
Coccyx, anatomy of, 9, *9*
Codeine, 106
Collagenase injection in intervertebral discolysis, 352
Collis lumbar discography table, 72, *71*
Compression, axial, tests of, on lumbar spine, 29–30,
    29, 30
Compression fractures, lumbar, 31
Contrast studies, x-ray, 58–76
Corset(s), dorsolumbar, 132, *132*
  low back, 130–132, *130, 131, 132*
    advantages of, 126–127
  lumbosacral, 130–132, *131*
  sacroiliac, 130, *130*
Corticosteroids, 110
  intrathecal use of, 110–111
Cortisone, intrathecal, in lumbar disc operations, 227
Cuatico needle, in myelography, 68, *68*
Cysts, sacral, myelography in, 337–338, *340–341*
  surgical removal of, 337, 338, *338, 339*
    case history of, 341–342

Darvon, 108
Demerol, 106
Depo-Medrol, following myelography, 110–111
  intrathecal, in lumbar disc disease, 177
Dermatomes, lower extremity, 45, *44*
Dilaudid, 106
Disc(s), intervertebral. *See* Intervertebral disc(s)
  lumbar, disease of. *See* Lumbar disc disease
Discogram, interpretation of, 74, *73, 74*
Discography, advantages and disadvantages of, 75
  basic principles of, 69–70
  Collis table for, 72, *71*
  history of, 71
  lateral approach in, 74–75, *75*
  midline lumbar, injection of contrast material in,
    74, *72*
    interspace identification in, 72–73

needle placement in, 73–74, *72*
  positioning in, 72, *71*
  preparation of patient for, 72
  postmortem, 75
  role of, 76
Discolysis, intervertebral, 350–352
  indications for, 351
Dolophine, 106–107
Dorsal column stimulation, 359–365
  contraindications to, 361
  equipment in, 363, *362, 363, 364, 365*
  indications for, 360–361
  postoperative care in, 363–364
  surgical technique in, 361–363, *364, 365*
Dorsiflexion, of great toe, testing of, *45*
Dorsolumbar corset, 132, *132*
Driving, proper posture for, 116, *116*
Drug(s), analgesic, non-narcotic, 107–109
  synthetic addicting, 106–107
  anti-inflammatory, 109–111
  muscle relaxant, 111
  therapy, for hypochondriac or malingerer, 92

Electromyography, in lumbar disc disease, 156–157
Embryo, after second week, 2, *2*
  amnion of, 3, *3*
  at 3 or 4 weeks, *3, 4*
  at 8 or 9 weeks, *4*
  neural groove of, 3, *3*
  notochord of, 3, *3*
    obliteration of, 5–6, *5*
  1-week-old, 2, *2*
  primitive groove of, 3, *3*
  primitive segments of, 3, *3, 4*
  somites of, 3, *3, 4*
Emotions, reactions to pain and, 79–80
Epiphyseal ring, 11
Erector spinae, 19, *19*
Ethoheptazine citrate, 108
Evaluation of patient, 38–76
  examination in, arterial pulses in, 48
    gait in, 42–43
    hip rotation in, 47–48, *49*
    inspection in, 41–42, *41*
    leg length in, 44
    lumbar mobility in, 43, *42*
    motor strength in, 45–46, *45, 46*
    reflexes in, 44, *43, 44*
    sensation in, 44–45
    spinal pressure in, 48
    squatting in, 43–44, *42*
    straight leg raising in, 46–47, *47, 48*
  history in, 38–41
    past medical, 41
  malingering, examination in, 91–92
  x-ray contrast studies in, 58–76
  x-ray of lumbosacral spine in, 49–58
Exercise program, adaptation of, to specific needs of
    patient, 118
  establishment of, 120
  evaluation of muscle strength and flexibility prior
    to, 118–120, *119*
  hip flexor elasticity exercises in, 121, *121*
  low back exercises in, 121–124, *121, 122, 123, 124*
  pelvic "uplift" in, 120–121, *121*

purpose of, 117
    relaxation exercises in, 120
    when to start, 118
Exercises, in chronic lumbosacral strain, 136, *136*
Extensor(s), foot, weakness of, inspection for, 42, *41*
    knee joint, strength of, testing of, 46, *45*
    of lumbar spine, 19–20
External oblique muscle, 20–21, *21*
Extremities, lower, dermatomes of, 45, *44*

Fabere sign, 48, *49*
Facet rhizotomy, 356–358
Fajerstajn well leg raising test, *47*
Fascia, body, and musculature through third lumbar
    vertebra, *23*
Femur, dislocation of, sciatic trauma in, 325
Fetus, spine of, 7, *7*
    twelve-week, *5*
Filum terminale, 241
Flexion, lateral, in lumbar disc disease, test of,
    151–153
    lumbar, annulus, nerve root and intervertebral
        foramina in, *96*
    in lumbar disc disease, test of, 151
Flexor(s), knee joint, testing strength of, 46, *45*
    of lumbar spine, 20–23
    plantar, weakness of, inspection for, 42, *41*
Foot drop, partial, 39–40, *39*
Foot extensor weakness, inspection for, 42, *41*
Foramen(ina), intervertebral, stenosis of, in lumbar
    disc disease, 159–160, *160*
Foraminal root compression syndrome, 161–163, *160,
    161*
Forceps, intervertebral disc rongeur, 197–198, *197*
Fracture(s), compression, lumbar, 31
Fulcrum-lever concept, and stress on spine, 28, *28*

Gain factors, secondary, lumbar disc disease and,
    142–143
    malingerer and, 90–91
Gait, in lumbar disc disease, 151
    of malingerer, observation of, 91
    observation of, in physical examination, 42–43, *41*
Gill procedure in isthmic spondylolisthesis, 286–287

Hamstring elasticity, evaluation of, 119–120, *119*
Headache(s), postspinal, Depo-Medrol in reduction of,
    110–111
    postspinal, following myelography, 59
Heat, as physiotherapy, 98–99
Hemangiomas of spine, incidence of, 307
    pathology of, 307
    signs and symptoms of, 307–308
    treatment of, 308
    x-ray findings in, 307, *308–309*
Hemilaminectomy, in lumbar disc disease, 177
    retractors, for lumbar disc surgery, 190–192, *188,
    189*
Hip(s), arthritis of, 332–333
    flexor elasticity, exercises for, 121, *121*
    rotation, assessment of, in physical examination,
        47–48, *49*

Hydrocortisone, intradiscal injection of, in
    degeneration of intervertebral disc, 352–353
Hydromorphone, 106
Hyperesthesia, area of, in lumbar disc disease, *164,
    165, 166*
Hyperparathyroidism, 293
Hypnotherapy, 112
Hypochondriac, 89–90

"Ice lollipop" massage, 99, *99*
Iliohypogastric nerve, anatomy of, 328
    mechanism of injury to, 328–329
Ilioinguinal nerve, anatomy of, 328, *329*
    mechanism of injury to, 328–329
Ilium-transverse process, pseudoarthrosis of, 333, *332*
"Imaginary" pain, 78–79
Immobilization in management of infection of lumbar
    spine, 298
Indocin, 110
Indomethacin, 110
Infection(s), interspace, refractory, 298
    intervertebral disc space, 297–298
    of lumbar spine, nontuberculous, in adults, clinical
        picture of, 301–302
            disc space abcess in, case history of, 303
            management of, 302–303
            x-ray findings in, 302
        in children, case history of, 299–300
            clinical picture of, 300
            management of, 301
            process of, 300–301
            x-ray findings in, 301
        subsequent to lumbar disc surgery, 296–299
        without antecedent operations on spine, 299–305
    soft tissue, 296–297
Injection(s), chymopapain, in intervertebral discolysis.
    See Chymopapain injection in intervertebral
    discolysis
    collagenase, in intervertebral discolysis, 352
    intradiscal hydrocortisone, in degeneration of
        intervertebral disc, 352–353
    in prolotherapy, 353–354
    sciatic nerve trauma from, 325
Internal oblique muscle, 21, *21*
Interspinalis, 20, *21*
Intertransversarii, 20, *21*
Intervertebral disc(s), biochemical changes in, 26
    biomechanics of, 26–28, *27*
    collapsed, instability of facet joint and, 356, *357*
    degenerative effects of living and, 6
    development of, 5, *6*
    discolysis of, 350–352
    lumbar, blood supply of, 17–18
        bone-disc ratio of, 10–11, *10, 11*
            and root compression lesions, 11, *11*
        degeneration of, intradiscal hydrocortisone
            injection in, 352–353
        excision of, in lumbar disc surgery, 196–199, *196,
            197*
        free fragments of, location of, *148*
            removal of, 199–201, *199*
        lesions of, spinal fusion in. *See* Lumbar spinal
            fusion

Intervertebral disc(s), biochemical changes in (*cont.*)
     massive extrusion of, 205–207, *201, 202–203*
          surgical technique in, 207–208, *207*
     midline protrusion of, transdural excision of,
          indications for, 208–209, *206*
               technique in, 209–210, *208, 209, 210*
     pressure measurements in, 33–35, *34*
     ruptured, Cloward technique in, articular facets
          in, 226
               disc removal in, 224–227, *223, 225*
               fascia incision in, 219–220, *221*
               instruments for, 226, *220, 221, 222, 223, 224,
                    225*
               ligamentum flavum and laminae in, 220–224,
                    226, *221, 222, 223, 224, 226*
               position and anesthesia in, 219, *219*
               skin incision in, 219, 226, *219, 220*
          interlaminar operation in, 218
     structure of, 11–12, *11, 12*
     traction and, 98, *97*
narrowing of, 58
protrusion of, nerve root compression in, 8–9, *8*
space, abscess in nontuberculous infection, case
          history of, 303
     infections, management of, 298
          signs and symptoms of, 297–298
     narrowing of, in lumbar disc disease, 157–158,
          158
and vertebrae, 6–7
Intra-abdominal vascular disease, low back pain in,
          324–325

Joint(s), amphiarthrodial, 10, *10*
     arthrodial, 10, 13, 14, *10, 13, 14*
     diastasis of, in pregnancy, 324
     facet, "over-riding," 356, *357*
     intervertebral, articular rootlets entering capsule of,
          357
          complete fibrous ankylosis of, in lumbar
               spondylosis, 265, *266*
          spondylosis of, in lumbar spondylosis, 264, *265*
     knee, extensor strength of, testing of, 46, *45*
          flexor strength of, testing of, 46, *45*
     of lumbar spine, 10–15
     lumbosacral, *9*
     pelvic-vertebral, 15–17, *16*
     sacrococcygeal, 17
     sacroiliac, 17
     vertebral arch, 13–15, *13*
     vertebral body, 10–13

Knee, joint, extensor strength of, testing of, 46, *45*
     flexor strength of, testing of, 46, *45*
Knight spinal brace, 124–125, 129, *128*

Laminectomy, in achondroplasia with stenotic lumbar
          spinal canal, 272
     in cauda equina syndrome, 207, *207*
     complete, reexploration following, 215, *214*
     in dorsal column stimulation, 361, *364*
     in lumbar disc disease, 177
     in posterior lumbar rhizotomy, 250, *250*
     in spinal cord tumors, 316–317, *316, 317*

Lasègue test, 46–47, *46*
Lateral bony recess, 8–9, *8*
Lateral femoral cutaneous nerve, *331*
     block of, 331–332, *331*
     neuralgia of, 330–332
Leg(s), length, examination of, in pain, 44
     passive straight raising of, in manipulative therapy,
          104, *105*
     straight raising test of, in lumbar disc disease, 156
          in physical examination, 46–47, *47, 48*
Leptomeningitis, aseptic, 60
Leritine, 107
Levo-Dromoran, 106
Levoprome, 108–109
Levorphanol tartrate, 106
Lifting, proper posture for, 116, *116*
Ligament(s), anterior longitudinal, composition of, 12,
          12
     capsular, 14, *14*
     interspinal, 15, *15*
          injection of, 269, *270*
     intertransverse, 15, *15*
     lateral vertebral, composition of, 13, *13*
     of lumbar spine, 10–15
     pelvic, 17, *16*
     posterior longitudinal, composition of, 13, *12, 13*
     relaxation, prolotherapy in, 353–356
     supraspinal, 15, *15*
     yellow, 14–15, *14*
Lordosis, lumbar, annulus, nerve root and
          intervertebral foramina in, *96*
     flattening of, and sciatic scoliosis, 149–151, *149,
          150*
     increased, *113*
          impacted spinous processes in, 269, *269*
          low back pain and, 57
     reduction of, 112–117
Low back, anatomy of, 2–23
     development of, 2–7
     dysfunction, psychology of, 78–92
     exercises. *See* Exercise program
     manipulation of, in lumbar disc disease, 170
     mechanics, 125
     musculature of, 19–23
Low back pain, conservative treatment of, 95–132
     eliciting history of, 38–39
     examination of patient with, 41–48
     experimental and unorthodox treatments for,
          349–366
     management of, evaluation of, 349–350
          nonsurgical, 95–117
     nonorganic. *See* Backache, nonorganic
     uncommon causes of, 323–342
Lumbar disc disease, 141–216
     ankylosing spondylitis and, 336
     degenerative changes as cause of, 158–160
     disc protrusion in, clinical differentiation of level
          of, 167t
          clinical pattern(s) of, *164, 165, 166*
          L1-2 level, *166*
          L2-3 level, *165*
          L3-4 level, *165, 172*
          L4-5 level, *150, 152–153, 154, 158–159, 164,
               170–171, 172, 174–175, 176*
          L5-S1 level, *146–147, 164, 172*
          T12-L1 level, *166*

electromyography in, 156–157
gait in, 151
history of trauma in, 143–144
intervertebral disc space narrowing in, 157–158, *158*
lesion in, side of, 177
level of, clinical differentiation of, 167t
management of, conservative, 168–171
    inadequate response to, 173
mobility of spine in, tests of, 151–153
motor dysfunction in, 156
    persisting, 173
myelography in, in location of disc protrusion
        levels, *146–147, 150, 152–153, 154, 158–159,
        170–171, 172, 174–175, 176*
    in location of free disc fragment, *148*
    normal, 177
other lesions simulating, 156
preexisting backache in, 141–144
radiculitis in, 148–149
reflex examination in, 153–155, *156*
rest in, 168
sciatic scoliosis in, 149–151, *146, 147, 148, 149, 150,
        153, 155*
sciatica in, 145
    absence of, 144–145
    distribution of, 145
sensory changes in, 155–156
signs of, 151–156
statistical analysis of, 141
surgery in, 177–203
    anesthesia for, 177, *180*
    contraindications for, 174–175
    development of interspace in, 192–194, *190, 191,
            192*
    failure of, causes of, 205
    historical development of, 177
    indications for, 173–174
    infections subsequent to, 296–299
    interlaminar, free disc fragment removal in,
            199–201, *199*
        inspection in, 195, *193*
        intervertebral disc excision in, 196–199, *196,
                197*
        root tension and, 195–196, *194, 195, 196*
        surgical judgment in, 201–203
        wound closure in, 203, *200*
    intervertebral discolysis as alternative to, 350–351
    operative report of, 204
    on physical laborer, spinal fusion and, 347
    position for, knee-chest, 178–179, *178*
        lateral, 178, *178*
        prone, 180, *182*
            equipment in, *179, 180*
            modified, 180, *181, 182*
        sitting, 179–180
    postoperative management in, 204
    postoperative pain following, causes of, 205
    repeat, indications for, 210–211
        results of, 215
        spinal fusion and, 346
        technical considerations in, 211–215, *211, 212,
                213*
    results of, 205
    skin incision for, 184–189, *186*
    skin preparation and draping for, 183–184, *183,
            184, 185*
        spinal fusion and, 345–346
        subperiosteal dissection in, 189–192, *187, 188*
            retractors for, 190–192, *188, 189, 190*
        surface landmarks for, 181–182, *183*
        vascular and visceral injuries during, 203–204
        with degenerative changes, spinal fusion and, 346
    symptoms of, 141–151
        activities and posture precipitating, 146–148, *145*
        intermittent, 173
        intractable, 173
        motor, 149
        primary, 144–151
        sensory, 149
    traction in, effects of, upon protruding fragment of
            disc, *168*
    treatment of, factors determining, 163–168
    vacuum phenomenon in, 157, *157*
    vertebral body alignment changes in, 158
    x-ray findings in, 157–160
Lumbar disc problems, exceptional, 205–210
Lumbar disc surgery. *See* Lumbar disc disease, surgery
        in
Lumbar elasticity, evaluation of, 119–120, *119*
Lumbar epidural block, 238–240, *239*
Lumbar lordosis. *See* Lordosis, lumbar
Lumbar spinal fusion, 344–347
    anterior interabdominal interbody, complications
            of, 345
        indications for, 345
    following surgery of spinal cord tumors, 318–319
    indications for, 345–347
        specific, 347
    lumbar disc excision and, 345–346
    lumbar disc excision upon physical laborer and,
            347
    lumbar disc surgery with degenerative changes and,
            346
    posterior, advantages of, 345
        disadvantages of, 344–345
        interbody, advantages of, 235–236
            bone grafting in, 231–233, *232, 233, 234*
            bone grafts for, 230–231, *231*
            disc removal in, 228–230, *228, 229, 230*
            instruments for, 232, *228, 229, 230, 232, 233*
            in isthmic spondylolisthesis, 287
            postoperative care in, 235
            prerequisites for, 227
            wound closure in, 233–235, *234, 235*
        materials for immobilization in, 344
    repeat lumbar disc excision and, 346
    spinal instability and, 346–347
    vertebral body, 345
Lumbar spine. *See also* Spine
    abductors of, 23
    anterior, relationship of major vessels and ureters
            to, *198*
    articulations and ligaments of, 10–15
    biomechanics of, 24–35
    blood supply of, 17–18, *17*
    bone-disc ratio of, *10*
        and root compression lesions, 11, *11*
    extensors of, 19–20
    flexors of, 20–23
    infections of, subsequent to lumbar disc surgery,
            296–299
        without antecedent operations on spine, 299–305

Lumbar spine (*cont.*)
  instability of, spinal fusion in, 346–347
  of malingerer, inspection of, 91–92
  mobility of, 24–25, *24, 25*
    assessment of, in physical examination, 43, *42*
  muscle groupings in flexion and extension of, *118*
  nerve supply of, 18–19
  Paget's disease of. *See* Paget's disease
  pain-producing structures of, study of, 18
  pressure, in physical examination, 48
  spinous processes of, impaction of, 269, *269*
  stress studies of, 28–31
    clinical verification of, 31
  tuberculosis of, 303–305, *304–305*
Lumbar strength, evaluation of, 119, *119*
Lumbar vertebrae, anatomy of, 7, *7*
  foramina of, 8–9, *8*
Lumbodorsal corset, 132, *132*
Lumbosacral corset, 130–132, *131*
Lumbosacral facets, asymmetrical, 58
Lumbosacral spine, x-rays of, 49–58, *51, 53, 55*
    in evaluation of lumbar disc disease, 157–160
    positions for, *50*
    radiographic abnormalities noted on, 57–58
    retrograde reasoning in, 49–57
    tracings of, *52, 54, 56*
Lumbosacral strain, acute, 137–138
    management of, 137–138
    signs and symptoms of, 137
  chronic, 135–137
    management of, 135–137
      Achilles tendon exercise in, 136, *136*
    pathophysiology of, 135
    signs and symptoms of, 135
  diagnosis of, inclusive, 134
  epidemiology of, 134
  other lesions simulating, 57

Malingerer, 90–92
  physical examination of, 91–92
  and secondary gain factors, 90–91
Maneuvers in manipulative therapy, 101–104, *102, 103, 104*
Manipulative therapy, arguments against, 100
  arguments for, 100–101
  contraindications to, 101
  in management of low back pain, 100–104
  maneuvers in, 101–104, *102, 103, 104, 105*
  preparation for, 101
  repetitive, 101
Marie-Strumpell disease. *See* Spondylitis, ankylosing
Massage, as physiotherapy, 99, *99*
Measurin, 108
Medication. *See also* Drug(s)
  in management of low back pain, 104–111
  in management of lumbar disc disease, 170–171
Mefenamic acid, 109
Meningiomas of spine, 315
Meningitis, aseptic and bacterial, following myelography, 59
  from postlumbar disc surgery infection, 298–299
Meperidine, 106
Mephenesin, 111
Meralgia paresthetica, diagnosis of, 330–331
  pathophysiology of, 330

signs and symptoms of, 330
  treatment of, 331–332, *331*
Metastatic disease of spine, incidence of, 311
  management of, 314
  and osteoporosis, differential diagnosis of, 293
  physical findings in, 312–313
  route of metastasis in, 311
  symptoms of, 311–312
  x-ray diagnosis of, 313–314, *312, 313*
Methadone, 106–107
Methocarbamol, 111
Methotrimeprazine, 108–109
Methyl methacrylate, in spinal fusion, 318–319
Methyl salicylate, 108
Methylprednisolone acetate, following myelography, 110–111
Mobility, of lumbar spine, assessment of, in physical examination, 43, *42*
Morphine, action of, 105
  side-effects of, 105
  synthetic derivatives of, 106
  therapeutic use of, 105–106
Motor impairment, 39–40
  in lumbar disc disease, 149
    test of, 156
Motor strength, of malingerer, test of, 92
  tests of, in physical examination, 45–46, *45, 46*
Multifidus, 20, *20*
Multiple myeloma, 293, 310
Muscle(s), external oblique, 20–21, *21*
  piriformis, sciatic nerve and, *325*
  spasm, paraspinal, palpation of, 153, *156*
Muscle relaxants, 111
Musculature, abdominal, 20–23
  body, and fascia through third lumbar vertebra, *23*
  in flexion and extension of lumbar spine, *118*
  low back, 19–23
    trigger points in, 99–100
Musculoligamentous pain, versus true sciatica, 40–41
Myelography, in achondroplasia with stenotic lumbar spinal canal, 271
  air, 58
  arguments for, 60–61
  care following, 69
  cisternal puncture in, 63, *63*
  Cuatico needle in, 68, *68*
  Depo-Medrol following, 110–111
  high cervical lateral puncture in, 63–64, *64*
  history of, 58–59
  incidence of error in, 59–60
  indications for, 61
  lipiodol, 58
  in location of disc protrusion levels in lumbar disc disease, *146–147, 150, 152–153, 154, 158–159, 170–171, 172, 174–175, 176*
  in location of free disc fragment, *148*
  lumbar puncture, anesthesia in, 65
    disposable needle in, 65
    needle position in, 64–65
    needle technique in, 65–66, *66*
    Pantopaque injection in, 66–67, *67*
    Pantopaque removal in, 67–68, *65, 67*
    site of puncture in, 65
    technical problems in, 68–69
  myelogram tracing in, 69, *70*
  needle placement in, 63–64, *63, 64*

normal, in lumbar disc disease, 177
objections to, 59–60
in Paget's disease, 273
Pantopaque, 58–59
patient apprehension in, 59
positioning for, 61, *60, 61*
preparation of patient for, 61
principle of, 59
in sacral cysts, 337–338, *340–341*
in stenotic lumbar spinal canal syndrome, 261–262, *260–261*
Myeloma, multiple, 293, 310

Neoplasm, metastatic, and low back pain, 38
Nerve(s). *See also* Specific names
block, lateral femoral cutaneous, 331–332, *331*
obturator, 326–327, *329*
recurrent sinuvertebral, 18–19, *18*
supply, of lumbar spine, 18–19, *18*
Nerve root(s), articular, entering capsule of intervertebral joints, *357*
compression of, in isthmic spondylolisthesis, 282–283, *283, 285*
compression syndrome, foraminal, 161–163, *160, 161*
lumbar, and cervical, lesions of, bone-disc ratio related to, 11, *11*
mechanism of, 8–9, *8*
damage, in lumbar disc surgery, 205
function of, transitional lumbosacral vertebrae and, 163, *162*
in lumbar disc disease, appearance of, 195, *194*
care of, 195–196, *195, 196*
lumbar vertebral foramina and, 8–9, *8*
pain, posterior lumbar rhizotomy in, 249–253
and sensory symptoms, 40, *40*
Neural groove, formation of, 3, *3*
Neurilemmomas of spine, 314–315
Neuritis, iliohypogastric, 327–330
ilioinguinal, 327–330
inguinal, 327–330
obturator, 326, *327, 328*
obturator nerve block in, 326–327, *329*
sciatic, 325–326
Neurofibroma of spine, 314–315
Neuropathy(ies), entrapment, 326–327
obturator, 326, *327, 328*
obturator nerve block in, 326–327
Nisentil, 107
Norflex, 111
Notochord, cells of, degeneration of, 6
formation of, 3, *3*
obliteration of, 5–6, *5*
Novocain, 111
Nucleus pulposus, composition of, 12
development of, 6, *5*
in intervertebral disc biomechanics, 26–28, *27*
in lumbar spondylosis, 263, 264, *263, 265*
and spinal compression, 30, *30*
Numbness, site of, and lesion, 40, *40*
Numorphan, 106

Obturator nerve, *328*
block of, 326–327, *329*

Occupational changes, in management of low back pain, 111–112
in management of lumbar disc disease, 171
Orphenadrine, 111
Osteitis deformans. *See* Paget's disease
Osteitis pubis, obturator neuritis and, 326
Osteoarthritis. *See* Spondylosis, lumbar
Osteoarthropathy, vertebral, 336–337
Osteomalacia, 292–293
Osteomas of spine, 308–309
Osteoporosis, causes of, 290–291
definition of, 290
laboratory data in, 292
postmenopausal, differential diagnosis of, 292–293
etiology of, 291
treatment of, 293–294
secondary to specific diseases, 292
signs and symptoms of, 292
x-ray diagnosis of, 291–292
Oxymorphone, 106

Paget's disease, diagnosis of, 274
laboratory findings in, 274
microscopic changes in, 272
myelography in, 273
pathology of, 272
signs and symptoms of, 273
treatment of, 274–275
x-ray changes in, 273
Pain, absence of, 82–83
area of, in lumbar disc disease, *164, 165, 166*
in arthritis of hips, 332–333
cycle, 104
and doctor-patient relationship, 79
during myelography, 59
evaluation of, diagnostic difficulties in, 84–85
"imaginary," 78–79
low back. *See* Low back pain
in lumbar disc disease, classifications of, 142
management of, 85–86
overtreatment in, 85
target fixation in, 86
in metastatic disease of spine, 312
musculoligamentous, versus true sciatica, 40–41
organic, 78–79
placebos in control of, 87
postoperative, following lumbar disc surgery, causes of, 205
protective function of, 80
psychology of, 78–88
reactions to. *See* Reactions to pain
receptors, 80
sciatic. *See* Sciatica
secondary gain factors in, 86–87
malingerer and, 90–91
secondary loss factors in, 86
sensory deprivation and, 83–84
in spondylolisthesis, causes of, 284
transmission of, gate theory of, 359–360, *361*
traditional concept of, 359, *359*
in vascular and cauda equina claudication, compared, 268
Pantopaque, 59
absorption of, 59
irritative effects of, 59
sensitivity, 60

Paraflex, 111
Paraspinal thrust in manipulative therapy, 101–103, *102*
Paravertebral block, indications for, 246
  technique in, 246–248, *247, 248*
Pars interarticularis, defects in, 58
  pseudoarthrosis at. *See* Spondylolysis
Patellar reflexes, examination of, 44, *44*
Patient, examination of. *See* Evaluation of patient
Patrick's sign, 48, *49*
Pelvic disease, low back pain in, 323
Pelvic sling, 324, *324*
Pelvic "uplift" exercise, 120–121, *121*
Pelvis, joints and ligaments of, 15–17, *16*
  rocking of, in manipulative therapy, 103–104, *105*
  rotation of, in manipulative therapy, 103, *103*
Pentazocine, 109
Periosteum, dissection below, in lumbar disc surgery, 189–192, *187, 188*
Phenacetin, 108
Phenazocine, 107
Phenylbutazone, 109–110
Physical examination. *See* Evaluation of patient, examination in
Physiotherapy, in lumbar disc disease, 169–170
  in management of low back pain, 98–99
Piriformis syndrome, 325
Placebos, double-blind method of testing, 87
  mechanism of action of, 88
  placebo effect and, 87–88
  "placebo reactor type" and, 88
  types of, 87
Plantar flexion, strength of ankle, testing of, 46, *46*
  weakness, inspection for, 42, *41*
Ponstel, 109
Posture, erect, "flattened low back," *112, 113*
  faulty, treatment of, 112–117
  in lumbar disc disease, sciatic scoliosis and, 149–151, *149, 150*
Pregnancy, low back pain in, 323–324
Pressure, measurements of, in lumbar discs, 33–35, *34*
Primitive groove, formation of, 3, *3*
Primitive segments, formation of, 3, *3, 4*
Prinadol, 107
Procaine hydrochloride, 111
Prolotherapy, complications of, case histories of, 354–356
  definition of, 353
  injection site for, 354
  injection technique in, 353–354
  present status of, 356
  proliferating solutions in, 353
Propoxyphene hydrochloride, 108
Pseudoarthrectomy, 279, *279*
Pseudoarthrosis, at pars interarticularis. *See* Spondylolysis
  ilium-transverse process, 333, *332*
Pseudospondylolisthesis, description of, 279
  types of, 279–280, *280*
Psoas, major, 23, *22*
  minor, 23, *22*
Psychosis, reactions to pain and, 82
Psychotherapy, 112

Quadratus lumborum, 19, *19*

Radiculitis, in lumbar disc disease, 148–149
  postmyelogram, 59
Radio frequency electrode in facet rhizotomy, 357–358, *358*
Radiographic position, A-P, *50*
  lateral, *50*
  left posterior oblique, *50*
Reactions to pain, adaptation and, 80
  athletics and, 81–82
  body area and, 82
  emotions and, 79–80
  psychosis and, 82
  socioeconomic and cultural factors in, 80–81
Rectus abdominis, 22–23, *22*
Reflex(es), assessment of, in lumbar disc disease, 153–155, *156, 164, 165, 166*
  in physical examination, 44, *43, 44*
  suprapatellar, examination of, *156*
Rela, 111
Relaxation exercises, 120
Rest, bed. *See* Bed rest
  limited activity program and, 95
  in management of low back pain, 95–97
  in management of lumbar disc disease, 168
  mattress for, 95
Retractor(s), for Cloward technique of disc removal, 219, 220, *220, 221*
  for lumbar disc surgery, 190–192, *188, 189, 190*
Rhizotomy, facet, 356–358
  principle of, 356
  technique of, 357–358, *358*
  posterior lumbar, patient selection for, 249
  procedure in, 250–253, *249, 250, 251, 252, 253*
  "provisional," 251–252
Robaxin, 111

Sacral canal, 9, 240–243, *9, 240*
Sacral cysts, myelography in, 337–338, *340–341*
  surgical removal of, 338, *336, 338, 339*
  case history of, 341–342
Sacral hiatus, 243, *243*
Sacroiliac corset, 130, *130*
Sacrospinalis, 19, *19*
Sacrum, *241*
  anatomy of, 9, *9*
  common anomalies of, *242*
  unroofing of, *336, 338*
Salicylic acid, derivatives of, 107–108
Sarcomas of spine, 309–310
Schmorl's nodes, 159
Schwannoma of spine, 314–315
Sciatic nerve, entrapment neuropathy of, 325
  piriformis muscle and, *325*
  trauma to, 325
  tumors involving, 326
Sciatica, 39
  confirmation of, 47, *48*
  in lumbar disc disease, 144–145
  nonsurgical management of, 95–117
  primary, 325–326
  true, versus musculoligamentous pain, 40–41
  uncommon causes of, 323–342
Scoliosis, low back pain and, 57–58
  sciatic, in lumbar disc disease, 149–151, *146, 147, 148, 149, 150, 153, 155*

Sensation, tests of, in physical examination, 44–45
Sensory changes, of malingerer, 92
Sensory deprivation, pain and, 83–84
Sensory impairment, in lumbar disc disease, 149
    test of, 155–156
    site of, and pain, 40, *40*
Shoe lift in lumbar disc disease, 171
Sitting, proper posture for, 115, *115*
Skeleton, as structural unit, 28
Skin, incision, for Cloward technique of disc removal,
    219, 226, *219, 220*
    for lumbar disc surgery, 184–189, *186*
    in surgery of spinal cord tumors, 315
    preparing and draping of, for lumbar disc surgery,
      183–184, *183, 184, 185*
Skin rolling massage, 99, *99*
Sleeping, proper posture for, 116–117, *117*
Sling, pelvic, 324, *324*
Sodium salicylate, 108
Soma carisoprodol, 111
Somites, formation of, 3, *3, 4*
Sphincter impairment, 40
Spina bifida, back pain and, 57
    spondylolisthesis and, 283–284, *283*
Spinal canal, cervical, stenotic, 257
    lumbar, stenotic. *See* Stenotic lumbar spinal canal
      syndrome
Spinal fusion, lumbar. *See* Lumbar spinal fusion
Spinal thrust in manipulative therapy, 101, *102*
Spine, cervical, bone-disc ratio of, *10*
    and root compression lesions, 11, *11*
    closed biopsy of, 314
    curves of, 7, *6*
    early fetal, 7, *7*
    extrinsic support of, 31–33, *32*
    hyperextension of, in manipulative therapy, 103,
      103
    lumbar. *See* Lumbar spine
    lumbosacral, x-rays of. *See* Lumbosacral spine,
      x-rays of
    mobility of, in lumbar disc disease, tests of,
      151–153
    rotation of, in lumbar disc disease, test of, 153
    thoracic, bone-disc ratio of, *10*
    torsion of, in manipulative therapy, 103, *104*
    tumors of. *See* Tumors, of spine
Spondylitis, ankylosing, examination in, 336
    lumbar disc disease and, 336
    symptoms of, 333–336
    treatment of, 336
    x-ray diagnosis of, 336, *334–335*
    lumbar. *See* Spondylosis, lumbar
    septic. *See* Infection(s), of lumbar spine,
      nontuberculous
Spondylolisthesis, description of, 277, 279
    isthmic, classification of, 280–281, *281, 282*
    establishing skeletal weight-bearing line in,
      282–284, *283, 284*
    management of, conservative, 286
      surgical, 286–287
    mechanical factors in, 281–282, *283*
    pain in, causes of, 284
    physical findings in, 285–286, *286*
    signs and symptoms of, 284–285
    x-ray findings in, 286
    reverse, 287, *287*

Spondylolysis, clinical features of, 279, *277, 278*
    description of, 277
    etiology of, 277–279
    treatment of, 279, *279*
Spondylosis, cervical, 262
    lumbar, 58
      diagnosis of, 262–263
      pathology of, 263
      progressive development of, 263–265, *263, 264,*
        265, 266
      with spinal cord of normal dimensions, 266–267
      with stenotic lumbar spinal canal, examination in,
        268–269
        history in, 267–268
        neurological deficit in, case history of, 267
        treatment of, 269
        x-ray changes in, 266
Squatting, in examination for location of pain, 43–44,
    42
Standing, proper posture for, 113–114, *113, 114*
Stenotic lumbar spinal canal syndrome,
    achondroplasia and, 270–272
    anatomical characteristics in, 257, *257*
    clinical characteristics in, 259–260
    historical data on, 256
    lumbar mobility in, 257–259, *259*
    lumbar spondylosis and, 262–269
    myelography in, 261–262, *260–261*
    plain x-ray changes in, 261
    radiographic characteristics in, 257, *258*
    stenotic cervical spinal canal and, 257
Strain, lumbosacral. *See* Lumbosacral strain
Stress studies, of lumbar spine, 28–31
Support(s), low back, fitting of, 126
    history of, 124–125
    and immobilization, 126
    low back mechanics and, 125–126
    in lumbar disc disease, 171
    purposes of, 126
Symphysis pubis, 17
Syphilis, tertiary, low back pain and, 336–337

Talwin, 109
Tandearil, 109–110
Taylor spinal brace, 124, 129–130, *129*
Tendon, Achilles, shortened, exercise for, 136, *136*
Tendon reflexes, deep, examination of, 44, *43*
Test(s), abdominal strength, 118–119, *119*
    hamstring elasticity, 119–120, *119*
    lumbar elasticity, 119–120, *119*
    lumbar strength, 119, *119*
Thigh, hyperextension of, in manipulative therapy,
    103, *103*
Thoracic cavity, as spinal support, 31–33, *32*
Thoracic spine, bone-disc ratio of, *10*
Thrombophlebitis, and bed rest, 98
Tissues, soft, infection of, subsequent to lumbar disc
    surgery, 296–297
Toe, great, testing dorsiflexion strength of, *45*
Torsion, tests of, on lumbar spine, 30–31
Traction, leg, 97–98, *97*
    in management of low back pain, 97–98
    pelvic, 97, 98, *98*
    in lumbar disc disease, 169
Trancopal, 111

Transversalis, 21–22, *22*
Trauma, in lumbar disc disease, classifications of, 144
Trichlorethylene, 111
Trigger points, in low back muscles, 99–100
    relief of pain at, in lumbar disc disease, 170
Trilene, 111
Trochanter belt, 130, *130*
Tropism, 58
Tuberculosis, of lumbar spine, management of,
        304–305
    signs and symptoms of, 303
    x-ray findings in, 303–304, *304, 305*
Tumors, involving sciatic nerve, 326
    of spine, benign, 307–309
        intradural, 314–315
        malignant, 309–310
        metastatic, 311–314
        surgery in, 315–319
            laminectomy in, 316–317, *316, 317*
            location of incision in, 315
            opening of dura in, 318, *318, 319*
            spinal fusion following, 318–319
            tumor excision in, *319*

Ureters, relationship of, to anterior lumbar spine, *198*

Vascular disease, intra-abdominal, low back pain in,
        324–325
Vena cava, inferior, relationship of, to anterior lumbar
        spine, *198*
Vertebra(ae), lateral displacement of, 288
    lumbar, anatomy of, 7, *7*
        foramina of, 8–9, *8*
    lumbosacral, transitional, and root function, 163,
        162
    pseudo, 6

transitional, low back dysfunction and, 57
    true, 6
Vertebral body(ies), alignment of, changes in, in
        lumbar disc disease, 158
    articulation of, 10–13
    fusion, 345
    precursors of, 5, *4*
    and spinal compression, 30, *30*
Vertebral column, cervical, curve of, 7, *6*
    lumbar, curve of, 7, *6*
    pelvic, curve of, 7, *6*
    thoracic, curve of, 7, *6*
    vertebrae of, 6–7
Vertebral osteoarthropathy, 336–337
von Recklinghausen's disease, 314–315

Walking, proper posture for, 113–114
Williams lordosis brace, 127–129, *127, 128*
Wintergreen, oil of, 108

X-ray(s), in ankylosing spondylitis, 336, *334–335*
    changes, in lumbar spondylosis, 266
        in stenotic lumbar spinal canal syndrome, 261
    contrast studies, 58–76
    in hemangiomas of spine, 307, *308–309*
    of lumbosacral spine. *See* Lumbosacral spine, x-rays
        of
    in metastatic disease of spine, 313–314, *312, 313*
    in nontuberculous infections of lumbar spine, in
        adults, 302
        in children, 301
    spinal, in osteoporosis, 291–292
    in tuberculosis of lumbar spine, 303–304, *304–305*
Xylocaine, in lumbar disc disease, 170

Zactane, 108